WOMEN DOCTORS IN WEIMAR ⌐⌐

Maternalism, Eugenics, and Professional Identity

Melissa Kravetz

Examining how German women physicians gained a foothold in the medical profession during the Weimar and Nazi periods, *Women Doctors in Weimar and Nazi Germany* reveals the continuity in rhetoric, strategy, and tactics of female doctors who worked under both regimes. Melissa Kravetz explains how and why women occupied particular fields within the medical profession, how they presented themselves in their professional writing, and how they reconciled their medical perspectives with their views of the Weimar and later the Nazi state.

Focusing primarily on those women who were members of the Bund Deutscher Ärztinnen (League of German Female Physicians or BDÄ), this study shows that female physicians used maternalist and, to a lesser extent, eugenic arguments to make a case for their presence in particular medical spaces. They emphasized gender difference to claim that they were better suited than male practitioners to care for women and children in a range of new medical spaces. During the Weimar Republic, they laid claim to marriage counselling centres, school health reform, and the movements against alcoholism, venereal disease, and prostitution. In the Nazi period, they emphasized their importance to the Bund Deutscher Mädels (League of German Girls), the Reichsmütterdienst (Reich Mothers' Service), and breast milk collection efforts. Women doctors also tried to instil middle-class values into their working-class patients while fashioning themselves as advocates for lower-class women.

(German and European Studies)

MELISSA KRAVETZ is an associate professor of history and co-chair of women's, gender, and sexuality studies at Longwood University.

GERMAN AND EUROPEAN STUDIES

General Editor: Jennifer J. Jenkins

MELISSA KRAVETZ

Women Doctors in Weimar and Nazi Germany

Maternalism, Eugenics, and Professional Identity

UNIVERSITY OF TORONTO PRESS
Toronto Buffalo London

© University of Toronto Press 2019
Toronto Buffalo London
utorontopress.com

Reprinted in paperback 2023

ISBN 978-1-4426-2964-6 (cloth)   ISBN 978-1-4426-2966-0 (EPUB)
ISBN 978-1-4875-5647-1 (paper)   ISBN 978-1-4426-2965-3 (PDF)

(German and European Studies)

Every effort was made to discover and contact the photographer who took the photos included in this book; if anyone believes they should be credited, University of Toronto Press and the author will be happy to do so in future printings or editions of the book.

Publication cataloguing information is available from Library and Archives Canada

Cover design: Heng Wee Tan
Cover image: Photo courtesy of the Stadtarchiv Erfurt Photo Archive
Printed and bound by CPI Group (UK) Ltd, Croydon, CR0 4YY
We wish to acknowledge the land on which the University of Toronto Press operates. This land is the traditional territory of the Wendat, the Anishnaabeg, the Haudenosaunee, the Métis, and the Mississaugas of the Credit First Nation.

University of Toronto Press acknowledges the financial support of the Government of Canada, the Canada Council for the Arts, and the Ontario Arts Council, an agency of the Government of Ontario, for its publishing activities.

**Canada Council
for the Arts**

**Conseil des Arts
du Canada**

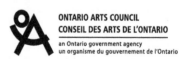

**ONTARIO ARTS COUNCIL
CONSEIL DES ARTS DE L'ONTARIO**
an Ontario government agency
un organisme du gouvernement de l'Ontario

Funded by the   Financé par le
Government   gouvernement
of Canada   du Canada

Canadä

Contents

vi   Contents

Illustrations

Acknowledgments

My parents, Rita and David Kravetz, instilled in me a sense of hard work and responsibility – qualities that were essential to getting me through the process of writing this book. They always supported my endeavours even when they did not understand them. Their love and continued encouragement have sustained me through every moment, and it is to them that I dedicate this book.

Jeffrey Herf has always been an exemplary model of how to write directly and honestly – qualities which I hope this work embodies. He has continuously supported my professional growth and accomplishments, even if they shifted far from his own, and for that I am very thankful. Sonya Michel helped me formulate some of my early key arguments in the book and guided me through the final chapter with her abundance of knowledge on gender and family and social policy. I also acknowledge her course on Gender, Women, and Modernity in the Americas for inspiring my initial interest in gender and eugenics. Tom Zeller always encouraged me to think about the important, big questions, and he fostered my interest in the history of science and medicine through his courses and a number of wonderful early teaching opportunities. The University of Maryland's history department at large provided a very supportive atmosphere in which to research and write the dissertation from which this book emerged.

Longwood University has provided me a wonderful home over the past five years, and my colleagues in the Department of History, Political Science and Philosophy make it a joy to come to work every day. Generous funding from the university and the department allowed me to return to Germany several times to complete the research and writing process. A grant from the Berlin Program for German and European Studies allowed me to undertake the initial research.

The isolation that research and writing bring was eased by the warmth of a number of friends and colleagues in Germany, including Karin Goihl, Mate Tokic, Renee Reichl Luthra, Matthew Conn, Friederike Menzel, and the *Mädels* of FC Schöneberg. The Institute for the History of Medicine in Berlin has always generously provided me with an office space and an academic community. Sabine Schleiermacher, Jutta Buchin, and Melanie Scholz were especially helpful, friendly, and welcoming as I navigated the Institute's collections, and Sabine became my adopted *Doktormutter* in Germany. The friendly archival staff at the Stadtarchiv in Erfurt made the final months of research a real pleasure, and the Director, Dr. Antje Bauer, kindly gave me permission to use the images in chapter 5.

The University of Toronto Press has made the publication process a seamless one. I would especially like to thank my editor, Stephen Shapiro, and the two anonymous reviewers. Several people read drafts of the chapters or commented on portions of these chapters at various conferences, in particular, Matthew Conn, Donna Harsh, Annette Timm, Amy Carney, Elizabeth Heinemann, Alice Weinreb, Heather Perry, Ann Taylor Allen, and Kirsten Leng. Rexford Jones diligently helped me complete the bibliography with a grant from Longwood's Office of Student Research.

My time as an academic has been enriched by the friends and colleagues I have collected over the years, either from college, grad school, conferences, or my previous jobs. In particular, I would like to thank Roger Recupero, Victor Nguyen, Lizzy Chapman, Jonathan Jenkins, Kate Padbury, Jenna Leventhal, Jeff Crawford, Richard Imamura, Mike Bell, Mark Villanueva, Melanie Calbow, Valerie Barro, Dusty Fox, Annie Dummett, Mike Markey, Lauren Kokernak, Naomi Coquillon, Sara Snyder, Courtney Michael, Melanie Prange, Keith Swaney, Cory Bernat, Mike D'Amato, Amy Rutenberg, Jeremy Best, Eric Ruark, Becky Ruark, Andy Palmquist, Mary-Elizabeth Murphy, Tess Bundy, Katlin Hampton, Melissa Byrnes, Lorinc Redei, Sarah Brackmann, Lauren Hammond, Jennifer Miller, Mattheis Bucholz, Mikkel Dack, Jane Freeland, John Miller, Yulia Uryadova, Lara Fergeson, Rachel Goodman, Julie Hunter, Lauren Work, and Carrie Collenberg-Gonzalez.

Becoming a mentor and teacher to several hundred students over the past seven years has allowed me to reflect on the people in my life who were passionate teachers and provided incredible guidance, even when I did not know I needed it. They include Harold Marcuse, Ralph Armbruster-Sandoval, Avinoam Patt, and Glenn Madrid, who instilled in me a passion for history, one I have never lost since the age of sixteen.

Megan Harris has always been one of my biggest cheerleaders and never doubted me or this project. Gladys Cisneros has been a constant source of love and support over the past twenty years. I am eternally grateful for her friendship, which has carried me through the years. Mike Nichols, whom I met and married in the final stages of this project, makes waking up every day blissful. I've been grateful for his continual interest in the project, his copywriting expertise, and his patient, encouraging demeanour. I am incredibly happy that I get to do life with him and that he witnessed the birth of this book alongside the birth of our son, Elijah.

Abbreviations

ADE	Archiv für Diakonie und Entwicklung, Berlin (Archives for Diakonia and Development, Berlin)
BArch	Bundesarchiv-Berlin (Federal Archives-Berlin)
BDÄ	Bund Deutscher Ärztinnen (League of German Female Physicians)
BDF	Bund Deutscher Frauenvereine (League of German Women's Associations)
BDM	Bund Deutscher Mädel (League of German Girls)
DDP	Deutsche Demokratische Partei (German Democratic Party)
DGBG	Deutsche Gesellschaft zur Bekämpfung der Geschlechtskrankheiten (German Society for Combating Venereal Disease)
DNVP	Deutschnationale Volkspartei (German National People's Party)
DVP	Deutsche Volkspartei (German People's Party)
FMS	Frauenmilchsammelstelle (breast milk collection facility)
JM	Jungmädelbund (Young Girl's League)
LArch-Berlin	Landesarchiv-Berlin (State Arhcive-Berlin)
NSDÄB	Nationalsozialistischer Deutscher Ärztebund (National Socialist German Physicians' League)
NSDAP	Nationalsozialistische Deutsche Arbeiterpartei (National Socialist German Workers' Party)
RAfMuK	Reichsarbeitsgemeinschaft für Mutter und Kind (Reich Working Group for Mother and Child)
RÄK	Reichsärztekammer (Reich Physicians' Chamber)

RGA	Reichsgesundheitsamt (Reich Health Bureau)
RGR	Reichsgesundheitsrat (Reich Health Council)
RJWG	Reichsjugendwohlfahrtsgesetz (National Youth Welfare Law)
RMD	Reichsmütterdienst (Reich Mothers' Service)
RMI	Reichsministerium des Innern (Reich Ministry of the Interior)
SPD	Sozialdemokratische Partei Deutschlands (Social Democratic Party of Germany)
StadtA-E	Stadtarchiv-Erfurt (City Archive-Erfurt)
VD	venereal disease
VsÄ	Verein sozialistischer Ärzte (Association of Socialist Physicians)

WOMEN DOCTORS IN WEIMAR AND NAZI GERMANY

Maternalism, Eugenics, and Professional Identity

Introduction

From the earliest days when the first breast milk collection facility was established in Magdeburg in 1919, Dr Marie-Elise Kayser, a pediatrician, enlisted her colleagues to support the collection of breast milk from mothers who produced a surplus for redistribution to sick, weak, or premature infants. In her recruitment efforts, Kayser stressed a "conviction that female physicians are particularly suitable to call and support institutions such as these in life." In her years as a pediatrician in Magdeburg, she "gained the belief that it would be particularly easy for us women as female physicians to persuade nursing mothers to cooperate in charity work that creates life-saving medicine for sick infants."[1] In her remarks, Kayser highlighted that there was something unique about women that allowed them to more easily influence other women to breastfeed and to donate surplus breast milk. In addition, her own unique experience as a mother who produced a surplus of breast milk when nursing her second child drove her decision to open the first facility.[2]

In her recruitment efforts and reflections as to why she initiated breast milk collection, Kayser employed rhetoric that appealed directly to women physicians' self-image as professionals; they were valuable and necessary and the most fitting people for this type of work because of their concurrent professional and domestic experiences. Kayser is emblematic of women doctors throughout Germany who were entering the medical profession in the 1910s and 1920s. As they professionalized with their own organization and journal, they sought to find a niche for themselves in what was then an overcrowded and inhospitable profession. Consequently, Kayser and many others like her crafted professional identities by claiming a unique ability to influence women's and children's health.

This book seeks to bring their story to light. Focusing primarily on those women who were members of the Bund Deutscher Ärztinnen (League of German Female Physicians, BDÄ), founded in 1924, I trace the rhetoric that politically active and professionally engaged female physicians used to maintain their presence and strengthen their significance in particular women's and children's medical spaces. During the Weimar Republic, they laid claim to marriage counselling centres, school health reform, and the movements against alcoholism, venereal disease (VD), and prostitution. In the Nazi period, they emphasized their importance to the Bund Deutscher Mädel (League of German Girls; BDM), the Reichsmütterdienst (Reich Mothers' Service; RMD), and Kayser's breast milk collection efforts. Women doctors populated new areas of medical practice – what I often refer to as new medical spaces because they were both actual and discursive – that were opened up primarily because of the policies of the Weimar state or through the emergence of Nazi state organizations, all of which were not of high status for male practitioners.

While female physicians sought professional status in medicine and equal medical care for their female patients, they relied on traditional notions of gender difference to secure and expand their presence within women's and children's medicine. They accomplished this primarily by adopting "maternalist discourses" – "ideologies and discourses that exalted women's capacity to mother and applied to society as a whole the values they attached to that role: care, nurturance, and morality."[3] Maternalism and the promotion of motherhood were by no means unique to doctors or to Germany in the 1920s and 1930s.[4] Yet women physicians there argued that because the caring and nurturing nature of their work was an extension of their domestic responsibilities, they were better suited to care for women and children than their male colleagues, and therefore could best serve the individual yet overlapping needs of the Weimar and Nazi states – both of which articulated concern for the social welfare of women and children, couched in the context of nation-building.

Charting the narrative of female physicians' discourse also means recognizing how class became a crucial category for understanding their position vis-à-vis the lower-class women they often worked with in Weimar society. The relational analytical categories of gender and class deserve more attention in medical histories of Weimar and Nazi Germany because they affected the way women practised medicine, especially how they treated their patients and how they built their careers.[5] The relationships created between middle- and upper-class doctors and their lower-class female patients augmented both the development of the confidential patient–doctor relationship in medicine as well as the personal and intimate contact among different classes in German society. At the same time, however, female physicians often sustained and expanded their careers at the expense of lower-class women.[6] The great majority of female doctors were from upper- and middle-class backgrounds. Many of them were the children of physicians or were married to physicians, with whom they often shared a practice. All of them clearly had enough privilege to study at a university, and in fact the vast majority of doctors had enjoyed a bourgeois lifestyle since the late nineteenth century.[7] And yet their patients – visitors to marriage counselling centres, students in vocational schools, or prostitutes – were predominantly working-class, especially during the Weimar period. These class differences did not escape female physicians, who taught lower-class mothers how to instil health habits in their children based on their own middle-class values or became advocates for working-class women who had "fallen" into prostitution. Their own upper-middle-class values accompanied them to work every day and seeped into their advising sessions, lesson plans, or conversations with their patients and students. They thus fit well within the larger German medical profession, which Paul Weindling says "played a part in defining the middle-class values which were associated with health and family welfare" and imposed these bourgeois values of cleanliness, fitness, sobriety, hard work, and order on the rest of the nation.[8]

The debate about continuity and change from the Weimar and Nazi periods has dominated those histories that focus on German social, family, and population policy. Historians have sought to determine continuity and/or change with regards to ideas, policies, practices, and professionals across the regime change in 1933. For example, Atina Grossmann sees 1933 as a definitive and irrevocable break for social medicine and reformers involved in the sex reform movement.[9] But in her specific work on female physicians, she notes the continued (albeit altered) professional existence of women doctors through both regimes.[10] Michelle Mouton sees sharp differences between Weimar and Nazi marriage and family policy.[11] Edward Ross Dickinson warns against overestimating the degree of continuity between Weimar and Nazi eugenic policy.[12] Laurie Marhoefer in her history of homosexual reform and Julia Roos in her history of prostitution reform unsurprisingly emphasize discontinuity, as the Nazi policies were generally a repudiation of Weimar-era progressivism.[13] By contrast, Cornelia Usborne posits strong continuity in terms of Weimar and Nazi population policies, including abortion.[14] Annette Timm, in her account of VD control and marriage counselling through four German regimes, agrees that "very similar population policies can be devised by very different political systems." She also recognizes continuity in Weimar and Nazi era experts and personnel serving in state and local welfare institutions.[15]

My work, while not focusing solely on population and family policy also seeks to address continuity and change by following a group of experts – female physicians – and how they contributed to these types of policies in Weimar and Nazi Germany. I argue for continuity in the rhetoric, strategy, and tactics of those doctors working under both regimes. The attention that female doctors paid to women's and children's medicine to create their professional identities demonstrates continuity between these two regimes. The language or strategy of employing maternalism to articulate their identities was also constant among these doctors from 1919 through 1945. Their tactics of working in similar types of spaces that catered to women and children and to then advertise the success of their work within the medical field and beyond endured, at least among the women who remained in the profession throughout both regimes and who are at the centre of this book. Lastly, women's complex relationships with their patients were consistent through both regimes. They aimed to treat the whole patient and claimed to build trusting relationships with women and children. Women doctors simultaneously made professional gains on the backs of their patients while demanding more rights and opportunities for them.

While the Weimar Republic and Nazi Germany were fundamentally different states and had divergent motivations for promoting maternal and childcare, they both offered space for female physicians to articulate their professional identities. The social and family policies developed during the Weimar Republic, hardly cohesive, were primarily voluntary, including marriage and sexual counselling, infant care, and VD counselling, and were aimed at rebuilding a nation devastated by war and alleviating fears about a number of perceived social crises resulting from that war – a birth crisis, higher divorce rates, and a rise in prostitution, VD, alcoholism, and youth criminality. During the Third Reich, the state developed compulsory programs dedicated to intervening in private life for the purposes of ensuring a racially valuable and exclusive community. Under Nazism, the scientific and medical intrusion into private life was most often rhetorical, but there were also some real possibilities for scientists and doctors to intervene, unlike the Weimar Republic when most of the discussion about managing people's private lives was discursive. Both states, however, devoted considerable rhetoric – even if this never came to fruition – to caring for women and children and suggested initiatives that promoted women's health. In the Weimar Republic, for example, the Reichstag debated whether to make marriage genetic testing compulsory, passed a National Youth Welfare Law, and passed a law in order to curb the spread of VD, which stipulated the need for female doctors to treat female patients in select states. The Nazi regime established organizations for mothers and girls, rewarded motherhood, and promoted nursing efforts for women who fit within the confines of its racial ideology. Throughout the Weimar and Nazi periods, the first and then second generation of women doctors operated in a German state that was deeply concerned about the health of women and girls and at least suggested policies to bolster their health, even if these did not always become a reality. Women doctors continuously had an actual and rhetorical space within which to advance their claim that they were needed to treat women and children; if anything, that space became bigger after 1933, but it did not fundamentally change.

Female physicians continuously appropriated the language used by these regimes to focus their professional goals primarily around women and children. Female physicians employed the states' rhetoric of marriage and motherhood to seek broader social and political changes for their women and youth patients, and, most importantly, professional growth for themselves, thereby "extoll[ing] the private virtues of domesticity while simultaneously legitimizing women's public relationships to politics and the state, to community, workplace, and marketplace."[16] Women doctors worked tirelessly to legitimize their public roles as professional physicians and also advised their women patients to be proper mothers and embraced this role themselves. Because their knowledge was grounded in real-life experience and they developed trusting relationships with their patients, women physicians claimed to wield more legitimacy among their patients but also more clout to sway patients when it came to state and political matters – something they believed helped them mobilize women for the goals of the Weimar and Nazi regimes.

For one, female physicians argued their experiences of womanhood and motherhood equipped them with unique identities and abilities that prepared them to care for women and children. While working in Weimar marriage counselling centres (chapter 1), they deemed their married colleagues who were mothers as the most suitable profession-als to advise women about marital or familial problems. In their posi-tions as school doctors (chapter 2), they tapped into their identities as women and mothers to provide adequate health lessons to schoolchil-dren when parents failed to do so. They discussed how alcohol affected nursing mothers or how venereal disease destroyed marriage and the family (chapter 3). Their experience embracing maternalist discourses before 1933 drew non-Jewish female doctors to the Nazi state – a state that deliberately championed motherhood – and thoroughly readied them for espousing similar rhetoric while teaching health to girls in the BDM, offering mothers' training courses for the RMD, and indoctrinat-ing women to join the movement to collect surplus breast milk (chapters 4 and 5). Women professionals used maternalism to aid the causes of both a social welfare, democratic state and a totalitarian regime, signify-ing that the term is perhaps more malleable than originally intended.[17]

The change in the BDÄ's larger understanding of medicine is the one point of discontinuity between the Weimar and Nazi Germany in this study. From the Imperial to the Nazi periods, professional experts and administrators were granted a broader scope in welfare organizations, but the aims and values of these organizations changed, according to Paul Weindling. Weimar pro-natalist organizations became focused on racial selection and the segregation of population groups deemed infe-rior under Nazism.[18] I would argue that the BDÄ also followed this pat-tern. The goals of the organization were largely still focused on caring for women and children, and women doctors had even more latitude to work in these fields, but the BDÄ promoted women's and children's medicine only insofar as the racial hygiene aims and total war effort of the regime could also be maintained. The BDÄ no longer supported a social welfare system that prioritized individualized health care or the public's well-being, for example in marriage counselling, youth welfare, and anti-alcohol and anti-VD measures. It now made fulfilling Nazi ideology a primary goal of medical practice, and that new form of medicine did not promote the well-being of all citizens. The BDÄ's elimination of all Jewish members of the organization during the *Glei-chschaltung* (coordination) of 1933 is one example of this. The fact that BDM doctors assessed the racial features of girls to determine which girls would be admitted is another distinctive racial aspect of the BDÄ's understanding of medicine. While the regime change did not, in fact, bring about an overall change in the type of work that women doctors were doing – that is, in women's and children's medicine – the venues of their work changed, as it shifted from a focus on the home, marriage, the family, and schools to workplaces, the home front, and the exclusive *Volksgemeinschaft* (people's community).

This story of female physicians is a history that privileges the nation-state and its traditional periodizations. Germany's turning points, namely 1918/19, 1933, 1939, and 1945, and the question of continuity in German history have dictated the types of questions asked here and elsewhere.[19] This book explains how and why women occupied particular fields within the medical profession, how they presented themselves in their professional writing, and how they then reconciled their medical perspectives with their views of the Weimar and later the Nazi state. The periodization driven by the political transitions between 1918/19, 1933, and even 1939 shaped the opportunities available to and seized by the women who stand at the centre of this book. The rhetoric of "the nation," especially national rebuilding and the preservation of national health espoused by both the Weimar and Nazi states consistently provided female physicians the language to legitimize their professional endeavours to both states. Both states came to depend on these non-state actors, most of whom worked part-time, voluntarily, or for private institutions because they were excluded from state institutions.[20]

Female physicians were by no means exceptional among professional groups – male and female – who made a seamless transition from democracy to dictatorship.[21] Reproduction and motherhood were at the core of the Weimar Constitution (Article 119) and the Nazi cult of motherhood, which was aimed at increasing the number of racially valuable births and raising the status of racially valuable mothers.[22] Because of this, women physicians were able to make this the focus of their professional work after the First World War, when the first generation of women was graduating from medical school and entering the oversaturated medical world. During the Weimar Republic, even if the federal and state governments did not always openly employ them to do so, female doctors presented themselves as instrumental in the enlistment of women's support for state-wide educational and social welfare policies focused on bolstering the family and the health of individuals and of the nation. Female doctors, in turn, appropriated the rhetoric of the burgeoning welfare state and the institutions created by the Weimar Republic in order to broaden their medical roles. The stark transition from democracy to dictatorship in 1933 hardly disrupted the two-thirds of non-Jewish women in the BDÄ, who could claim that the state that championed motherhood (even if the state expanded and contracted its definition of that role depending on its needs) now needed them more than ever.[23] Even in the face of legislation that prohibited female secondary wage-earners in the civil service (the *Doppelverdiener* law), forbade married women whose husbands had adequate income from working for the elite health insurance practices, and limited the number of women entering medical school, women's and children's health could remain their calling. Their authority over patients proved to be especially crucial under Nazism, as the Reichsgesundheitsamt (Reich Health Bureau; RGA), the BDM, and the RMD recognized that women physicians could be much more effective than men at recruiting women to support the regime's ideology. In turn, women doctors adopted the rhetoric of the Nazi regime, asserting authority through their contributions to women's health, motherhood, the *Volksgesundheit* (people's health), and the total war effort. After 1939, doctors like Marie-Elise Kayser, for example, could fashion herself as strengthening the nation during war through the collection and redistribution of surplus breast milk.

To a lesser extent and less consistently than maternalist arguments, female doctors also occasionally employed eugenic principles to justify their presence in Weimar and Nazi medical spaces, especially those that were already infused with eugenics. Eugenics was an offshoot of social hygiene, which had emerged as a distinct specialty in the late nineteenth century and was focused on population management and reforming state welfare.[24] Eugenics, the study and practice of improving humans and future generations through selective reproduction, had become popular in Germany and several other countries through the support of prominent scientists and physicians who wanted to use "science" to improve the health and welfare of their populations. Positive eugenics encouraged those individuals who were considered "valuable" (*hochwertig*) or who possessed "desirable" traits to marry and reproduce through incentives like tax breaks, motherhood awards, and improved societal status. Negative eugenics discouraged and sometimes prevented procreation of individuals deemed "inferior" (*minderwertig*) through proposed measures like marriage restrictions, compulsory abortion, and sterilization. Positive and negative eugenics were and are complex, ambiguous concepts that can both be used to help the public's needs and desires in a positive way or to go against those needs and desires in the service to larger ideological and nationalistic causes.[25]

During the Weimar period, scientists and doctors followed a broad discourse of eugenics that connected social ills, such as alcoholism, criminality, and poverty, to a person's genetic makeup and sought to prevent the propagation of these "inferior" genes. The eugenically inclined, from both the right and left, discussed fitness for reproduction and intelligence in ways that correlated with their class biases due to eugenic fears that the wealthiest and best educated were producing far fewer children than the poorest and least educated.[26] People who feared that the higher birth rates of the lower classes created a significant threat to the future of the German race often referred to eugenics by its German variant, racial hygiene, coined by Alfred Ploetz and his Racial Hygiene Society, founded in Berlin in 1905.[27] The eugenics movement drew its support from several different groups in society, including the middle and upper classes, professional groups, scientists, and women, but it was physicians, particularly those working with people suffering from mental diseases or disorders, who were remarkably strong supporters of eugenics because social medicine was such a strong element of professional duty in Germany.[28] The social hygiene movement had also redefined the doctor's role in society to focus on the improvement and health of the nation rather than individual treatment.[29] Women physicians' work in public health positions – marriage and sexual counselling centres, welfare offices, and school health – led them to become some of the strongest supporters of interwar eugenics.[30] In these spaces, they witnessed social misery among desperate women and thus sought scientific solutions to help their patients. For the most part, they were acting out of humanitarian motives to help their individual patients and society as a whole; rarely did they make a distinction between eugenics and social welfare or elaborate the genetic rationale for their beliefs.[31]

In the Weimar era, compulsory, harsher eugenics practices often faced much resistance, especially on the national level, and were often never implemented, as evidenced by discussions over the exchange of marriage health certificates in chapter 1. As a result, eugenics often became associated with "welfare-oriented measures, including improved public housing, state-supported maternal and infant health care, and readily accessible contraception, to improve individual lives and national health."[32] Whereas before 1933, eugenics policies were non-invasive, voluntary or suggested policies focused on health education, after the Nazis came to power, they became compulsory, racially motivated programs propped up by the national government.

In the Weimar era, some influential women physicians' eugenic beliefs were closely tied to their class biases, as they sought to isolate the "civilized" or upper classes from social problems understood to be genetically transmissible. Besides attempting to prevent the spread of these traits among middle- and upper-class people, some women physicians also intervened to hinder the lower class from spreading these traits. For example, as seen in chapter 1, in marriage counselling centres, some women physicians endorsed birth control or suggested additional advising sessions for their lower-class patients, who they claimed failed to use contraception correctly. As we will see in chapter 2, in youth welfare their class biases were less blatant, but female physicians still focused on preparing women to be "fit" mothers and admonished working-class mothers for the lack of attention to their children's health. As discussed in chapter 3, in the anti-alcohol movement – a movement founded by eugenicists – female doctors like Agnes Bluhm called attention to the destructive effects of alcohol on the German gene pool, and others involved attempted to prevent the spread of alcohol among the upper classes. While female doctors did not necessarily call for the sterilization of lower-class members of society, they used language that indicated an awareness that certain groups in the population were "unfit" to reproduce and laboured to intervene and assist them whenever possible. Their eugenic leanings allowed certain opportunistic doctors who had contributed to wider Weimar-era discussions about eugenics to more easily transition to and accept the radical eugenics of the Nazis. Dr Ilse Szagunn, a school doctor who also worked in a marriage counselling centre, was a perfect if not exceptional example here, as she was involved in eugenics spheres prior to 1933 and then became a leader in the Nazified BDÄ after. Chapter 4 discusses how, at Alt-Rehse, the Nazi racial hygiene training camp for physicians, BDÄ members not only participated but also expressed their utmost joy and optimism that the ideology of the regime had been successfully implemented. Moreover, they insisted that they could, and did, in fact, enlist other women to become believers in Nazi racial hygiene in the BDM. Chapter 5 describes how another resourceful doctor, Dr Marie-Elise Kayser, saw the benefit of receiving recognition from the regime and promoted the collection of breast milk from Aryan women only, demonstrating how the BDÄ's understanding of medicine took on an ideological face after 1933.

Women's entry into medical schools and the medical profession in Germany occurred relatively late in comparison with other European countries and the United States. Germany was, in fact, the last major European country to admit women to medical study and permit them to receive medical certification. Michael Kater attributes this to "the vehement opposition of misogynist medical professors ... aided by the conservative bureaucracy."[33] Patricia Mazón corroborates Kater's claim that male physicians and professors, who felt the new threat of women medical practitioners, expended much energy protesting women's access to higher education, often stressing how studying would negatively affect women's attractiveness, health, and reproductive development.[34] These disputes delayed women's entry into universities for several years. It was not until the first decade of the twentieth century that most German universities opened their doors to women – decades after institutions such as Oberlin College in the United States (1833), the Sorbonne in France (1860), and the University of London in England (1878) welcomed women.

The medical profession in Germany followed a similar course to that in many other countries that had industrialized in the nineteenth century, with doctors establishing themselves as "experts with professional autonomy" based on their specialized scientific training at a university or similar academic institution. However, the primary difference between medicine in Germany and in other Western countries was that, like almost all German professions, it was state-sponsored. Not only did medical training occur in government-controlled and -funded institutions, but state-appointed boards administered examinations and doctors had to take professional oaths. No professional organization of physicians controlled licensing, training, or conduct, as they did in England or the United States.[35] The profession considered itself indispensable to the state, whether it was under the Wilhelmine, Weimar, or Nazi periods.

During the mid-nineteenth century, German women who wanted to study medicine had to travel abroad. The first German female doctors, Franziska Tiburtius and Emile Lehmus, were, in fact, Swiss educated. Both practised medicine in Berlin beginning in 1876–7. Between 1865 and 1873, Zurich University became a haven for women from all over Europe (including 10 Germans and 148 Russians) who wanted to pursue degrees in the natural sciences and medicine.[36] German female physicians who were trained abroad were not allowed to receive medical certification in Prussia until 1899, the year they also won the right to study medicine and establish medical practices under the protection of a Reich ordinance. Between 1900 and 1908, universities across Germany opened their doors to women on a state-by-state basis: Baden in 1900, Bavaria in 1903, Württemberg in 1904, Saxony in 1906, and Prussia and Hesse in 1908. The first German woman graduated with a medical degree in Freiburg in 1901.[37] The first woman to receive her licence in Germany was Ida Democh-Maurmeier, who had started her training in Switzerland but completed her state exam in Halle in March 1901. She became the first German woman to become a licensed doctor.[38] By comparison, the first woman physician in the United States, Elizabeth Blackwell, received her medical licence in 1859.

After this long struggle to gain admission to universities, the first generation of female doctors finished medical school during or right after the First World War. In the Weimar period, the professionalization of women in medicine intensified. In 1925, women made up 5.4 per cent of all doctors (2,572 of 47,904). Women comprised 8.6 per cent of the medical profession (or 4,367 of 51,067 total doctors) by 1933. By 1939, women composed 9.5 per cent of all doctors, or 6,280 of a total of 65,780.[39] In 1942, 12.4 per cent (or 9,426) of Germany's 75,960 total doctors were women, meaning that between 1925 and 1942, the number of women in medicine more than doubled.[40]

It was during this same period that they founded and grew a professional organization, the BDÄ, and an accompanying journal, *Die Ärztin* (*The Female Physician*). Although *Die Ärztin* never focused overwhelmingly on any of the women's and children's issues covered in this book, it was the BDÄ's main platform for openly discussing prominent issues of the time and clearly guided the framework of the chapters that follow. The BDÄ was founded in 1924 by 300 women from Berlin; by 1926, the organization claimed to have over 600 members.[41] In 1930, the organization declared it had 799 members.[42] They came from a variety of political and religious backgrounds; the majority of them were Protestant, about 10 per cent were Catholic, and before 1933, approximately one-third were Jewish.[43] As a result of their divergent backgrounds and work experiences, women doctors in the BDÄ were not always unified in their views on eugenics, birth control, and abortion. The question of whether to provide birth control in marriage counselling clinics was certainly a point of division among female doctors, who often formed their beliefs based on their exposure to women in desperate circumstances and eugenic ideas. In vocational schools, doctors disagreed over their purpose there; some highlighted the need for female physicians to comfort young women going through menstruation, while others thought they were needed to develop physical education programs that suited women's bodies and needs. In the anti-alcohol campaign, doctors openly disagreed over the use of alcohol for medicinal purposes. Regardless of their differences, they all claimed to have some sort of "gender-based authority" in discussing these issues.[44]

In its 1924 bylaws, the BDÄ had espoused neutrality on issues of politics, religion, and race. Many women doctors, too, conformed to these early requirements. Hertha Nathorff, for example, recounts how she was asked her position on Paragraph 218 (the law that forbade abortion) when she applied for a job in family and marriage counselling, but disapproved of all political concerns in the medical profession. Moreover, when recalling how her patients would bring their political moods to consultations, she reasserted that she was a doctor who had no interest in politics.[45] The majority of BDÄ members belonged to no political faction.[46] The umbrella organization for all organizations of German women, the Bund Deutscher Frauenvereine (League of German Women's Associations, BDF) had members who primarily belonged to the German People's Party (Deutsche Volkspartei; DVP), the German Democratic Party (Deutsche Demokratische Partei; DDP), and the German National People's Party (Deutschnationale Volkspartei; DNVP) during the Weimar period.[47]

Although the association proclaimed itself to be politically neutral in theory, the BDÄ was hardly apolitical in practice.[48] In addition to its efforts to secure women access to birth control in marriage counselling centres, it worked to equalize school health programs and VD medical treatment during the Weimar era. In these instances, female physicians identified that women faced inequalities in their medical access and should have fundamental rights as women and patients. The attempt to include women in the medical profession was also in itself a political undertaking that started in the 1920s and spanned both regimes.

With the rise of Nazism in 1933, the organization and the journal's editorial staff purged themselves of Jews, Communists, and other political opponents while appointing Nazi sympathizers to leadership positions. There was a generational changeover in the BDÄ, similar to its parent organization, the BDF, in which many younger women joined Nazi women's organizations.[49] The BDÄ very much mirrored the trend of liberal feminists, which showed affinity towards National Socialism in terms of social welfare, universal health care, and a more progressive attitude towards women controlling their own reproduction, but opposed Nazi attempts to dissuade women from university study and remove them from public and professional life.[50] By the end of 1936, the regime had taken over the ideological leadership of the BDÄ and *Die Ärztin*. The themes of the articles changed after 1933, focusing on achievements of the new state, the questions of sterilization and abortion, the prevention of "genetically diseased offspring," or other reports on racial hygiene.[51] Under the new regime, German women doctors became overt political actors who participated in Nazi programs, indoctrinated others to Nazi ideology, assisted with the war effort, and endorsed Nazi policies in *Die Ärztin*.

While there was certainly a shift in membership demographics after 1933, this study highlights those women who worked for either one or both regimes.[52] Because the BDÄ was the first and only organization exclusively dedicated to women doctors during the Weimar and Nazi periods, it can be seen as representative of professionally and politically active female physicians of this time period. Thus, this project draws primarily on women doctors' own interpretations of their work in *Die Ärztin*, and also utilizes the publications, personal papers, and memoirs of its members. Through a close reading of their writing, we can determine the professional, political, and intellectual interests of female physicians during the Weimar and Nazi periods.

While the Weimar Constitution guaranteed women's full professional equality by removing all discrimination against them in public service (which included large numbers of teachers as well as doctors and lawyers), the promises made by the Constitution did not reflect reality in the medical field.[53] Women often found it more difficult than their male colleagues to gain coveted state positions, whether in hospitals, prisons, or courts. The elite health insurance funds also favoured male doctors.[54] Male doctors, hoping to maintain the exclusivity of their profession, were fearful of and emasculated by professional competition from women, who they thought were threatening to replace them in the workforce.[55] Weimar medical authorities often issued warnings to medical students regarding the overcrowded profession.[56] The Law Governing the Legal Status of Female Civil Servants and Public Officials, passed in 1932, stated that married women who were second wage earners could be dismissed from public service, which included medicine. That same year, German Chancellor Heinrich Brüning put a 5 per cent cap on women entering medicine.[57] In December 1933, the new regime put fixed quotas on the number of women who could be admitted to universities each year.[58] That same month, Gerhard Wagner, the Reich Physicians' Leader (Reichsärzteführer) publicly declared that the Nazi party intended "to rid the nation gradually of all female doctors by curtailing university (medical) training for women." In January 1934, Wagner barred married women doctors whose husbands had adequate income from working for official health insurance organizations. This was an extension of the law against married women civil servants who were second wage earners. While few married women doctors actually suffered in the end, the ban remained on the books, even if it was only theoretical after the war started. Wagner also attempted to clarify his position later in 1934, and his threats to throw women out of the profession never materialized, but his strong rhetoric left many women in doubt.[59] Conservatives and Nazis believed that women were becoming de-feminized in their pursuit of academic and professional work, a matter of grave concern because women were now deemed "spiritually and physically unfit for motherhood."[60] The male medical profession welcomed women in peripheral roles, where they would primarily treat women and children, citing the need for their "feminine qualities of maternal empathy and warm-hearted kindness."[61] Women physicians appropriated this maternal rhetoric and claimed that it was precisely these qualities that made them better doctors for female patients and students.

The profession at large victimized women physicians, who were compelled to limit their own careers because of the social expectations and assumptions attached to their gender. Simultaneously, female physicians seized upon what they considered their unique insights as women and mothers to launch and sustain their professional careers. The women who are the focus of this book had a precarious position as women and practitioners, which begs the question of social control – who *really* had it? As Cornelie Usborne states, "the recasting of the relationship between state and society both entailed an unprecedented intervention into individual women's bodies and also provided a new discursive space for women to voice their concerns about their bodies."[62] These women doctors were both participating agents of the larger profession (and the states they worked in), and also arrogating power within the space(s) provided.

The profession's bias against women, as well as the widespread belief that they should treat only women and children, which dated back to the nineteenth century, led women to also appropriate particular medical fields. If they had a private practice, most women served as general practitioners in large cities or specialized in pediatrics or gynecology. Since the Victorian era women had been using the language of reticence about sexual matters to claim they were more fit to be gynecologists.[63] In the late 1920s, over half of women doctors were in general practice, and of those who specialized, almost half were in pediatrics and another

15 per cent were in women's specialties.[64] This trend was also the norm in the early 1930s, when there were twice as many female general practitioners than female specialists, nearly 60 per cent of whom specialized in children's illnesses or women's ailments.[65] Entering private practice offered flexible hours to combine family duties and professional work but remained a distant option for many female medical graduates, who had less of a chance to establish themselves compared with their male colleagues, and if women did go into private practice, it was often with their husbands. They also sought out the burgeoning fields of public health and welfare work in spaces such as schools and counselling centres – supplementary positions that were part-time, that did not pay very well, and that their male colleagues eschewed. In many public health and welfare jobs, female physicians were employed exclusively on an hourly basis and had no job security.[66] It was in these fields, however, that they could balance their professional and family lives – an important factor to the high number of women who were wives, mothers, *and* doctors.[67] Single doctors, too, had the autonomy to balance work in a number of different public health and social work roles. Both married and single doctors benefited from their middle-class status, which allowed for financial freedom, domestic help, and adequate childcare.[68]

In all of these female-dominated spaces, they could stress their special gendered contributions to the profession, not only through treating female patients and students with more care and empathy than their male colleagues, but also by disseminating rhetoric and developing programs that specifically targeted women's bodies and domestic spaces. They participated in debates about reproductive rights in marriage counselling centres, women's proper physical education curriculum in schools, and the effects of drinking, VD, and prostitution on women and the home. During the Nazi period, the politicization of reproduction, and therefore women as the nation's reproducers, endured. Women physicians intervened in cases where they could teach women to be good mothers in the RMD, where they could train and mould young women's bodies in the League of German Girls, and where they could literally use the body and its reproductive elements – breastfeeding – for national purposes. Women doctors may have consigned themselves to the sphere of "women's work" in order to maximize their influence in the medical profession, but this certainly did not minimize their political influence within these spaces. Those who worked in Nazi medical spaces like the BDM, the RMD, and breast milk collection – all of which promoted the regime's ideology – do not fall so neatly into a category of perpetrators or agents, but they can be considered actors under Nazism and most certainly opportunists.[69]

Highlighting their gender, including their feminine abilities of care and empathy and their "natural" roles as mothers and caretakers,[70] provides one example of how women successfully and strategically entered the scientific professions, including medicine.[71] These women physicians suggest that there was as a female style of practising medicine, characterized by greater empathy and greater concern for context.[72] Margaret Rossiter has noted a trend among women in what she called "marginal fields" of science to spend their careers in "womanly" areas of employment, which were less often recognized and on the periphery of scientific professions.[73] In this story, however, women's and children's medical spaces like marriage counselling centres, female vocational schools, VD clinics, the BDM, the RMD, and breast milk collection facilities, were not considered marginal to Weimar and especially Nazi authorities. These were the very spheres where the state and its agents – in this case, the female physicians at the centre of this study – could exercise power by managing reproduction and regulating, disciplining, improving, and shaping individual bodies and the collective national body. Michel Foucault refers to this governmental regulation of practice, institutions, and ideas for the purpose of controlling both individual bodies and entire populations as biopolitics.[74] Biopolitics could be productive as well as repressive; the state could intervene and steer individuals in directions that benefited the state as well as the individuals themselves.[75] Female physicians, as the state's agents, heralded their contributions as improving the health of the German nation and simultaneously as assisting overburdened mothers, aiding young girls, or advocating for women's rights, including their own. They bolstered nationalism through crafting girls' physical education policies that were focused on producing healthy German mothers, while creating a health program that fit women's bodies and abilities. They sought to eradicate social ills such as alcohol, venereal disease, and prostitution that threatened Germany's national prominence, while encouraging women to remove them from their own families and homes. They promoted the collection and redistribution of surplus breast milk to improve Germany's infant mortality rate and thereby its national status, while guiding women to breastfeed, which they deemed healthier for women and their babies. Their concerns, which were sometimes overlapping and interchangeable, were primarily their patients and students, secondarily, themselves, and thirdly, the nation.

The complicated layers of these women, the mixture of modernity and tradition in their individual identities and professional lives, and, apropos to this, the blending of eugenics, class biases, and social justice in their rhetoric have sustained my own interest in them for several years. In many ways, they mirrored a constant tension between conservatism and progressivism or tradition and modernity that governed Weimar and then Nazi politics and social and cultural movements. Female physicians embodied the same doctrine of the German women's movement at large, which Ute Frevert has described as "confused and contradictory."[76] They were, as Jeffrey Herf might label them, reactionary modernists.[77] They accepted the nineteenth-century notion that the female body was physically weaker and more delicate than the male body and thus warranted a separate gymnastics program. They simultaneously demanded things like an equal physical education program for female students and insisted that the curriculum of such a program should be suited to women's differing dispositions – namely, their biological ability to bear children. They promoted equal medical treatment for women with venereal disease by affording them access to physicians of the same sex, and also pointed out that women's differences merited their separate treatment by female physicians. Women doctors, in other words, adopted a rhetoric that insisted women were different *and* merited equal treatment.[78] In physical education reform and then the League of German Girls, they specifically encouraged girls to prepare their bodies for motherhood, illuminating the paradox of professional women compelling women on to non-professional paths. In the breast milk collection movement, Dr Kayser scientized, publicized, and modernized the once private and natural realm of breastfeeding.

The experiences of women doctors based primarily on the accounts presented in their professional journal and discourse demonstrates that the career choices they made were both voluntary and swayed by political pressures and temptations. Their professional and personal identities also influenced their decisions. German women doctors employed their identities as mothers to practise medicine by focusing on the comprehensive care of women and children and by developing trusting relationships with their patients and students, which allowed them to simultaneously indoctrinate them to Weimar social welfare programs and later Nazi politics. Ultimately, their story illuminates how women in scientific and medical professions strategically used their identities to gain professional legitimacy, to aid women and women's causes, and to influence policy.

1 Promoting Marriage, Motherhood, Eugenics, and Comprehensive Health Care in Marriage Counselling Centres

In August 1931, a journal article described the early morning scene in a counselling centre of the Internationale Arbeiterhilfe (International Worker's Aid). The women were waiting on the female physician, expected to arrive at 7:00 a.m., and they primarily visited this clinic for birth control.[1] The article, which clearly advocated women's access to birth control, also claimed "there [were] still too few counselling centres."[2] The article suggested that it was a novelty for these patients to be waiting for a *female* physician and for a *woman* doctor to be distributing information about birth control. By 1931, women doctors had become involved in the dissemination of birth control information in public counselling centres. This role was a new one for female physicians, as was staffing new municipal, religious, and private marriage counselling clinics, which emerged as a result of the long-standing rhetoric about a population "crisis" and calls from Weimar authorities to intervene in marriage and reproductive choices.[3] This chapter highlights the maternalist discourse that female doctors elaborated to lay claim to marriage counselling centres and bolster their work within them. It also demonstrates how these doctors articulated their own concerns within this medical space in order to broaden their medical roles and provide comprehensive health care for women.

Various municipal, private, and religious counselling centres opened throughout the Weimar Republic in an attempt to address population experts' claims of a crisis of marriage and a decline in fertility (*Geburtenrückgang*) that followed the First World War. Whether it was intended or not, all three types of marriage counselling clinics became involved in debates about the distribution of birth control to their primarily lower-class clients – an indication of the ways in which the duties of the clinics adapted to the needs of advice seekers. Female doctors, who found space working in all three types of clinics as a result of discrimination in the medical field but also because they highlighted their natural suitability to these centres, became involved in distributing birth control. Women doctors were hardly united in their opinions about birth control, but all referred to their gender in making authoritative statements about the distribution of birth control in clinics. Some female physicians exhibited biases against the primarily working-class women who visited the municipal centres, suggesting that the living conditions or problems arising from their economic status led to the failure of these women to properly use birth control, getting pregnant over and over again and causing further burdens for society. Sometimes the female physicians who subscribed to eugenic views by advocating birth control or even sterilization couched their beliefs in the view that they were helping the community at large and alleviating overburdened lower-class women. Their eugenic beliefs were closely tied to their class biases and were sometimes mixed up with genuine concerns for patient welfare and a confused sense of social justice.

Women doctors recognized that the majority of advice seekers were women – as high as 95 per cent in one study – and that these women were searching for particular types of advice that centred around birth control, birth prevention, marriage problems, social questions, and sexual questions.[4] They suggested that their maternal experiences lent them privileged insight into their patients' lives as they sought to create and strengthen their leadership roles within the field of marriage counselling. Female physicians claimed their "womanly" and "motherly" roles proved why they were better suited for work in marriage counselling, especially through their abilities to build trusting relationships with advice seekers. They also championed marriage and motherhood as qualifications that afforded counsellors the most success in serving their patients. In this sense, they pioneered a unique path for themselves in what was the primarily male-dominated world of medicine. Marriage counselling was one of the paths of least resistance for these women, and their work in these centres was, in fact, widely welcomed.

Treating primarily women for women-centred issues in marriage counselling clinics was a practical way for women doctors to balance their own professional and personal aspirations. The minimal office hours of clinics, for one, allowed them to pursue motherhood in addition to employment. They were also able to convey their own interests in women's social and political issues within the professional sphere of marriage counselling, thereby broadening their roles within these clinics and calling for comprehensive health care for women – something that they criticized their male counterparts for not offering. In this new gendered medical space, they fashioned themselves as the best providers of educational, moral, legal, practical, and personal advice for women.

This chapter begins with a discussion of policy debates regarding the exchange of marriage health certificates. It was in these discussions that officials first emphasized the need for female physicians to care for female patients – rhetoric that the doctors themselves would later arrogate for their own employment purposes. Next, it charts the establishment of three different types of marriage counselling centres, their outlined duties, and what they did in reality, which primarily entailed distributing birth control. The next section examines female doctors' discussions about distributing birth control to visitors. It was in their debates about birth control that they initially claimed the marriage counselling centre space as one they were particularly suited for – the subject of the next section – largely because of the overwhelming number of female visitors and the types of woman-centred questions these visitors were asking. Once female doctors had created a woman-centred space, the next section shows how they pushed the boundaries of what medical care entailed for these women. Finally, the last section focuses on how women doctors adopted eugenics discourse in their rhetoric about marriage counselling centres.

Wartime and Interwar Debates over Marriage Health Certificates

Municipal, religious, and private marriage counselling centres would eventually become the sites where Weimar government authorities and various organizations and individuals would intervene in the institutions of marriage, but prior to this, there were debates about the exchange of premarital health certificates. The discussion over marriage health certificates shows the early Weimar government's attempts to expand its authority over marriage, which paved the way for the establishment of municipal marriage counselling centres and women doctors' employment within them. The government's hope of curtailing experts' claims of a falling birth rate and declining national health served as motivation for intervening in marital choice and focusing on couples planning to procreate. A eugenic undercurrent dominated these early discussions, and female physicians working in these centres later adopted this rhetoric.

Demographers, social hygienists, and politicians had been warning of a population collapse since the late nineteenth century. Couched under the enduring ideology of *Bevölkerungspolitik* (population politics), this rhetoric proliferated in the twentieth century with the growing popularity of Social Darwinism, the professionalization of medical and scientific specialties, and the loss of millions of young lives in the First World War.[5] By the 1920s, the German birth rate was lower than that in any other European nation, with the exception of Austria.[6] Fear of Germany's enemies and "the other" was often what drove population policies that focused on encouraging higher birth rates at home in the interwar era.[7] The large demographic imbalance as a result of the war – perhaps over two million more women than men in Germany – led many to fear that marriage was in crisis because women would under no circumstances be able to find a marriageable male and would be "condemned to singleness."[8] Rising divorce rates were also a concern, causing people to fear the breakdown of the institution of marriage and, as an extension, all of society, and they continued to blame the First World War as "the great destroyer" of marriage.[9] The cumulative social effects of the First World War – the declining birth rate, increasing divorce rates, and marital problems – added to an "atmosphere of pessimism and panic about the nation's future," which Annette Timm claims became intensified in the postwar period as a result of Germany's losses (demographically, financially, and militarily), but also because most German citizens were shocked to learn of their defeat when the war ended.[10]

These discussions moved beyond just questions of quantity; increasingly, conversations about population politics also began to centre around the quality of Germany's population. Under an overarching ideology of population politics, the once private, individual choices about marriage, sexual partners, and family size became further couched in the context of duty to one's nation in the postwar era.[11] Scientists and physicians had these same concerns prior to the war when eugenics was first being articulated in mainstream, professional settings, but after the war, these efforts became much more extensive, especially as government officials began parroting such views.[12] The Reichsgesundheitsamt (Reich Health Bureau; RGA), demographers, racial hygiene experts, doctors, and population policy associations and journals emphasized the importance of upholding the institution of marriage and offspring, now deemed the cornerstone of the family, society, and nation.[13] Such rhetoric often became embedded in language suggesting that it was in Germany's best interest to be concerned with the quality of its population.[14] In a context in which "the trauma of war" was used "as a justification for more state intervention into the everyday lives of German citizens," marriage became a site of intervention.[15]

In September 1917, the Berlin Society for Racial Hygiene sent a petition to the Reichsministerium des Innern (Reich Ministry of the Interior; RMI) calling for an amendment to be added to the original 1875 marriage law recommending the exchange of marriage health certificates based on premarital health exams. The Berlin Society for Racial Hygiene recognized the loss of many "valuable and above-average men" in the Great War and promoted marriages between "capable" individuals (*Tüchtige*) and discouraged marriages between "less valuable" individuals (*Minderwertige*). This measure was necessary to produce the "highest quality offspring possible" and to prevent individuals from entering marriages when diseases or "inferiorities" could potentially be passed to healthy spouses or offspring.[16] The Reich Health Bureau and its president, Franz Bumm, were also committed to this plan, citing the fact that health restrictions on marriage had already been discussed in Germany and implemented in places like the United States and Sweden.[17]

It was in the conversations about marriage health certificates that officials first stressed the need for women doctors. Radical feminists in the Bund für Mutterschutz (League for the Protection of Mothers) had advanced demands for marriage certificates even prior to the First World War.[18] In wartime discussions about the issuing of marital health certificates, representatives from the Medical Society for Sexual Science and Eugenics and Alfred Blaschko, chairman of the German Society for Combating Venereal Disease, cited the issue of women's modesty, arguing that women should be given the possibility of refusing the premarital medical exam or of choosing a female doctor. After all, the secret of their "virginal status" (*Deflorationsgeheimnis*) had to be protected. Similar considerations of women's modesty did not appear after the war. Blaschko was an early opponent of premarital health certificates and of recommendations that informational leaflets encouraging marriage candidates to undergo these exams be distributed in registry offices. He thought leaflets and even examinations would do little to curb the spread of VD and might even, in fact, spread VD through extramarital sexual activity if infected persons were prevented from marrying. He concluded that rather than leading to an improvement of the race, premarital health exams might possibly lead to a "deterioration of the race" because only "intellectually and morally superior individuals" would be dissuaded from marrying, while "less valuable" individuals would continue to propagate themselves in illegitimate relationships.[19] The eugenically inclined, no matter their political backgrounds, discussed intelligence in ways that correlated with their class biases, which were unmistakable in early debates about premarital health certificates and a theme that female physicians would adopt later.

Early hopes of implementing marital health requirements ended in February 1918 when the RMI temporarily quashed the initial proposal to distribute informational leaflets and require individuals to undergo premarital health exams, citing "the population's underdeveloped understanding for racial hygiene claims." Implementing such "premature" measures would undoubtedly cause people to regard health restrictions on marriage as a "sensitive infringement of personal freedom."[20] After the war, in the population politics–obsessed Weimar Republic, health experts and government medical officials again began demanding the distribution of informational leaflets and the exchange of premarital health certificates. Representatives of the Sozialdemokratische Partei Deutschlands (Social Democratic Party of Germany; SPD) were among the first to pressure the Prussian Ministry of the Interior to respond to the idea of distributing educational health leaflets. The Prussian Ministry was reluctant to take a stand on the issue, fearing that the public would view the certificates as a type of moral suasion and reject them. By February 1920, the Reich Health Council (Reichsgesundheitsrat; RGR) began to re-examine the idea of premarital health certificates. Dr E. Schubart, a judge and an active member of the Berlin Society for Racial Hygiene, was a strong proponent of voluntary premarital health exams, but he thought a law for men only would be easier to pass.

After several letters and petitions to the Reich Ministry of the Interior, the Ministry of Justice, and the Prussian Ministry of the Interior, the RGR discussed Schubart's draft law, as well as guidelines formulated by Prof. Dr Abel, a government medical administrator in Jena, in a meeting on 26 February 1920.[21] Abel's guidelines insisted that marriage health certificates were essential to ensure a future healthy population, that medical restrictions on marriage were necessary to prevent racial degeneration, that the public should be educated on genetic disorders, and that a law should be instituted requiring marriage candidates to undergo medical exams. The RGR accepted Abel's guidelines with only minor revisions, and the majority voted for the obligatory exchange of marriage health certificates. It did not favour Schubart's male-only plan though, instead advocating that both men and women be subject to these policies. The strict stance of the RGR and the SPD on forced exchange has led historian Paul Weindling to call this meeting a "turn-ing point in official acceptance of the desirability of eugenic controls on marriage."[22]

The RGR sent the guidelines to the Reichstag with the stipulation that if the Reichstag could not reach a decision regarding the obliga-tory exchange of certificates, then measures should be taken to ensure a voluntary exchange. However, typical of the indecisiveness that it was constantly plagued by, the Weimar coalition government, under the leadership of the SPD, could not pass the proposal – the suggestion for voluntary exchange of certificates. Instead, it passed only a law for the obligatory distribution of premarital health leaflets in registry offices. These educational leaflets, which "outlined the dangers of venereal dis-ease, tuberculosis, and other unnamed afflictions to future generations and warned prospective marriage partners of their duty to inform each other of any health problems before they married," received positive response from several associations, especially women's organizations.[23]

Prussian authorities were much more accepting of the February 1920 guidelines and made another attempt to suggest the immediate imple-mentation of the voluntary exchange of marriage health certificates in 1922. Other states, however, objected to any legal regulation of marriage health certificates. As a result, the RGA, in May 1922, temporarily put an end to national discussion of the matter, asserting that it was not the right time to institute legal measures governing the exchange of health certificates. Nevertheless, the Prussian Racial Hygiene and Population Policy Committee continued to debate the matter and pushed the Reich Ministry of the Interior towards enforcing an obligatory exchange of marital health certificates for engaged couples. Another RMI meeting on 9 March 1923 led to similar objections about enforced exchange and determined that nothing could be accomplished at the Prussian (or state) level without changing the federal civil status law. The obliga-tory exchange of marriage health certificates remained the most con-troversial issue debated among health experts and state and federal politicians. The federal government never wavered from its consistent opposition to forced exchange and never supported any sort of ban on marriage. Prussian efforts finally succeeded to some extent in February 1926 when the federal government issued a memo recommending a voluntary exchange. That was as far as the federal government would go though, and after this, the Prussians turned their attention to the establishment of marriage counselling clinics – a realm over which it had more control.[24] Marriage counselling, in general, now became much more significant for municipal and religious authorities, as it seemed more feasible to implement because precedents already existed.

The Establishment of Marriage Counselling Centres and Their Duties

A few different types of marriage counselling centres were established during the Weimar Republic, and female physicians played a significant role in all of them. At the state level, Prussia turned its full attention to marriage counselling in 1926. On 19 February, the Prussian Minister for the People's Welfare, Heinrich Hirtsiefer, crafted guidelines for the establishment of medically led marriage counselling centres in all municipalities and counties in Prussia. These were in accordance with the guidelines outlined in the RGR's meeting from February 1920 and followed the advice of the Prussian Health Council's (Landesgesundheitsrat) Committee for Racial Hygiene and Population Policy. Adopting portions of the 1920 RGR guidelines, the "Hirtsiefer Decree" (as it became known) recommended the appointment of doctors as marriage counsellors who would, after an examination, issue certificates on the health condition of marriage candidates. By that point, private marriage counselling centres already existed in many major German cities and a state-sponsored counselling centre had opened in Vienna in 1922. This memo was the basis for the creation of Prussian municipal clinics and provided instruction as to what doctors should be looking for – namely, the health compatibility of marriage candidates as well as the presence of genetic dangers and the degree to which they threatened the marriage or future children. In order to avoid any conflict with the federal government, marriage counselling would be voluntary.[25] Doctors played an advisory role by recommending against marriage if they suspected genetically unhealthy offspring or by suggesting the marriage be postponed until the conclusion of medical treatment.[26] While individuals did not necessarily have to take this advice, doctors sought to instil in the population a larger sense of responsibility regarding marriage choice. They aimed to inform citizens that choosing a partner was no longer a private, individual decision; Germans also had what Timm perceives as "eugenic responsibilities" towards the health of their families and future generations, and towards the "enhancement of the *Volksgesundheit*."[27] This blurring between the individual and the nation, or the once private and public spheres, especially in terms of marriage and reproduction, was a phenomenon characteristic of the ideology of *Bevölkerungspolitik* (population politics) that dominated this era.[28]

The impact of the Prussian ordinance spread quickly. There were 129 such centres by 1927.[29] Between 1926 and 1928, twelve municipal counselling centres were set up in Berlin. By the early 1930s, Prussia had 200 of these municipal clinics. Outside of Prussia, the movement for municipal marriage counselling centres took hold only in Saxony, Brunswick, and the Hansastädte in northwest Germany (Lübeck, Bremen, and Hamburg). In southern Germany, the idea of state-authorized marriage counselling centres hardly emerged.[30] In 1932, forty-nine of the ninety-eight German cities with more than fifty thousand inhabitants had marital counselling centres.[31]

The choice of doctors as the leaders of municipal marriage counselling centres was logical considering physicians would administer physical examinations and medical questioning prior to issuing marriage health certificates. In addition to their extensive medical training, doctors had gained an increased level of public trust and prestige since the professionalization of medicine and the growth of eugenics as a scientific discipline in the early twentieth century.[32] They were considered "experts" when it came to determining if a disease or a predisposition to disease existed that would make marriage unadvisable.[33] Medicine was also a profession focused on caring for people, which coincided with the aims of municipal counselling to maintain the welfare of the *Volk* through guidance about marriage choice.[34] The calls for medically led clinics, however, extended beyond the requirement for doctors to take a leading role. Prussia also stipulated that these leaders be trained in genetics, which corresponded to the clinics' goals of determining whether marriage candidates were eugenically fit and compatible enough to marry.[35] Female doctors were considered suitable enough leaders to be included in Hirtsiefer's guidelines. In fact, by 1931, women led five of the sixteen municipal clinics in Berlin. Female doctors were leaders in municipal marriage counselling centres in Friedrichshain, Neukölln, Reinickendorf, Wedding, Charlottenburg, and at the Registry for Engaged and Married People (Vertrauensstelle für Verlobte und Eheleute) in Charlottenburg.[36] Kirsten Reinert differentiates the Vertrauensstellen from municipal clinics, which primarily served the working class, by the fact that middle-class women's organizations founded them and they targeted primarily middle-class women in large cities.[37] According to at least one welfare journal, educated women, with their mature and composed personalities, were especially suitable for issuing marriage advice, which required extreme reliability, tactfulness, and a rich knowledge of people.[38]

In addition to municipal clinics, a number of sexual counselling centres already existed in Germany. These centres had independent sponsors, especially from women's organizations, the sexual reform movement, and the workers' rights movement.[39] They provided sex education, advice on partners and sex, and guidance on the types and usage of birth control and how to prevent unwanted pregnancy. Magnus Hirschfeld (1868–1935), a physician and sexologist who advocated homosexual rights and was a leader of the sexual reform movement, established the first sexual counselling centre in 1919, the Berlin Institute for Sexual Science (Institut für Sexualwissenschaft). Hirschfeld's institute was one of a number of early private sexual counselling centres that emphasized the genetic quality of parents and offspring. In 1924, he added a private marriage counselling centre to his institute, which determined marriage candidates' health and sexual compatibility as well as "their eugenic suitability for parenthood." It also offered counselling for already-married couples experiencing marital problems.[40] Feminist sex reformer Helene Stöcker's (1869–1943) Bund für Mutterschutz also opened private marriage and sex counselling centres in 1924 in Hamburg, Frankfurt, Mannheim, and later in Breslau and Berlin. Following Stöcker's own eugenic inclinations, the Bund initially wanted these clinics to centre on premarital counselling that would prevent the spread of VD and the perpetuation of undesirable offspring, but instead it ended up focusing its efforts on solving the marital problems of couples and providing them with birth control for social, eugenic, and population policy reasons.[41] Kristine von Soden, in her account of sexual counselling centres in the Weimar Republic, estimates that between 1919 and 1932 over 400 sexual counselling centres were founded, with almost 40 of these in Berlin. In addition, there were about 100 travelling counselling centres (*fliegende Beratungsstellen*), for a total of over 500 clinics.[42]

Drawing the line between private marriage and sexual counselling centres and municipal marriage counselling centres has not always been straightforward, especially because the majority of individuals who visited clinics sought information about birth control and diaphragms and these clinics often ended up adapting to visitor desires even if that was not their intended purpose. Distinguishing between clinics was especially difficult because, as Timm demonstrates, "eugenic thinking also permeated progressive thinking" in the Weimar Republic; such stark distinctions between eugenically oriented municipal clinics and progressive, left-wing sexual counselling centres cannot be made, as individuals from both the left and right used eugenics rhetoric to support government intervention in order to improve individual and national health.[43] Female physicians, through their endeavours in municipal, private, and even religiously sponsored clinics, were no exception to this rule. Their analogous work in several different types of centres attests to the fact that the ideological boundaries between them were quite fluid.

The distribution of information about birth control and abortion in private clinics was more or less a given. Not only were they privately sponsored and thus exempt from state regulations, but it was a well-known fact that most visitors who came to the private sexual and marriage counselling centres sought birth control and abortion. For example, Max Hirsch, a Berlin gynecologist, reported that in 1926, 79 per cent of the 630 women who visited the Bund für Mutterschutz clinic in Hamburg were seeking advice about pregnancy, and one-fourth asked specifically about abortion.[44] Dr Rabe, a medical assistant at a sexual counselling centre in Hamburg, confirmed that the vast majority of people seeking advice – he estimated 85–90 per cent – came to prevent unwanted pregnancy.[45] Given the activities of private marriage and sexual counselling centres like the one in Hamburg, the RGA feared that the public would come to view them as abortion centres.[46]

Municipal clinics also debated the distribution of birth control because the majority of visitors to municipal centres were not engaged couples seeking premarital counselling and concerned about the quality of their prospective offspring, but unmarried couples seeking birth control. The fact that many of these couples wanted to avoid having babies has led Edward Ross Dickinson to question whether municipal clinics actually achieved what they intended.[47] Certainly, the issue of whether or not to disseminate birth control and advice on how to prevent pregnancy was more ambiguous in these centres, with groups from different sides of the religious, political, and professional spectrum weighing in. In his ordinance, the Prussian Minister for the People's Welfare warned against marriage counselling centres that limited their activities to disseminating birth control information.[48] Conservative factions, disturbed by the public's access to birth control in such clinics, launched a campaign against dispensing it in private and municipal centres.[49] Communists, at the other extreme of the political spectrum, demanded that counselling centres teach women about the various ways to prevent pregnancy.[50] They thought clinics should provide contraception, information about how to end unwanted pregnancy, and free advice to people entering marriage about their health conditions and any possible genetic weaknesses, as well as free legal help regarding marriage and divorce.[51]

Religious circles expressed dismay that contraception was widely available at marriage counselling centres. The predominantly Catholic Centre Party objected to sexual counselling and widespread access to contraception in any clinic.[52] The Protestant Church and its welfare arm, the Inner Mission, became incensed by the lack of clarity about whether it was the responsibility of marriage counselling centres to distribute birth control and advice on pregnancy prevention. Hans Harmsen, the leader of the Inner Mission, complained about the large disconnect between Hirtsiefer's Decree, which explicitly stated that it was not the duty of marriage counsellors to deal with the question of contraception, and the massive distribution of birth control happening on a day-to-day basis in state-run marriage counselling centres in Prussia. Harmsen thought the municipal clinics were too similar to the sexual counselling centres set up by sexual reformers like Magnus Hirschfeld and Helene Stöcker. He sought to create a strict divide between the two realms, suggesting that marriage counselling should focus on issuing marriage certificates and that sexual counselling centres handle questions of contraception. He cautioned, however, that sexual counselling clinics not only contradicted Paragraph 184 (which forbade the distribution and advertisement of contraceptives), but they conflicted with the moral values of the majority of people. If sexual counselling centres had to be established, he suggested that only certain types of clinics – namely religious ones – take up the issue of birth control. This nearly year-long discussion within the Inner Mission and petitioning of the Prussian state concluded with Harmsen asking Hirtsiefer to consider the disparity between his original ordinance and the daily operation of marriage counselling centres, and to make Protestant sexual counselling centres available.[53] The Inner Mission, with the support of the Catholic welfare organization Caritas, continued to petition the federal government on this issue throughout the Weimar Republic.[54]

Timm's overview of the network of Catholic and Protestant marriage counselling centres demonstrates how much they had in common with municipal centres, even if they opened in an attempt to counteract the liberal views on contraception held by municipal clinics. Both Catholic and Protestant centres had eugenic undertones and in some cases distributed birth control, even if they proclaimed to be against it. The Catholic

Church's marriage counselling centres advised engaged couples on issues of economic, legal, and health compatibility, and helped married couples stay together. They combined "eugenics with religious ethics," setting themselves against the profit-making private sexual counselling centres (which they thought contributed to society's ethical downfall) by claiming to be countering the threat that "proletarian radicalization" posed to marriage and the family. These centres refused to provide information on birth control, even if many clients, according to counsellors, continued to request contraception. Timm concludes "that despite the emphasis on spiritual counselling, actual practice, even in Catholic marriage counselling, occasionally adapted pragmatically to patient needs."[55]

The Protestant Church had set up seven marriage counselling centres across Berlin by 1930, and more in cities like Potsdam, Kassel, Stettin, Düsseldorf, Munich, Stuttgart, Königsberg, and Hamburg.[56] In the hopes of attracting parishioners back to the church by offering spiritual marriage counselling as well as legal advice, these centres always included a female pastor and female lawyer on staff in addition to a female doctor for consultation.[57] In reality, people sought guidance on a number of other issues – alcoholism, psychological illness, divorce, fertility, abortion, and matchmaking.[58] Its welfare arm, the Inner Mission, still struggled to determine the appropriate means to reconcile their religious beliefs with the social needs and wants of visitors to their marriage counselling centres. Harmsen, a controversial figure who supported both the repeal of Paragraph 218 (the law that forbade abortion) and birth control for the "unfit" masses, again found himself occupied with the question of birth control in Protestant marriage counselling centres in 1932.[59] In a letter informing a pastor about an anticipated meeting of all the leaders of Protestant marriage counselling centres, Harmsen asserted that "the biggest practical difficulty" the Inner Mission faced was "the fact that the leading personalities had an unclear position regarding sexual ethics issues, primarily the distribution of birth control." Therefore, he called for a general meeting in which the leaders could share their experiences on fundamental issues.[60] Moreover, in an attempt to assess various doctors' positions on birth control in marriage counselling centres, Harmsen asked a few doctors in Berlin about whether they were fundamentally opposed to giving contraceptive advice or if they issued advice on a case-by-case basis. All doctors – male and female – working within these Protestant marriage counselling centres agreed that they gave (or would give) such advice based on the conditions of each case, demonstrating that they were more or less following the policies of municipal clinics.[61] Harmsen also recognized the limited appeal of Protestant clinics, which working-class populations would reject for not offering birth control.[62] This comment elucidated the class background of the majority of visitors to marriage counselling centres – something that middle- and upper-class female physicians would come to take advantage of.

The fact that so many municipal marriage counselling centres were dispersing birth control and sexual counselling advice led to the formation of the Association of Public Marriage Counselling Centres (Vereinigung öffentlicher Eheberatungsstellen) in June 1927. Timm argues this organization showed just how far municipal clinics had strayed from their intended purpose to examine and advise marriage candidates on genetic compatibility. The Association sought to incorporate all marriage counselling centres that adhered to the eugenic goals outlined in the original 1926 Prussian decree. Although the Association excluded progressive sexual reformers like Stöcker, it never took a strict stance against sexual counselling and some of its members still promoted access to birth control.[63] At a meeting of the Association in Leipzig on 9 September 1928, it became evident that some of these supporters of contraception were female physicians. At the meeting, Alfred Grotjahn, the founder of the German social hygiene movement, gave a presentation on "Marriage Counselling Centres and Birth Prevention" in which he argued that municipal marriage counselling centres should under no circumstances distribute birth control but should instead be concerned with the maintenance of the *Volk*. Käte Frankenthal, a Social Democrat, and Minna Flake, a Communist, both practising doctors in Berlin, disagreed with this view, revealing the general stance that women doctors took on the question of contraception in marriage counselling centres. Frankenthal described birth control as an "essential duty" of marriage counselling centres, which she otherwise saw as "worthless." Flake, who asserted that economic hardships were the main cause for the decline in fertility, advocated for marriage counselling centres to push birth control in order to combat the "inevitable alarming increase of abortions."[64] Frankenthal and Flake were not alone in their calls for birth control to be distributed in marriage counselling centres.

The Distribution of Birth Control

While female doctors, as a group, were primarily in favour of expanding women's access to birth control in marriage counselling clinics, some were more extreme than others. Hertha Nathorff, the director of a Berlin family and marriage counselling centre, agreed that "female doctors in [their] double role as women and doctors [had] the utmost duty ... to educate women about rational birth control."[65] Although municipal marriage counselling centres had not taken an official position on birth control in 1928, Hermine Heusler-Edenhuizen argued that it should be the duty of these clinics to advise women about rational birth control on a case-by-case basis. Heusler-Edenhuizen was the first president of the Bund Deutscher Ärztinnen (League of German Female Physicians; BDÄ) and wrote a short history of marriage counselling in *Soziale Praxis*. She, like Flake, viewed birth control as the only successful method for preventing an increase in the number of abortions. Heusler-Edenhuizen was sympathetic to the fact that having a large number of children exacerbated the hardships people were already facing in interwar Germany. She had faith that providing information about birth control in marriage counselling centres would not, in fact, result in a further decline in population, as many people feared.[66] Because she claimed to know "the strong motherly instinct of women," she was certain women's desire to have children would return as soon as their life difficulties were minimized.[67] Heusler-Edenhuizen, a mother of two, used her own experience to fashion herself as having a strong understanding of what she perceived to be a motherly instinct innate in all women. While she may have shared a commonality with female advice seekers in their interests to reproduce, she certainly lacked an authentic understanding of how the economic adversity of the Weimar-era affected their decisions about procreation. Instead, she assumed that these primarily lower-class visitors to municipal marriage counselling centres shared her middle-class values about prioritizing having a family.

Dr Josephine Höber, a marriage counsellor who worked in a municipal clinic in Kiel, also called for counselling about birth control, especially in certain cases. These included cases in which families had several children, one of whom was handicapped, or when fathers were almost permanently unemployed. She thought birth control counselling was "certainly called for" in these cases because without counselling, the risk of criminal abortion was too high.[68] Höber's own eugenic leanings were reflected in her wish to push birth control among the handicapped, but also among families who were struggling financially. She was likely motivated by a desire to alleviate the burden of her patients, who faced having more children when they were already overwhelmed by economic troubles and caring for several children. Simultaneously, she could have also been driven by a desire to ease the burden these families would be on the marriage counselling centre and society.

While Heusler-Edenhuizen and Höber supported birth control on a case-by-case basis, Lotte Fink and Hertha Riese, who led the Bund für Mutterschutz's marriage and sexual counselling centre in Frankfurt, took a more extreme view. Fink and Riese were among some of the most active campaigners for birth control, but they also recognized the shortcomings of some of their lower-class patients in successfully using contraception, resulting from either their "despair" or "obtuseness."[69] The debate about contraception in marriage counselling, this example revealed, centred not only around *when* (in which cases) it should be issued, but also around *who* should be receiving it. As historian Atina Grossmann shows, female doctors believed that the lower classes could not always be trusted because they were generally assumed to be irresponsible when it came to sexual hygiene. Doctors thus recommended different contraceptive devices for "intelligent" women and "unintelligent" women, using eugenics terminology that divided women into the responsible worthy and the irresponsible unworthy.[70] The debate over birth control in marriage counselling centres, therefore, led to larger questions over *which* women should be seeking and receiving birth control and *whether* certain women were even capable of using it, as concerns about the "inferior" overrunning the "superior" were still imperative in many circles.

In their demands for birth control, female doctors undoubtedly played on the public's fears of a growing abortion rate, yet many of them also called for the elimination of Paragraph 218. To some, questions of birth control and abortion could not be separated.[71] Flake and Frankenthal, both members of the radical Verein sozialistischer Ärzte (Association of Socialist Physicians; VsÄ), were quite political in their demands for the abolition of Paragraph 218, often shifting the discussion from one about morality to one about women's individual health, independence, and sexual happiness.[72] Cornelie Usborne has argued that "despite these remarkably emancipatory sentiments," women doctors like Flake and Frankenthal "shared the preoccupation of the time with a qualitative population policy," which, she notes, "implied an infringement of the very rights that they expressly demanded for every woman." She criticizes female physicians, in other words, for speaking out "as feminists" while also subscribing to abortion on eugenic grounds, like those members of the VsÄ.[73] Rather than viewing this as an inherent contradiction, I view women doctors' endorsement of birth control and abortion within the context of marriage counselling centres as strategic, as it legitimized their careers by offering them an area of expertise serving the primarily female clientele in clinics on these matters.

Claiming Their Work Space

The debates about birth control in marriage counselling centres help to explain part of the story of how women doctors came to take an interest in this new medical field. There were also practical reasons that led female physicians to argue for their presence in this space – the flexibility of the clinic hours and the high number of female visitors to the clinics. In addition, female physicians claimed that in this woman-centred space, they offered a valuable confidante to the primarily female clientele because they, as women, had similar needs and concerns. Their analogous life experience was also why they promoted a particular type of married female doctor to counsel visitors – something doctors claimed that their clients wanted.

By working in marriage counselling clinics, where they generally had office hours only twice a week, women could straddle their professional and domestic roles. Many women doctors were also mothers, and in fact, *Die Ärztin* reported in 1933 that the average number of children of married female doctors (1.65) was higher than female civil servants (1.02), which Dr Grete Albrecht claimed countered the constant accusation (seen, for example, in articles in *Deutsches Ärzteblatt* from that same year) that female doctors were having fewer children than the national average.[74] Sabine Schleiermacher also maintains that a disproportionate number of female doctors during the Weimar period were married and had children.[75] Working in counselling centres, then, proved desirable since it offered flexible hours to combine family duties and professional work. As the needs of clients multiplied, however, the reality of these more flexible employment opportunities waned. Women often worked in marriage counselling centres in addition to having their own practices, and sometimes worked more than the necessary hours at marriage counselling centres, or even out of their own homes. Ilse Szagunn was one example of these overworked physicians. She worked in an infant and mother counselling centre in Charlottenburg (1914–1927) and then in the Protestant marriage counselling centre in Friedenau (1927–1943). She simultaneously worked as Germany's first vocational school doctor starting in 1918 and developed health lessons for the women's school of Alice Salomon in Berlin (1919–1931). Meanwhile, she served on a number of committees, including the Prussian Health Council's Committee for Population Politics and Committee for School Health Care (1927–1933). She also had a husband and two children of her own.[76]

Another practical concern for women physicians in their claims to occupy this space was the predominantly female clientele who visited marriage counselling centres. Through its premarital educational leaflets, the RGA encouraged women to initiate marriage counselling, thus leading to a large majority of female visitors, whom women physicians claimed they could better serve. Estimates of how many people visited marriage counselling centres within their first few years are difficult to determine, as not all municipal, private, or religious centres kept precise records. Based on those that did, it appeared that between two-thirds and three-quarters of the visitors were women. The Information Centre and Registry for Marriage Questions and Marriage Crisis (Auskunfts- und Vertrauensstelle für Ehefragen und Ehenot) in Berlin-Steglitz, established in February 1928, claimed that in a seven-week period immediately after its opening, the clinic saw 61 people, 75 per cent of them women.[77] The popularity of the clinics, especially among women, flourished even after the Nazis came to power. After 1933, the Nazis immediately closed the private marriage and sexual counselling centres and closed municipal clinics or converted them to counselling centres for genetic and racial health (Beratungsstellen für Erb-und-Rassenpflege).[78] This has led Paul Weindling to see Weimar municipal clinics as precursors to the Nazi clinics, for both had eugenic objectives at their core.[79] The Protestant marriage counselling centres remained open and active during the Third Reich, and thus Szagunn kept her job and sought opportunity in promoting this counselling.[80] These centres did not cease to attract women. In the 1932–5 annual reports from the Protestant Marriage Counselling Centre in Berlin-Friedenau, which opened in 1932, the number of advice seekers rose from 105 in 1932 to 190 in 1933, to 315 in 1934, and to 369 in 1935. The number of female visitors in these four years never dipped below 70 per cent, demonstrating the consistency with which women sought help from the centre. Moreover, Dr Szagunn reported that the percentage of people among the total visitors who sought her medical advice remained around 50 per cent for all four years. Within this group, women again made up two-thirds to three-quarters of those in search of medical advice specifically.[81] Similar figures regarding the number of women visitors held true for other municipal and religious marriage counselling centres.[82]

In light of the large majority of women who visited marriage counselling centres, female doctors rallied for their presence in these spaces
because they thought they would be more effective at building trusting relationships with these patients. Creating a space where patients
could trust their doctors was one of the new expectations of marriage
counselling, as outlined by the RGA in its educational health leaflet.[83]
An open, trusting relationship between advice seeker and advice giver
was certainly an essential component of the success of clinics. Female
doctors' discussions of trust between physicians and patients revealed
their opinions regarding the shortcomings of their male colleagues and
provided a means for them to forge new ground in the discussion about
the relationship between practitioners and patients.

Dr Margarete Riderer-Kleemann, in her discussion of the effects of
internal disease on pregnancy and childbirth, stressed that because
female doctors were confidantes for women, they could provide
encouragement and education to their women patients.[84] Women visitors came to counselling centres sometimes with very difficult, embarrassing questions, noted Dr Helene Fritz-Hölder, a strong proponent
of marriage counselling as one of the specific duties of female physicians. Male doctors, according to her, had not "risen to the occasion,"
so instead she encouraged women advice seekers to turn to female
doctors, whom they could go to "with trust." She thought that talking
to male medical advisers was too difficult for women. Speaking to a
male doctor was embarrassing and frightening for a woman who could
hardly admit a marital or health problem to herself and dreaded being
misunderstood by a man. Some problems were so new to recently married women that they lacked the vocabulary to describe them. Beyond
advocating for marriage counselling to be the "loftiest" (*vornehmsten*)
duty of her colleagues, Fritz-Hölder was especially critical of her male
colleagues for abandoning women in their time of deepest need and not
understanding the intricacies of female reproduction. They did not, for
example, understand that intercourse within the first month of pregnancy could be harmful, or that abstinence should be advised within
the few weeks prior to delivery because of the dangers of infection.[85]
Female physicians unquestionably recognized such consequences
because they were familiar with the female reproductive system and
the dangers associated with pregnancy – something that Fritz-Hölder
seems to imply women doctors would naturally already know.

Highlighting the advantages of same-sex counselling for the female
patients who visited these centres allowed women physicians to further

justify the need for their work in counselling centres and to promote the essential role they played in their success. Since the majority of female patients visited marriage counselling centres to ask about birth control or other personal questions, such as marital problems or how their offspring might be affected by genetic diseases, many women professionals suggested that it was a good thing to have female doctors on hand. Women clearly had an easier time talking to their "same-sex companions" (*Geschlechtsgenossin*) than male doctors, especially about taboo topics like birth control, marital problems, and genetic diseases.[86] These doctors suggested that female patients would be more likely to disclose personal information about themselves to a woman because they understood that the female practitioner shared with them the experiences and tribulations of marriage, pregnancy, and childbirth. Because "their own experience unquestionably increases the understanding for the experience of others," Dr Heusler-Edenhuizen demanded that counselling centres exclusively employ female doctors to advise women and male doctors to advise men.[87]

In addition to the practicalities of flexible work schedules and handling primarily women, women doctors laid claim to marriage counselling by fashioning a certain type of woman doctor as better equipped to work in this field. The married woman doctor who was also a mother became the model worker in marriage counselling because she could best empathize with the experiences and needs of visitors. Thus, female doctors called for marriage counsellors with specific backgrounds. Dr Anne-Marie Durand-Wever, leader of the Registry for Engaged and Married People in Charlottenburg, recommended that counsellors be married and have their own families so that they could fully understand the difficulties and conflicts of their patients. In her opinion, purely theoretical preparatory training was sufficient for issuing marriage health certificates, drawing up marriage contracts, or determining reasons for divorce, but it was not adequate for helping people with individual needs – needs that, she claimed, went far beyond that of mere counselling before marriage. Durand-Wever underlined that only an "embarrassingly small percent" of people sought advice before marriage, instead coming with questions about sexual form, ways to limit the number of children, divorce, and economic concerns. Their questions were so wide-ranging, in fact, that one male doctor found himself unable to be of much help based on his training.[88] Marriage and parenthood gave female counsellors a privileged insight into their client's lives, according to Durand-Wever and other female doctors, meaning that they could be much more effective counsellors. Dr Heusler-Eden-huizen agreed that doctors working in marriage counselling centres should themselves be married because this increased their understanding of other people's marital experiences.[89] Experience had shown that visitors to the Kiel municipal marriage counselling centre, where Dr Josephine Höber worked, shied away from seeking advice from the young, unmarried female doctors employed at the clinic; instead, it made a great difference for a woman to pour her heart out to an older, married woman and mother – that is, someone just like her.[90] Marriage counselling centres certainly benefited from employing older, married doctors who were also mothers. Interestingly, this already marginalized group of female physicians perpetuated similar discrimination against their unmarried, childless female peers. By upholding women's responsibilities to be wives and mothers *first*, female physicians demonstrated how strongly they adhered to mainstream beliefs about the appropriate roles for women. However, this was also a means for them to strategically endorse women's domestic expectations alongside their aspiring professional careers and to bridge that gap in their own lives as well.

Women doctors claimed marriage counselling centres as their space for practical reasons, and they also promoted the married mother as the best type of doctor to serve the primarily female clientele seeking trustworthy confidants to discuss concerns that could be perceived as embarrassing. Usborne has asserted that female physicians "felt a mission to tend to women patients whose special needs and sense of propriety they felt were often badly served by male members of the profession," and we certainly can see how this was the case in marriage counselling clinics.[91] Their assertion that they more aptly served the needs of patrons in marriage counselling clinics came both as a criticism of the male profession but also as a desire to avoid competing with their male colleagues by serving primarily women. On the one hand, female physicians adhered to a traditional belief that they were different from their male colleagues because of their special feminine abilities. And yet, on the other hand, despite the fact that their gender coerced them down certain paths, that they were subject to larger societal discrimination and expectations of the time, or that they held their own personal preferences, women promoted themselves and, to a certain extent, worked as equals with men in the field of marriage counselling. Even more importantly, they gained the opportunity to follow their own individual agendas to provide comprehensive health care for women within this gendered space.

Rallying for Comprehensive Health Care for Women

Marriage counselling centres came to be a predominantly female space – in terms of both visitors and issues discussed. Women doctors working in these clinics benefited by working in what came to be a unique womanly space. They not only justified their presence in this women's realm, but also expanded the duties of marriage counselling centres to include their own agendas. Grossmann has argued that women actually profited from exclusion within the medical field. She demonstrates, for example, that in sex and marriage counselling centres, women doctors could balance their complicated lives as working mothers and wives due to limited hours, teamwork, and support from female colleagues. In addition to these advantages in their personal lives, their professional lives benefited too, as they were able to network with other women professionals and speak with women of other classes. This, according to Grossmann, allowed them to develop a professional identity that they could be proud of and control these centres as women's spaces, and it led them to be far more radical than they might have been otherwise.[92] This was most apparent in marriage counselling in the ways women doctors became advocates for women's equal and comprehensive access to medical care.

While emphasizing their unique insights as mothers, wives, and women to serve female patients, female physicians simultaneously criticized the impersonal, unfriendly, large clinics and the way in which cold, unsympathetic doctors treated their patients, instead stressing their "holistic 'woman-oriented' approach to medicine."[93] Ilse Szagunn, a doctor working in the Protestant Marriage and Family Counselling Centre in Berlin-Friedenau, in fact, described the positive aspects of counselling advice seekers in "totality," noting that in her counselling centre, a female minister, doctor, lawyer, and welfare nurse were always present at the same time. This type of cooperation between different specialists, she asserted, proved to be helpful.[94] The holistic approach to medicine, in marriage counselling centres more specifically, allowed women doctors to consider all things: the medical, legal, religious, ethical, political, and technical aspects of marriage, sex, and birth control. Marriage counselling, to women doctors, meant much more than the simple issuing of a marriage health certificate; their duties encompassed not merely the scientific, but the social too. Because they were dealing with intimate questions coming from primarily female patients, it was essential for them to have a humane social approach to medicine.

This became one of the main ways in which female doctors differentiated themselves from their male peers and articulated the broadening of their roles in marriage counselling centres.

Female doctors took control of the marriage counselling centre space by using it as an opportunity to provide more to women than mere medical exams and marriage health certificates. It was no longer a place where women would come only to get advice about whether they were fit enough to enter marriage; they could also come for all types of medical, legal, and, in some cases, religious advice before and during marriage. Experience showed that people rarely came for advising prior to marriage, but instead for questions about birth control, sexual needs, marriage problems, social needs, and abortion. In fact, Dr Durand-Wever admitted that one of the reasons for the founding of the Vertrauensstelle für Verlobte und Eheleute, where she worked, was because so few people came to clinics for premarital health advising. At these private clinics, women could get counselling on a number of other matters.[95] Dr Höber reported that in ten months' working at a municipal marriage counselling centre in Kiel, she saw five unmarried and sixteen married women for the following reasons: the desire to have a child, birth control, sexual questions, marriage disputes, depression, and premarital health certificates (only two unmarried and one married women came in for this reason).[96] In one of the private clinics of the Bund für Mutterschutz in Frankfurt, Dr Fink reported that in the five years since the clinic opened there had been an estimated 7,675 counselling sessions, 66 per cent of which handled questions of birth control. From the remaining third, 60 per cent of the advice seekers came for prevention, 20 per cent for social questions, 10 per cent for sexual issues, and 10 per cent for marriage counselling.[97] The understanding, according to some female physicians, was that this type of counselling could serve the individual needs and wants of women who encountered a variety of difficulties in marriage. As a result, some marriage counselling centres employed a variety of specialists from different fields. Durand-Wever said that the Vertrauensstelle für Verlobte und Eheleute not only had one adviser available, but offered a variety of doctors, lawyers, pastors, and economists free of charge, all of whom held regular office hours. The Protestant marriage counselling centre in Friedenau also employed a number of different specialists, as Szagunn noted above.[98]

What fell under "marital problems" came to encompass a broad range of concerns, namely alcoholism, domestic violence, unemployment, homelessness, disease, disloyalty, abortion, contraception, sterilization, property rights, and divorce. External circumstances like these some-times caused marital difficulties or several of these problems often coincided with or caused one another. Take, for example, one of the couples that Szagunn saw in the Friedenau Protestant counselling cen-tre. The pair, who had been married for nineteen years, came to see Sza-gunn because they were having marital problems. They had originally been pressured by their parents to marry because they were expect-ing a child. The husband was a drinker, had a venereal disease, and also had difficulty controlling his temper, having broken house and kitchen appliances several times. Their two children were also affected. The elder son, who was eighteen, was a severe psychopath, lied, and stole, while the younger was very disrespectful. This example, Szagunn asserted, showed just how much was masked behind the idea of a "dis-rupted marriage." Moreover, this couple was not an exception; accord-ing to Szagunn, alcoholism, extramarital relations, or sickness caused most marital problems, and frequently economic need or the husband's unemployment exacerbated problems, making the marriage unsustain-able.[99] Since, as Szagunn stated in an annual report, practically no one came in for advice about their health condition before marriage, doctors like her, trained in medicine, claimed to offer much more than merely medical advice, which concurred with their overall holistic view of medicine.[100] They did not seek to treat individual patients as "cases," but examined them wholly by considering their individual and social circumstances along with their medical concerns.[101] This was why, as Grossmann argues, they identified themselves as clinicians rather than scientists – an approach that allowed them to both criticize the male members of the profession and distinguish themselves from their male peers.[102]

Female doctors suggested that working at a marriage counselling centre was an opportunity to assist women in a number of other ways, thereby further expanding their medical roles to include the pedagogi-cal, legal, and moral. Beyond insisting that these clinics be a space where women could receive information about contraceptive options or, in some cases, possibilities for abortion, Durand-Wever also felt these cen-tres should be a source of legal information.[103] She contended that mar-riage counselling centres had to educate women regarding the basic idea that they did, in fact, have certain legal rights in marriage, but that these rights had always been in the hands of men. Therefore, she saw it as one of the goals of the privately funded Vertrauensstelle für Verlobte und Eheleute to declare and expose grievances and give suggestions for the legal regulation of marriage rights.[104] Providing legal knowledge was one means to grant women comprehensive care in these spaces.

In addition to stepping out of their medical roles to fashion themselves as legal advisers for visitors, some women doctors viewed marriage counselling clinics as an appropriate place to become women's moral guides. In light of the value placed on leading a successful marriage, which depended greatly on the mental and physical ability of women to balance their household responsibilities, caretaking obligations, physical and emotional relationships with their spouses, and perhaps even employment, Dr Riderer-Kleemann recognized the importance of educating young girls about their marriage responsibilities. Because she sought to strengthen this sense of responsibility in young girls, she saw it fit to act as more than just a medical leader by warning them against the current fad of having unhealthy sexual relations in large cities. Moreover, she passed moral judgment on this fad, suggesting that "unhealthy" and "unclean" activities had to be stopped.[105] In addition to her medical goal of raising a generation of healthy women, Riderer-Kleemann alluded to the fact that women doctors were concerned with moral issues that emerged from the growing number of single women living in urban centres, including sex outside of marriage, prostitution, back-alley abortions, and the spread of venereal disease. Dr Nathorff also appeared to follow a moral agenda, preaching to her young, single female patients, who were very sexually emancipated. She gave more than just doctorly advice to her married patients, even advising one patient to preserve her marriage by giving her tips on cunnilingus.[106] Other doctors used discussions of marriage counselling to argue against free-love advocates, claiming that a sexual commitment without love, whether or not there was a marriage certificate, was nothing more than prostitution.[107] Presuming they were acting in their patients' best interests, these female doctors evidently felt it was acceptable for them to intervene on issues of an ethical nature. The class divide that existed between doctors like Riderer-Kleemann and Nathorff and their advice seekers accentuated this, leading them to greatly overstep their professionally defined medical boundaries. By assuming they understood what were the most appropriate sexual norms for their supposedly sexually scandalous lower-class patients, Riderer-Kleemann and Nathorff displayed a clear maternalist attitude in passing judgment on them and attempting to guide them to an upper-middle-class sense of morality.

Education and enlightenment also fell under the purview of marriage counselling. Female physicians were most explicit about the medical *and* pedagogical goals of this type of counselling in an article from their journal *Die Ärztin*:

> The goal of marriage counselling is two-fold: Pedagogically, it should edu-
> cate people to have a higher sense of responsibility towards their own health,
> the health of their marriage partner and of their offspring, and it should
> supply them with the absolutely necessary physiological and hygienic edu-
> cation of all sex opportunities available. In the practical medical sense, it
> should preserve the health of those who are healthy, expose the apparently
> healthy as sick, care for the sick or prevent the transmission of their disease
> and finally the burden of inheriting their inferior dispositions.[108]

In this outline of the educational goals and medical expectations of marriage counselling centres, the eugenic thought behind both was apparent. The BDÄ certainly understood the implications of marriage choice on the genetic makeup of the future *Volk*, thus revealing the rea-son the organization educated visitors to take more responsibility in terms of their own health and that of their partners. By publishing the above piece in their journal, the BDÄ was undoubtedly subscribing to the eugenic duties of municipal marriage counselling centres, setting one of its medical goals as the prevention of "inferior" traits.

Engaging with Eugenics

While women doctors sought to expand the duties of the marriage counselling centre and create a unique woman-to-woman space in which issues previously considered private and taboo like abortion, birth control, and divorce could be publicly discussed, a select number of them also openly supported eugenics discourse that aimed to limit reproduction among certain members of the lower classes. Their actions and words revealed a sincere belief in alleviating society of the burdens that resulted from unhealthy offspring, advocating marriages only for capable individuals and dispensing birth control to individuals in the less-worthy classes. At the same time, they showed a desire to lessen the load of their already overburdened patients, who often came to them because they were in desperate situations.

The founding principle of issuing marriage certificates only to individ-uals who were "fit" enough to marry – the intended duty of municipal clinics even if this did not always come to fruition – coincided with the Weimar eugenics agenda. Those women doctors who worked in (and sometimes even directed) municipal centres also supported their eugenics objectives by issuing marriage certificates that either permitted or prevented individuals from getting married and producing offspring based on their health fitness. Certain female physicians, however, were sometimes more forthright about the eugenic mission of their work in these clinics. In a 1927 article, "The Racial Hygienic Duties of Marriage Counselling Centres," members of the BDÄ acknowledged that the primary duty of marriage counselling centres was to awaken the masses to the fundamental ideas of eugenics by clarifying the difference between normal, superior characteristics and abnormal ones – "in short: racial hygiene instruction." They saw it as their secondary task to test each marriage candidate for the presence of a "eugenically questionable disposition."[109] In their writing, doctors who worked in municipal centres fully understood that racial hygienic and eugenic considerations governed the founding of these centres, and they were well aware that offspring had become the highest priority of marriage, which Dr Durand-Wever described as "no longer an individual matter, but a matter of the state."[110] Dr Höber, who worked in a municipal clinic outside of Prussia, admitted that "population policy views in the sense of racial hygienic marriage restoration" had influenced the founding of municipal marriage counselling. She defended the existence of such centres in spite of the lack of a eugenic consciousness among marriage candidates, and claimed that experience had shown that prevention was better, cheaper, and more successful than healing, and that the current centres could be considered "the root for a racial hygienic one of the future."[111] Aspiring to fulfil the state's paramount goal of ensuring healthy offspring, Höber directed her eugenic rhetoric primarily toward her lower-class patients.

Doctors like Heusler-Edenhuizen, in typical maternalist fashion, attempted to teach the art of marriage to her lower-class advice seekers and suggested that this was a main duty of the clinics. Heusler-Edenhuizen recognized that marriage choices and the mistakes of parents ultimately had an impact on children because these factors determined the household atmosphere in which children were raised, and thus she thought that teaching a couple how to lead a healthy marriage was essential. Parents often underestimated the impact of their marriage disputes on children, or they assumed that children could not sense a tense household environment. As a result of these disharmonious marriages, according to Heusler-Edenhuizen, children often suffered mental trauma, which proved to be a danger to society because more criminals came out of this group.[112] Her reasoning for teaching the art of marriage, then, embodied a eugenic belief that "inferior" elements of the population – in this case criminals – resulted from children seeing their parents in bad marriages. Criminality, which eugenicists considered a heritable trait, was something that Heusler-Edenhuizen wanted to prevent, inspiring her to teach her advice seekers how to lead happy marriages.

Heusler-Edenhuizen believed that what she was doing was in the best interests of her patients as well as society at large. To her, marriage counselling was a scientific means of solving the practical problems of her patients, but also of lessening the social burdens that mental illness and criminality caused. She noted, for instance, the costs of housing mentally ill children in welfare institutions or prisons.[113] Heusler-Edenhuizen, therefore, reflected the attitude that was common at the time: eugenic measures were necessary in order to spare society from further social burdens. Weimar Germany was already facing a number of problems – massive inflation, unstable governments, a crisis of marriage, a decline in fertility – and the last thing it needed was to spend additional money and effort on accommodating criminals, asocials, or unhealthy individuals. In other words, the state was already overburdened with welfare obligations it could not fulfil, and Heusler-Edenhuizen did not intend to add any more.

Heusler-Edenhuizen fit the model of female physicians who, as Grossmann and Schleiermacher argue, supported eugenics based upon their experiences working in public counselling centres, where they saw primarily working-class female patients. Observing bad living conditions, unemployment, and poor people led women doctors to form their social and political views of medicine; they witnessed firsthand, for example, how oversized families living in small or inadequate housing became linked to criminality, drunkenness, and sickness.[114] The experiences of Szagunn, who worked in a religiously sponsored marriage counselling centre, demonstrated that most patients who visited these clinics had several interconnected problems. In an annual report from 1931, she claimed that four of the seven women who came to her asking for an abortion lacked housing and were in severe economic need; in three of these cases, their husbands were unemployed. All four women suffered from a serious health handicap too.[115] In addition, Szagunn had surely seen how the bad marriage choices of parents, as well as their unhealthy genetic dispositions, attributed to so-called "asocial" behaviour and degeneration in their children. As indicated in the above description of a family who visited her clinic, the couple's marital disputes and other troubles had led to mental illness and problems in their offspring (just as Heusler-Edenhuizen would have predicted).

Szagunn, who was likely confronted by desperate pregnant women like this all the time, also became an advocate of eugenics.[116] Although not necessarily a proponent of eugenically indicated abortion, she supported abortion for medical and economic reasons, noting that she had an obligation to advise a woman to have an abortion when pregnancy posed a threat to the mother's life. She also followed up on three cases in which women requested abortions for medical or economic reasons by advising them about birth control or a more "responsible birth outcome." Szagunn, who held extra advising sessions to encourage these women to use birth control, clearly advocated the use of birth control in cases where there were too many health or social problems, that is, in cases where such problems could be passed on to offspring, resulting in a higher number of inferior elements in the population. In all three cases, she had previously encouraged these women to take birth control, but they had failed to do so, demonstrating why some women doctors became involved in a debate over which women should use birth control.

Szagunn was only one example of women doctors who were concerned about poor women who were not able to use contraception properly and became pregnant over and over again.[117] The underprivileged visitors to marriage counselling centres often did not ask for birth control until the situation became dire. Szagunn noted that during 1932, only one woman, who had had twelve pregnancies in seven years, sought her advice about birth control.[118] Dr Riese reported that women came for birth control only after their fifth or sixth child and sought abortion advice only after their sixth, seventh, or eighth.[119] Women were often unable to use particular forms of birth control due to their living circumstances. As Grossmann explains, most of these women lived in overcrowded housing, which led to "poor health and sexual disturbances." Beyond the fact that "many women were irresponsible about sexual hygiene," the "effective use of a diaphragm necessitated privacy, running water, and [a] detailed, patient explanation" from a doctor – luxuries that poor women did not always have.[120] And it was not simply that lower-class women lacked the physical space to use certain types of contraception; some women were simply incapable. Dr Elizabeth Prinz, the leader of a municipal marriage counselling centre in the Berlin working-class neighbourhood of Friedrichshain, for example, complained that working-class women could not be trusted to use contraception regularly and continued to visit counselling centres to beg for abortions.[121] Dr Fink complained about the same issue in her private clinic in Frankfurt. Severely sick mothers with too many children, who failed to use contraception properly because of either their own ignorance or social despair, constantly found reasons to return to the centre to ask for abortions. Fearing that this would be a never-ending cycle, Fink and Riese recommended sterilization for a large number of women. Fink estimated that they suggested sterilization for women who requested an abortion for medical reasons in 59.4 per cent of the cases for married women and 21.2 per cent of the cases for unmarried women. The social milieu of these married patients was quite poor, with 70 per cent of them having unemployed husbands. The unmarried women were often from a much wider array of social backgrounds (students, welfare workers, children's nurses, domestic servants). In total, Fink and Riese sterilized 435 women in five years.[122] For those women who requested abortions and remained unsterilized after the fact, Fink and Riese continued to encourage birth control (in 83 per cent of the cases). Of those who were not using contraception, 10 per cent got pregnant again within two years. In one case, a woman got pregnant three times within a year and her reasons for wanting an abortion remained unchanged and she finally had to be sterilized.[123]

Motivated by both eugenic considerations as well as a philanthropic desire to help their patients, Fink and Riese demonstrated how birth control and sterilization were a means for women doctors to simultaneously regulate and help their patients.[124] On the one hand, these female physicians often recommended birth control or sterilization based on the woman's intelligence level, showcasing the eugenics dogma that made a distinction between those deemed superior and worthy and those considered inferior and unworthy. Their focus on intelligence was often a reflection of class ignorance and did not account for the fact that for some women, contraceptive failures were due not to intelligence, but to living circumstances. Advocating birth control and sterilization became a way for doctors to regulate both the number and quality of individuals in society, especially those "asocial" elements in the lower classes. On the other hand, these women doctors saw first-hand the hardships faced by poor women with too many children and wanted to both alleviate their problems and comply with their requests. Fink even admitted that she could not in good conscience advise single mothers to carry out new pregnancies, especially knowing the difficulties they would face trying to support the child.[125] Riese was also sympathetic to her socially disadvantaged patients who were trying to cope with life's realities.[126] In the former case, these women sought to protect the community; in the latter, they desired to protect their own patients, but there was no reason they could not do both. As practitioners, they understood the burden these women created for marriage counselling clinics and the community at large, and as women, they recognized how much of a burden a child could be, especially when compounded by other difficulties.

Beyond debates about whether certain people were capable enough to manage contraception, some women doctors deliberated about whether everyone should be getting married. For Dr Helene Fritz-Hölder, it was not only a question of who was fit enough to marry based on a medical examination; she claimed certain individuals might not be prepared for the larger responsibilities that came with marriage. She criticized male physicians, whom she labelled irresponsible for continuing to prescribe marriage or pregnancy as cures for abnormal conditions of the body or mind. Marriage, in her opinion, was not simply a "medicament" but rather a "holy and high and difficult duty" – one that was not ultimately about personal happiness, but instead mutual growth and reproduction. In fact, being able and willing to bear the nation's future offspring was so essential to marriage that she professed that "whoever is not fit (*geeignet*) for the noble duty of reproduction should not get married." Fritz-Hölder believed that some people were clearly more qualified for marriage and childbearing than others, asserting that it was the duty of female doctors to explain to women coming to marriage counselling centres that under some circumstances, remaining single was acceptable. Young women, she thought, should have enough courage to value their personal lives over marriage without fearing that they would be forever deemed "inferior" for not marrying. After all, "spiritual degeneration (*Seelenverkümmerung*) [could] also develop as a result of marriage." In addition, Fritz-Hölder thought women doctors had to explain "that singleness may be a social duty, that we [society] are responsible to the unborn."[127] She suggested that singleness was not only acceptable, but also perhaps an obligation. In other words, under certain circumstances, it was better for some people to remain unmarried and childless.[128] Simply to enter a marriage to cure an abnormal condition or to fill a gap in one's life demonstrated just as much irresponsibility as the male doctors who prescribed this as therapy because it would have detrimental consequences for offspring, creating further social burdens for all. Fritz-Hölder made a distinction between those who were capable of getting married and having children and those who were not, and she also subscribed to the belief that bringing children into the world in unhappy marriages or unhealthy circumstances would be a disservice to the nation.

Conclusions: Reconciling Differing Agendas and Creating a Gendered Space

Eugenic discourse sometimes fuelled discussions about who should be receiving birth control and who should be getting married. In municipal, religious, or private clinics, female doctors inserted themselves in these debates about birth control. In all three settings, many women medical leaders pushed their lower-class patients towards birth control (or suggested doing so) after recognizing the burden they caused to society and the difficulties they would have caring for additional children. Ilse Szagunn in the Protestant marriage counselling centre, Elizabeth Prinz in the municipal clinic, and Lotte Fink and Hertha Riese in the private Bund für Mutterschutz clinic in Frankfurt represented the spectrum of women doctors who complained about the abilities of their lower-class patients to use birth control, spent extra time encouraging them to do so, and even sterilized some patients when they failed to use contraception properly. They were simultaneously interested in alleviating society from the burden of caring for unhealthy individuals and easing the problems of their distressed patients.

Alongside this class-biased eugenics dogma, women doctors negotiated a separate space for themselves within the medical profession by fashioning the important role that they as women *and* doctors would play in marriage counselling. One practical concern was that most of the advice seekers were women. In addition, women patients could confide in women doctors in a way they could not with male physicians, and patients often found that women physicians fulfilled their needs better because they had experienced similar problems and needs.[129] Thus, female physicians proclaimed to expand the offerings for their patients in this space, allowing their patients to express much more than their uncertainties before marriage. The trusting relationships created between patient and doctor allowed women doctors to provide comprehensive treatment for women's medical and social problems.

Likewise, because women doctors had the trust of their female patients, they claimed to provide much more than premarital health exams, often giving women counselling on a wide range of topics. Female physicians, then, saw themselves as potentially having an extremely powerful impact on their patients. Szagunn, for one, recognized her ability to affect patients, noting that she enjoyed the most confidence from her patients when, in addition to being a doctor, she was an expectant mother.[130] Szagunn understood that young mothers who came to her while she was pregnant felt an instinctive connection because of their shared experience, and it was in this pivotal moment that she gained their full trust and could be influential, even when it came to non-medical issues. In this regard, Szagunn and her colleagues saw themselves as assisting the Weimar state in promoting the goals of marriage counselling. Because of the intimate nature of most discussions, women doctors, as trustworthy and nurturing advisers, could encourage female clients to visit counselling centres for premarital health certificates or other problems before marriage. Weimar's marriage counselling centres, then, became what Timm has called the "nexus of exchange" between doctors and patients, between the individual and state.[131]

Lastly, as part of their calls for comprehensive health care for women, some female physicians used their experiences in marriage counselling centres to justify certain rights for underprivileged women. Hertha Nathorff is an example of how female doctors used their experiences to extend social and legal rights for working-class women. Her work in a Family and Marriage Counselling Centre in Charlottenburg, she said, led her to the view that women needed to be educated about birth control options. She came to understand the importance of making contraception accessible to women who had multiple children and already faced difficult circumstances. Her experiences of witnessing the tragedy of unwanted children and the problems and needs of the poor and unmarried led her to demand accessible contraception and information about birth prevention for women, as well as the right to abortions. This right, in her opinion, would be the most effective measure for preventing unwanted pregnancy because it would stop women in abject circumstances from turning to quack abortionists, thus further risking their own lives and their ability to have children in the future. Overturning the law against abortion would also help doctors fulfil the requests of their patients without risking criminal penalties.[132] In her calls for comprehensive legal and social protections for unmarried mothers and their children, and her demands for basic life necessities – nourishment, clothing, housing – for all, Nathorff demonstrated how women physicians were political advocates for their patients in the field of marriage counselling. Women doctors would continue this political work in schools as they became involved in discussions about reforming girls' physical education curriculum.

2 Preparing Girls for Motherhood: School Doctors, Youth Welfare, and the Reform of Girls' Physical Education

Women physicians working in schools and the youth welfare movement employed similar tactics as their colleagues in marriage counselling centres, widening the scope of their medical practice to become experts about and activists for adolescent women's health. Like their colleagues in marriage counselling, they highlighted their abilities to make unique contributions to women's health. In schools, they claimed they could support their female students as they confronted menstruation, insisting that young girls with these embarrassing adolescent concerns would be more eager to turn to female school doctors because they offered both a scientific and personal approach. Women doctors, they argued, could develop trustworthy, maternal, and nurturing relationships with students, providing them advice on a wide range of issues and a source of solace during an uncomfortable time. By advocating a new type of physical education program – one that considered the needs of women and brought women's issues like menstruation into the curriculum – women doctors developed a new form of public health. This connected them to the ongoing international work in public health and the physical fitness of men and women.[1] Female physicians made marriage, motherhood, and women's domestic lifestyles the foci of their new health rhetoric – an approach that allowed them to transpose their experiences as mothers into their professional lives and one that afforded them entrance into medicine.

While they generally followed the direction that male doctors channelled them into, they buttressed their roles as doctors through discourse. Their rhetoric highlighted the benefits of their femininity and maternal instincts in their work in schools. Often the maternal discourse women doctors employed in school health reform revealed their class biases (tinged with eugenics) against working-class students and their mothers, and they made professional advancements at their expense.

Female medical practitioners also fashioned themselves as educational activists, demanding separate yet equal physical education attention, funding, facilities, and curricula for girls in German vocational schools. They refused to have their students treated like second-class children in matters of health simply because their bodies were different. Rather, they argued that their dissimilar bodies merited a unique gym program for girls – one that was more important than boys' programs because of the increased risks girls faced in adolescence and because of the crucial role women held as the mothers of Germany's future generation. In other words, female physicians demanded educational equality for girls precisely because the nation needed healthy mothers after the losses suffered during the First World War. These doctors placed their arguments in the context of German national interests, as they portrayed themselves as devoted to advancing the objectives of Weimar youth welfare – now an issue of national concern. The first president of the BDÄ, Dr Hermine Heusler-Edenhuizen, for one, largely blamed the First World War for the postwar deterioration of Germany's youth and thought the issue of youth welfare merited national attention.[2] "Health and fitness movements proliferated in Weimar Germany," according to historian Erik Jensen, and building girls' physical education became an arena for women physicians to overhaul both the national body and individual bodies.[3] The biopolitical nature of their work had complex effects. On the one hand, women doctors presented themselves as displaying authentic maternal concern for female students, arguing for their educational equality at a time when youth health was also in the interests of the nation. On the other hand, this was mixed with rhetoric about what was best for women and their bodies, as well as social interventions into their students' lives, because it was deemed best for the national body. This rhetoric later translated conveniently to analogous work some of them did in the Bund Deutscher Mädel (League of German Girls) after 1933.

This chapter initially highlights the pre-war rhetoric about youth, especially female youth, as the propagators of the next generation. Much of this discourse was focused on the pubescent years because this was when youth were most vulnerable. Women doctors like Dr Alice Profé became involved in the pre-war period, calling for more attention towards female youth, in particular to their clothing choice and how it might affect physical movement. She also started demanding equal physical educational opportunities for boys and girls – a concern that other female physicians took up again after the First World War. The next section focuses on the post–First World War period when, in light of wartime losses, there was even more of a focus on youth welfare with the creation of the National Youth Welfare Law. Female physicians built on this momentum and the Weimar Constitution's new mandatory vocational educational clause, calling for school health curriculum to accommodate girls. This happened both at the 1925 Conference on the Physical Education of Women and in female physician's rhetoric about their role in vocational schools – the topics covered in the next two sections. Doctors centred their lectures at the conference and in their writings on building a separate gendered curriculum for female students by strengthening a woman's body for pregnancy and birth. Some of them cited this new curriculum as a reason for their presence in the nation's vocational schools, while others claimed that issues of confidentiality and trust dictated the need for female physicians in schools. Often, their request for a stronger presence of female physicians was tied to their feelings about the lack of sex education at home, and thus, female school doctors expanded their work (at least rhetorically) to the home. They also focused on discussions of birth control, how to educate abnormal and asocial children, and how to tailor a curriculum to women's bodies, needs, and abilities during menstruation or before and after childbirth – all included in the last section.

Pre-war Concerns about Adolescent Female Youth

During the first decades of the twentieth century, German government authorities, scientists, and social reformers expressed concerns that the adolescent population was at risk and in crisis for a number of reasons, rooted in a plethora of social circumstances, including low fertility rates, urbanization, industrialization, higher divorce and abortion rates, and a perceived crisis of the family. After the First World War, German authorities pointed most directly to the "harmful" impacts of the war, most notably the uneven gender ratio and poverty. This perceived threat of a "youth problem" in the early twentieth century reflected a middle-class consensus that working-class youth, especially, presented a new set of problems that required intervention.[4] Elizabeth Harvey has argued that working-class adolescents bore the brunt of changing economic, political, and social conditions in Germany, especially because they usually left school and entered the workforce or vocational school at the age of fourteen.[5] The majority of female doctors' discourse and work centred on vocational and secondary schools and their discussion of girls' health focused on puberty, the stage between eleven and eighteen years of age.[6] These adolescents were primarily from working- and lower-middle-class families, based on their enrolment in vocational schools and higher girls' schools. Women doctors did not work at the more academic *Gymnasium*, which fed into universities. Middle- and upper-class doctors did, however, consistently apply middle-class adolescent norms to working-class individuals.[7]

Conversations about the physical education and health of adolescents, primarily female adolescents, began prior to the First World War among Reich health officials and policymakers at the state and regional levels. For example, in the 1911 Prussian decree for *Jugendpflege* (the fostering of youth), which allocated funds for the care of youth and encouraged a national network of youth organizations, broad-based discussions about female youth and their unique needs first surfaced.[8] One journal harshly criticized the Prussian Ministry's "exclusion of female youth" and advocated that the systematic development of youth welfare should also apply to young girls, and to an even higher degree than young boys because "the health of the future generation rest[ed] primarily on the health of the female part of the population."[9] The journal equated the good health conditions of female adolescents to a vigorous and resilient *Volk*, and more specifically to its next generation. The Prussian state's attention toward "moulding girls" before the war, offering funds for home economics training and physical recreation, for example, was often motivated by its desire "to create healthy, competent, and patriotic wives and mothers."[10] The Prussian Central Office of People's Welfare similarly viewed the care of female youth as particularly important, creating an entire department devoted to supporting Germany's adolescent girls.[11]

Perhaps unsurprisingly, women doctors were some of the earliest advocates for more attention to female youth. Doctors had also already taken prominent roles as physical educators in the Jungdeutschland-bund (Young Germany League), a nationalist organization founded in 1911 and backed by the Kaiser that was dedicated to the health improvement of youth living in the countryside.[12] Physicians, in general, recognized the vital role they could play in caring for the nation's youth. Female physicians, in particular, argued that girls' health should be highlighted in conversations about youth welfare. Their early work identifying the unique health needs of adolescent girls marked only the start of their long careers devoted to discourse on the physical development and abilities of young girls. In the Weimar era, this ultimately resulted in their arguments that female physicians were the most suitable individuals to undertake the care of adolescent girls, especially in schools.

Racial hygienist and doctor Agnes Bluhm was one of the first female physicians to recognize the importance of girls' health to the future of the *Volk* in her 1913 article "Female Youth Welfare and the *Volksgesundheit* [people's health]." According to her, "the health of the next generation [was] to an even greater extent dependent on that of the mother than that of the father because any impediment to the maternal organism [could] damage the development of the best-laid offspring." Bluhm emphasized the treatment of adolescent girls precisely because this was the time when their reproductive organs developed. This period, generally considered to be between the ages of fourteen and twenty for girls, was when a woman became physically prepared for motherhood, and therefore, Bluhm regarded "this age [as] crucial for the later motherly-productivity of a woman" – rhetoric that her colleagues would echo in later years as well. Bluhm argued that female youth welfare, especially during the developmental years, should be one of the most important duties of *Volksgesundheitspflege* (people's health care), for this would "guarantee the *Volk*'s productivity and vitality."[13]

In addition to women's important responsibility to the reproductive process, Bluhm also noted that disease and death afflicted adolescent girls more seriously than boys. Bluhm documented that although girls got sick less frequently than boys, their illnesses were more severe and they were less resistant to disease during adolescence.[14] According to Bluhm, when disease threatened the individual health of girls, it also affected the overall productivity of the *Volk* because girls produced the future generation. In addition, certain diseases resulted in infertility, thus also endangering the vitality of the *Volk*. Bluhm emphasized that the health condition of the mother during pregnancy influenced the resilience of offspring. She also thought the development of secondary sex organs, namely female breast glands, was crucial for nursing – widely believed to be essential to good infant health, as we will see in the last chapter. An "undisturbed female adolescence," Bluhm concluded, clearly had extensive meaning for the *Volksgesundheit*, proving just how critical female youth welfare was.[15] Helping young girls avoid the dangers developed during adolescence was a skill that female doctors like Agnes Bluhm came (and would later come) to pride themselves on.

Dr Alice Profé was one of the earliest crusaders for the improvement of girls' physical education and health. After her medical studies in Straßburg and Freiburg, she settled in Berlin, where she practised medicine from 1905 until her death in 1946. She quickly became involved in what would become her life's work: health education for adolescent girls. She taught health classes at one of Berlin's municipal girls' vocational schools, held lectures on "the health of children's education" for the Berlin Association of School Health Care, and in 1908 she reported on the health of girls at the higher girls' schools at the annual meeting of the German Association for School Health Care in Darmstadt.[16] In addition, she participated in various international congresses for school health in Nuremberg (1904), London (1907), and Paris (1910).

In her numerous publications, Profé focused on girls' and women's sports, female clothing, and the equal physical education of girls and boys. In a 1914 article, for instance, she emphasized that girls should not wear restrictive clothing, echoing Bluhm's arguments that restrictive clothing could impede the growth of the chest and, therefore, "become fatal for the development of the reproductive system."[17] Profé described women's clothing as neither comfortable nor rational, for it did nothing to enhance women's health but instead restricted the body and prevented its natural movement. Profé's arguments parroted those in the life reform (*Lebensreform*) movement, who in the face of an increasingly urbanized, industrialized society, sought to expose the body to more "natural" ways of living. This included nudism, vegetarianism, abstinence from alcohol and nicotine, natural healing, and dress reform that was focused on liberating the body.[18] Profé thought the modern, urban, middle-class woman with her uncomfortable shoes, tight skirts, and long, narrow coats was unable to walk sturdily and properly, and she often had to swing her arms in an awkward fashion because of muffs, long furs, handbags, or umbrellas, which further minimized her movement. The trendy clothing of the day, according to Profé, even affected a woman when she was sitting because corsets bunched around her waist, preventing a comfortable sitting position. Corsets also paralysed the flexibility of the breast, abdominal wall, shoulders, diaphragm, and the pelvic floor, resulting in unnatural heavy external breathing, as well as feelings of fullness even if a woman had not eaten very much. One experiment, for example, showed that an increase in stomach pressure led patients to eat 8 per cent less on average during periods in which they were wearing a corset because they felt full faster. The removal of suffocating clothing cured young girls who lacked a desire to eat.[19]

Moreover, Profé noted that confining clothing had a negative influence on blood consistency, blood flow, and most importantly, on the reproductive organs, which became compressed from the pressure of the corset pushing against the pelvic floor.[20] Profé's arguments echoed those of her predecessor Dr Anna Fischer-Dückelmann, a German physician educated in Switzerland, who deplored women's fashion such as confining shoes and corsets, which she claimed restricted movement and weakened women.[21] Like Fischer-Dückelmann and Bluhm, Profé was concerned about maintaining strong and healthy offspring, thereby preserving the *Volk*, and recognized just how greatly something as simple as clothing could affect the people's health.

While condemning women's restrictive clothing because of its harmful effects on women's health and, by extension, the vitality of the *Volk*, Profé also offered a critique of modern society and even of the modern woman. She disapproved of the urban elite who spent all day in their sitting rooms withering away because they lacked ample air, light, and movement, which helped enhance one's well-being. Showing her class bias against the lower-classes as well, Profé negatively depicted an image of the urban poor, who were "to some extent prisoners of their own homes" since they lived in cramped apartments. She also thought young, single women on the go were "unnecessarily ... prisoners of their suffocating clothing." Uncomfortable shoewear, tight skirts, long coats, and a number of the new fashion accessories that modern women carried restricted their fast-paced stride, as described above. Their use of public transit also created new challenges and further endangered their health: "The strange hat accessories force[d] the poor creatures to hold their heads in oppressive positions if they did not want to permanently bother their neighbours with feather plumes."[22] These independent women on the move exemplified the growing number of females in the workplace in metropolitan cities. But, according to Profé, their health certainly suffered from living in rapidly developing urban spaces and attempting to keep up with trends of the time. Other feminists in the *Lebensreform* movement agreed that contemporary fashion was incompatible with the independent woman.[23]

This pre-war modern woman was the predecessor of the Weimar New Woman, who faced even more health consequences as she battled the challenges of increasing industrialization and urbanization (including the growing use of public transit) and the expectation to dress fashionably during this golden era for women.[24] Doctors like Profé sought to help these free-spirited, single, working women, while conservatives and eugenicists feared they threatened the foundations of society and the future of the *Volk* by starting careers, thus delaying marriage and family. In this sense, Profé displayed a maternalist attitude, proclaiming that she knew what was best regarding the working women's attire. She also took a more practical, scientific approach to fashion based on her own work experiences. Often married, women physicians, like their single counterparts, were overburdened, fulfilling obligations in their own practices, in a number of women's and health organizations, and as teachers in schools or advisers in clinics for a few additional hours each week, in addition to balancing their responsibilities as wives and mothers. Women doctors, in other words, were the quintessential modern urban women, yet Profé disapproved of this type of lifestyle because of its consequences for women's health. One would hope that she at least took her own suggestions for clothing options seriously. Perhaps her own urban working experiences, however, made her more aware of how to help other women in this regard. And because clothing choice ultimately affected health, medical practitioners like Profé felt they were the appropriate people to determine what was best for adolescent girls and women when it came to their dress selection.

Profé also called on her colleagues in the medical profession to enlighten women about how harmful their clothing could be. She saw it as the "duty of doctors to show women that they [made] themselves sick through their dress," noting that the popular clothing of the time minimized the movement of the body, which could result in disease.[25] Doctors, Profé thought, should teach women that the first requirement of beauty was maintaining a healthy body. Doctors could follow the example of school authorities who had already placed restrictions on wearing confining clothing, such as corsets, during gym class. Proclaiming that such measures alone would not suffice, Profé called for dress regulations for young girls outside of gym class as well. She suggested that gym exercises for the back and stomach muscles were futile when those same muscles, which were essential for women's reproductive abilities, were only paralysed and dwarfed by wearing a corset. By checking for pressure marks on the skin when their female patients undressed, doctors could confirm the appropriateness of clothing. Profé even recommended certain types of clothing and advised that people contact the Association for the Improvement of Women's Clothing for further suggestions. Above all, doctors, along with teachers, played a critical role because they served as good examples to their students by wearing appropriate (read: healthy) clothing themselves. According to Profé, "comprehensive and absolutely effective physical education [was] not possible unless a basic reform of women's clothing [was] implemented at the same time."[26] She saw clothing as crucial to her campaign for the reform of girls' physical education, which she thought deserved a status equivalent to that of boys.

Profé viewed the reform of women's clothing as just one facet of a larger movement that demanded equal health educational opportunities and services for boys and girls. Profé believed that state officials did not pay serious enough attention to girls' education. For example, she noted that Prussia spent seventeen times more on the education of boys in the higher schools than it did for girls. The city of Berlin alone deferred 12,500 Marks for sports for boys in the higher schools and only 2,200 Marks for girls, according to a 1912 city report. Its municipal schools had eleven playgrounds for boys and only six for girls. And although Profé did not have accurate statistics from the other states, she suggested that the situation did not fare much better throughout the rest of Germany.[27] This led Profé to suggest that girls were "second-class" children when it came to education. They faced blatant discrimination at both the state and municipal levels, and also in everyday activities. The state and municipalities covered some of the costs for higher boys' schools but did not treat the higher girls' schools equally, meaning these schools had to find private funding from people or institutions or make cuts elsewhere, such as on school equipment or on the school spaces themselves. As a result, compacted schools offered only minimal movement for students and their insufficient air, light, and benches surely took their toll on girls' health. Administrative decisions also discriminated against women. For example, a Kiel public girls' school had enough money and enthusiasm to establish a rowing team for the upper classes, but the administration forbade it, citing the girls' lack of experience.[28] Moreover, in their daily regimen of school activities, girls faced more subtle discriminatory measures. For example, the public swimming pool in Charlottenburg was available to girls only at inconvenient hours, such as 6:30–8:30 a.m. or 2:00–4:00 p.m. – an especially disadvantageous time since the school day ended between 2:00–3:00 p.m. Thus, girls were forced to eat their lunches en route between school and swim lessons, clearly not the best alternative if one considered the health consequences of eating too quickly or eating directly prior to exercising.[29]

In her unfavourable review of the funding and services that government authorities set aside for girls, Profé had to remind her readers that "our children are our *children* and not our *boys*." She pled for higher schools to create an exercise or play space for girls, or at least allow girls to use the boys' fields. Directors of public higher girls' schools often lacked the time, space, and money to hold individual gym classes for each grade, instead clumping students of all grades into a small gymnasium at the same time. Profé petitioned her colleagues to take gym class and sports seriously because it did no good to teach these subjects when the students' authority figures did not make them a priority.[30] Fischer-Dückelmann went so far as to state that women had smaller and weaker muscles than men because of their lack of a physical exercise regimen.[31] The practical financial and space requirements of girls' physical education were, in Profé's opinion, insufficient and ineffective, but she also had problems with the curriculum.

Profé disapproved of the "absurdity" of the physical education curriculum that did exist for girls in the pre-war era.[32] She found the primary theoretical goal of girls' physical education – to build charm and grace (*Anmut und Grazie*) – to be both illogical and confusing. Because female physical education did not at all focus on developing physical strength, promoting physical and mental health, or providing a balance to health problems induced by the adversities of school life, Profé claimed that "girls' physical education, as it is today, hardly represents a benefit for any organ in a child's body" and only "burden[ed] the brain through its heavy use of attention and memory." Physical education, then, was not at all a recreational activity for girls, but only caused more stress.[33] It also failed to prepare girls for the future. As Profé stated, these women were not training to be acrobats, but rather wives and mothers who could balance the physical and mental demands of domestic life.[34] In fact, Profé found it astonishing and "a testament to the powerful life force present in the woman's body" that women were able to achieve such efficiency later in life despite their total lack of physical education as adolescents.[35]

In Profé's view, girls' physical education was much more pertinent and necessary than boys'. Girls faced a greater number of risks because of their unhealthy clothing choices, the lack of movement in their domestic lives, and their malnutrition.[36] Profé, like Bluhm, prioritized the treatment of female youth prior to the First World War. On the one hand, female youth (including girls' physical education) did deserve special treatment because women were the primary guarantors of a healthy future population – something that Germany definitely needed in the face of a building war. And on the other hand, doctors like Profé likely bolstered the importance of girls' physical education in the pre-war era because of the new employment opportunities it offered to her and her colleagues in schools. Profé even admitted that one could not resist smiling when he/she thought about teachers conceiving of exercises that corresponded to the "female nature," or that adapted to both the "female body" and the "female spirit," which men had not yet envisioned.[37] With this comment, she suggested not only that there were particular "feminine" exercises that were better tailored for women's bodies and minds, but also that women were more capable of determining what these were. She emphasized the differences between girls and boys, which would thus merit a separate program for girls' physical development. This did not mean, however, that girls' physical education programs should be any less equal than boys'. Profé and others who followed her after the war no longer wanted their students to be treated like second-class citizens when it came to physical education and they demanded that authorities develop a distinctive, yet comparable, health curriculum for girls.

Facilitating Weimar Youth Health Education

Profé's extensive campaign for young girls' proper and equal physical education and health was truly exceptional in the pre-war period. It was not until the end of the First World War and especially into the mid-1920s that female youth and their health education reached the forefront of discussion among government authorities, pedagogues, and the medical profession. In light of the losses, failures, and disappointments of the First World War, the preservation of Germany through the strengthening of its youth became a national rallying call. The creation of the National Youth Welfare Law (*Reichsjugendwohlfahrtsgesetz*; RJWG) and concerns about fostering the family and providing comprehensive welfare for women became couched in the context of a national rebuilding campaign and the perceived chaos in the aftermath of the First World War. While discussions of physical education, sex education, and sport were not unique to Germany during the interwar era, the impetus for such social welfare programs arose in light of the devastating effects of the Great War on marriage, the family, and fertility rates, and the increasing spread of alcohol use and venereal disease.[38] As Erik Jensen claims, Germany was among dozens of countries in the interwar period focused on physical bodies and fitness, which were a means of rehabilitating populations and restoring national health. Germany tended to demand more than other countries because of its catastrophic military defeat, which called for "a complete overhaul of society, culture, government, and even the body itself."[39] In addition, the Weimar era was typified by fears of a rise of sexual promiscuity among youth, increasing illegitimacy and higher divorce rates among parents, and the rise of women in the workforce and therefore a shift away from the home – all of which led to the perceived breakdown of the family and a growing population of neglected youth. In his social history of the Weimar Republic, Detlev Peukert argues that the word *Jugend* (youth) itself implied the total breakdown of social control and traditional ties. Peukert shows that public concern regarding youth not only involved the individuals themselves but also equated to a problem of control in all of society.[40] Even Richard Bessel, who highlights the hyperbolic character of the perceived moral collapse of society, underlines its importance in framing public debates during the first years of the Republic.[41]

The RJWG was the state's means of overseeing all youth-related concerns, and women doctors, newly professionalized in the first years of the Weimar Republic, facilitated youth health education as potential administrators of this new law. Beginning with the newly ratified 1919 Weimar Constitution, national legislation guaranteed the systematic and comprehensive provision of youth welfare.[42] The Reich Ministry of the Interior circulated initial proposals for the RJWG in April 1919, and discussion about the law began in the Reich Council one month later. The RJWG, which eventually passed in June 1922, was couched in the context of Germany's national crisis, rationalized by "the unspeakable mental and physical sufferings of the war, the great crisis of the revolution and the harsh peace treaty."[43] After establishing the basic rights of children and the duties of the family, the law determined that the role of public welfare was to intervene in the interests of the child when the family could not adequately provide an education. This struck a similar chord as the Weimar Constitution. The RJWG, after much debate and compromise, became effective through an emergency decree in February 1924.[44]

These postwar concerns about youth welfare, justified through Germany's perceived crisis, provided women doctors an opportunity to make girls' physical education a central part of this agenda. As nascent managers of new national policies, they demanded the extension and modification of a physical education curriculum for girls through conferences and journal publications, showing that they were also reacting to a more conservative RJWG than originally anticipated – one that gave more power to state and local authorities and made a number of the initially planned duties of state public welfare optional.[45] In other words, even though the RJWG initially provided for girls, by petitioning for the inclusion of girls' physical education in vocational schools, women doctors were reacting to a biopolitical discourse generated by the RJWG, taking things into their own hands by insisting on the expansion of public youth welfare.

Female physicians harnessed the progressive spirit of reform. Their demands for a school health curriculum to accommodate girls reflected a "time of exuberant pedagogical innovation and optimistic plans to reform the stratified educational system in the name of democracy and social justice," which Marjorie Lamberti argues characterized the Weimar Republic.[46] Lamberti describes how elementary school teachers, organized in the German Teachers' Association, advocated to overturn Germany's rigid school system, which, patterned after the stratified class structure of society, limited access to secondary and higher education for those students who were not of a particular economic class. In addition to the national attention toward youth welfare, this reformist atmosphere of the early 1920s significantly animated the campaign to change school health curricula. The reformers' modern schools, for one, provided a model for women doctors because they offered a gymnastics and sports curriculum that promoted physical fitness and self-confidence for both boys and girls.[47] Women physicians' attempts to fashion an identity through reforming girls' physical education very much benefited from the myriad reforms to the educational system, initiated by the German Teachers' Association alongside the German Democratic and Social Democratic Parties. Because educational reform was already an issue of domestic politics and controversy, this likely encouraged women doctors and left room for them to work their way onto the public scene. Following in the footsteps of their progressive pedagogical predecessors, they could frame their arguments for girls' access to suitable doctors and for their equal opportunities in school health as attributes of a democratic welfare state. The possibilities suggested by Weimar democracy, whether real or imagined, gave female physicians a legitimate platform to make demands for the health education of women and thereby forge a place in the profession for themselves.

1925 Conference on the Physical Education of Women

With the growing national focus on youth welfare, collaborative discussions among women, gym teachers, pedagogues, and female doctors about what female physical education should entail emerged in the mid-1920s. At a German Gymnastics Association event in Leipzig in 1925, these various groups sought to clarify women's physical education and the work women needed to do in this regard. Dr Profé, still engaged with the issue of women's physical education and school health care, was a central figure in these talks. Alongside Paula Buché-Geis, who received her medical training in the early 1900s in Bonn and worked as a practising physician focused on the issue of women and sports for many years in Dresden, they drafted a set of guidelines that demanded no restrictions for women in gymnastic and sport organizations, as well as in track and field, swimming, and lawn games.[48] That same year, the Bund Deutscher Frauenvereine (League of German Women's Associations; BDF) and the Deutscher Reichsausschuß für Leibesübungen (German National Committee for Physical Exercise; DRL), the umbrella-organization for sports in Germany, organized the First Public Conference on the Physical Education of Women to discuss the form and goals of female physical education.

The conference, which took place 22–4 March in Berlin, addressed women's physical education and its importance to the population, which the organizers claimed had thus far received little notice from the German women's movement and the BDF.[49] This was, in fact, the first public forum to discuss the physical education of girls – a concern for members of the female medical profession since before the First World War and one that the organizers certainly thought would merit national consideration in the future.[50] After months of planning between BDF leaders, DRL leaders, pedagogues, doctors, and members of various education organizations like the German Female Teacher's Association (Deutsche Lehrerinnenverein) and the German Gymnastic Teacher's Association (Deutscher Turnlehrerverein), the conference was very popular, attracting some 900 participants.[51] The organizers recognized the increasing urgency and significance that physical education of women had for national rebuilding efforts. Theodor Lewald, the president of the DRL, in his opening remarks, noted the "enormous importance of the event in view of the weakening of national strength throughout the war and postwar years."[52] The organizers also insisted that women determine the direction and goals of women's physical education, based on their "precise knowledge of the physical and mental conditions for [women's] development."[53] The large number of female participants in terms of preparation for and attendance at the conference, as well as the overwhelming majority of female voices in the conference report and subsequent publication, substantiate the organizers' call for women to be involved in guiding the objectives of women's physical education.[54] The conference included lectures from several different points of view – medical, pedagogical, and governmental – as well as a practical demonstration of appropriate exercises or games. A small conference exhibition featured healthy and tasteful women's gym and sports clothing, showing that Profé's pre-war treatise on the health consequences of women's clothing had become a legitimate health concern by 1925.

Overall, female doctors had a strong presence at the 1925 conference. Initially, Dr Hermine Heusler-Edenhuizen was scheduled to speak, but another woman doctor, Dr Bertha Sachs, replaced her. Sachs had completed her medical training in 1918 and practised medicine in Freiburg, where she worked as a sports doctor. She was also a member of the BDÄ's Committee for Physical Education. In her lecture, Sachs proclaimed that the goal of women's physical education was "the strengthening of health and the preservation of vitality." She emphasized the importance of hiking and afternoon play sessions, noting the significant impact of sports on childbearing.[55] In fact, most of Sachs's lecture addressed the issue of physically preparing women for the tasks of motherhood and childbearing, demonstrating that women's domesticity became the primary language behind female doctors' discourse at the 1925 Conference on the Physical Education of Women.

Sachs relied on an argument of gender difference in her assessment of physical education. It was reasonable, she thought, for men to engage in physical education because they had to be prepared for military service and life's struggles. Women's work as mothers and as domestic caretakers, however, suggested that women's physical education was not necessary, not even desirable. At first, Sachs claimed, women "appear[ed] to be much too weak and too delicate to be able to carry out invigorating physical exercise without health risks." But she acknowledged that the First World War had demonstrated that a healthy woman could undertake a surprisingly large amount of physical activity. If and when health problems did arise, they could be attributed to a woman's lack of physical education or to the excessive demands on her body, rather than "female ineptitude." In the postwar period, the mental and physical demands on women grew substantially. For one, working women had to mobilize their strength to care for their relatives, children, and themselves after a long day at the office or factory. Wives and mothers, too, had to fulfil a multitude of responsibilities under considerably more difficult conditions.[56] Sachs, perhaps reflecting her own experience, perceived that women were generally the primary breadwinners, if they did work, or the heads of their households, if they did not, and oftentimes both due to the deaths or handicaps of their husbands. The postwar social and economic problems only compounded women's concerns. Regardless of whether or not they were employed, though, Sachs thought that physical education should prioritize women's domestic tasks and motherly responsibilities. Sachs recognized that women had to strive to enhance their stamina and productivity through physical exercise in order to fulfil their at-home obligations. She also noted that it was crucial for the state to have healthy, capable mothers who could produce healthy children. In advocating girls' physical education, Sachs highlighted the concerns both of individual women facing the daunting task of caring for their families on their own in the postwar period and of a larger German state encountering new social and economic problems during the same time. Her discourse shows that she was motivated by a desire to help her patients and the German state.

In her concluding remarks, Sachs acknowledged the significance of women's physical and mental strength for Germany's future. She stated that "the foundation for Germany's re-emergence (*Wiederhochkommen*) is a healthy *Volk*. We can only expect this from a physically and mentally powerful and strong female sex, who is able to bear healthy children for us and who is educated in the healthy German sense."[57] Sachs, like her predecessors, turned her attention towards strengthening women because they were Germany's direct link to a healthier offspring. In this sense, she also dabbled in the popular 1920s population politics discourse that focused on maintaining and perpetuating a qualitative healthy *Volk*. In light of Germany's declining international significance, government officials, policymakers, and those in medical and scientific circles (from both the right and left) thought that the state's re-emergence as an international powerhouse was directly connected to the physical capabilities of its people. The war had left Germany with fewer and weaker men than its neighbouring nations, and the fear that the unfit were overrunning the population increased with each additional crisis (real or perceived), whether it be the rapidly declining birth rate; the rise in poverty, prostitution, alcoholism, abortion, and venereal disease; the growing population of unwieldy youth; or the mounting divorce rate – all characteristic of the Weimar period.[58] As Paul Weindling has argued, eugenics and its goals of improving the quality of the population gained more prestige, especially during times of crisis.[59] Focusing on the physical education of adolescent girls, then, was one way to bolster a national ideology focused on a fit and efficient body politic and devoted to its future generations.

In her demands for a separate physical education curriculum for women, Sachs criticized the current state of women's physical education and suggested alternatives. Sachs viewed women's current curriculum as men's physical education, albeit in a "weakened form." Although she thought the basic goals of physical education were the same for men and women – a healthy development of the body and mind – Sachs demanded that women's physical education be built from the physical and mental character of a woman, not a man. While Sachs and other doctors called for more attention and funding to be paid to women's physical education, they also emphasized that they were not asking women to match the physical productivity or muscle strength of men. This, she claimed, would be "senseless" and "futile." Instead, Sachs simply wanted women to fully develop their naturally given physical bodies in order to be able to "fully and totally cope with the demands of life."[60] Physical education, she argued, could be beneficial only if it did not exceed the limits of one's given constitution. This was why it was essential to have different curricula for men and women, and to prescribe individual doses of exercise to each woman. The same exercise, naturally, had different effects on different people, and thus, Sachs suggested that doses be increased only when the particular character of a woman (or a man) allowed for it.

Sachs further underscored gender difference by highlighting women's unique physical structure and mental capabilities. Anatomically, women and men had distinct external sex characteristics, but they differed in the build and form of their bodies. For example, women's bone structure was smaller and more delicate, and the female extremities and body angle were generally shorter. Their shoulders were narrower, their hips were wider, and their bodies were longer. Sachs drew attention to these distinct physical differences in order to bolster her argument for a separate women's curriculum. Dr Heusler-Edenhuizen, whose intended lecture was included in the post-conference publication, agreed that in light of anatomical variation, girls and boys should not do the same gym exercises during puberty.[61] Women doctors like Sachs and Heusler-Edenhuizen eschewed the male paradigm, but still insisted on equalizing physical education opportunities between the sexes. The pubescent period for girls was earlier and quicker (ages twelve to fourteen) than it was for boys (ages thirteen to sixteen), and Sachs noted that such rapid development of girls' bodies could result in additional problems. Because of the physical strains of puberty, Sachs emphasized that daily physical exercise for girls was an urgent matter, certainly more so than boys'.[62] Like her predecessors, her rhetoric privileged women's needs.

In addition to the anatomical differences between men and women that Sachs thought merited a separate physical education program, she underlined a number of physiological differences as well. The most important, according to her, were those connected to women's occupation of motherhood. Certain organs had to develop specifically for this physiological task. Sachs argued that gymnastics and other physical exercise could disrupt menstruation, pregnancy, and childbirth. Thus, she thought it was "the noblest duty of female physical education to find the appropriate type and form of physical exercises for the development and functioning of these organs."[63] Sachs stressed women's primary life responsibility to be motherhood, thereby putting her among others in her cohort who equated womanhood and motherhood. Sachs and her colleagues drew on rhetoric that was familiar to them because of their own personal experiences with motherhood, and that could be perceived as non-threatening to other men and women in the profession. Even as health professionals, they relied on a language of women's natural-given abilities as mothers to advocate for women's improved and equalized physical education – a similar strategy employed in marriage counselling when doctors privileged marriage and motherhood in their positions as counsellors.

Even though she could not speak at the conference, Dr Heusler-Edenhuizen's lecture further confirmed that female physicians generally supported marriage, motherhood, and domesticity as the natural and proper roles for women. Speaking from her experiences as a gynecologist, she emphasized that women's physical education should have different goals than men's, namely that women needed to be strengthened "for their specific function – giving birth (*Gebärtätigkeit*)."[64] Heusler-Edenhuizen's remarks indicated that childbearing was women's primary function. It was most certainly the primary reason why she thought women deserved their own physical education curriculum, for this curriculum would be centred around reproduction. This was not, however, the only instance in which Heusler-Edenhuizen highlighted motherhood as the natural role for women. She also referred to "the strong motherly instinct of women" in debates about how the distribution of birth control in marriage counselling centres might lead to a population decline.[65] It appears, then, that whether she was campaigning for women's needs and rights in physical education or marriage counselling centres, she consistently linked them with motherhood.

In this sense, doctors like Sachs and Heusler-Edenhuizen adopted the views of the mainstream medical and scientific communities, which viewed women's domesticity as a priority.[66] Their detailed explanations of what components should be included in a women's physical education curriculum highlighted women's preparation for motherhood and domestic lifestyles. Heusler-Edenhuizen's proposed physical education regimen focused entirely on strengthening women's muscles for the birthing process. Not only did women need tight, firm stomach muscles, but also strong back muscles. Good chest muscles were also essential because during pregnancy a woman's abdominal respiration was hindered, meaning she had to breathe with her thorax. She thought achieving a balance between developing the back, stomach, and chest muscles was the "main value" (*Hauptwert*) of physical education for "our girls." She advised that this curriculum should be introduced to girls in early childhood and consistently implemented through their entire time in school.[67] Furthermore, Heusler-Edenhuizen suggested that exercises for the stomach and perineum muscles should begin on the third or fourth day of the postpartum period and should become a part of a woman's daily routine even after postpartum, especially if she was not playing sports. Heusler-Edenhuizen personally felt that with better physical preparation and the attendant feelings of strength and confidence, women would experience "considerably greater joy in reproduction."[68] The whole goal of her physical education agenda for young women, in other words, was to enhance the birth process and to toughen women in order to prevent the inevitable consequences that appeared after pregnancy – a raised stomach, a twisted back, saggy breasts, and stretch marks. Heusler-Edenhuizen claimed to be looking out intensely for "my young women" to ensure that they achieved beautiful bodies despite multiple births.[69] Such infantilizing language showed Heusler-Edenhuizen's maternal instincts surfacing in the workplace – a trend that became more common with the debate over women's physical education in schools.

Although Sachs did not centre her entire lecture on strengthening a woman's body for pregnancy and birth, she agreed with Heusler-Edenhuizen that this should be an important component of the physical development of women. A firm abdominal wall was critical for holding the womb in the correct position and for preventing excess hanging skin. The pelvic floor needed to be strong and elastic in order to allow for the easy passage of the baby without tearing. A robust pelvic floor was also necessary in the postpartum period, leading Sachs to discourage women from lying on their backs. Instead, she recommended they get up as soon as possible to exercise. In addition, exercise and sports had a positive influence on problems that emerged as a result of pregnancy, such as varicose veins, hemorrhoids, and constipation. Sachs emphasized that although these physical education efforts naturally had a positive influence on younger girls, they also benefited older women. After all, "exercise, daily walks, or short hikes offered the necessary balance to the monotonous movement which accompanied domestic work or a sedentary way of life."[70] While she encouraged women of all ages to undertake proper physical exercise, Sachs clearly restricted women's physical preparations to motherhood, housewifery, or sedentary jobs in an office or factory. She omitted any discussion of training women for other jobs, despite the fact that during the Weimar period women demanded full professional equality and entered the workforce at higher numbers than ever before.[71] Women doctors viewed childbearing and domesticity as women's primary tasks, at least in terms of their instructions for women's physical regimen. They located women's principal responsibilities in the home even if they did not always adhere to that standard themselves. Therefore, they extolled domesticity for their patients while simultaneously legitimizing professional paths for themselves, which Koven and Michel view as typical for maternalist discourses.[72]

Their discussion of the strictly female conditions of menstruation, pregnancy, and childbirth at the 1925 conference was also a means for women doctors to take ownership over a specific field within the youth welfare movement. They could, in other words, demand a particular type of physical education for women based on the special needs that women had or the specific tasks (like motherhood) that they encountered later in life. By focusing, for example, on what was appropriate in gym class for women preparing for pregnancy, they in essence created a space in which they claimed superior knowledge, thus promoting themselves as indispensable in the discourse on physical education for women. While their opinions about women's physical education were certainly limited to women's traditional roles as mothers, such views fit within their overall strategy of pushing women's issues to the foreground of the medical field. This allowed them to participate in the profession's discourse on youth physical education and even elevated their role within the movement because it offered them more job opportunities and their opinions became essential to crafting and monitoring adolescent girls' physical education.

Justifying Female School Doctors in Vocational Schools

If the 1925 Conference on the Physical Education of Women was the discursive space in which female physicians exerted their feminine influence on the discussion surrounding youth physical education curriculum, the higher schools became the physical places in which they put these ideas into practice. By the mid-1920s, the growing number of female physicians began to take advantage of the national focus on youth welfare, as they rallied for female doctors to treat female students and for a separate gendered curriculum for these students in the nation's vocational schools (*Berufsschule*). Female youth, in particular, became the concern of social reformers and female physicians in light of the biopolitical consequences that women's health had for the future of the *Volk* since women were considered the guardians of the next generation.[73]

Health education already existed in the German elementary schools, as was the case elsewhere in Europe, where school doctors provided children with a general introduction to physical education up to the age of fourteen.[74] In German primary schools, male and female doctors had instructed boys and girls, respectively, in sexual and moral education since around the turn of the century, when pedagogues, the women's movement, and the medical profession began advocating for biological, moral, and ethical education for youth on matters of sexuality.[75] During the First World War, members of the medical community voiced concerns that doctors also needed a presence in the higher schools, namely the vocational schools, as this was a crucial period (ages fourteen to eighteen) in terms of the schooling of Germany's working-class adolescents who learned a trade.[76] It was during puberty when young girls and boys experienced new psychological and physical changes and were the most susceptible to peer pressures that could negatively affect their upbringing. The war, marked by changing conditions and attitudes around sex, only expanded the need for doctors in schools, but their funding was delayed.[77] "The uneven and haphazard growth which had characterized the development of vocational education before 1918 was a thing of the past," as Article 145 of the Weimar Constitution introduced compulsory vocational education until the age of eighteen. The postwar period initiated a new sense of economic urgency to develop vocational education and it was also the time when the children of working-class families began to attend vocational schools en masse. State officials crafted a program to modernize German industry through technological and organizational innovation, which necessitated a mass of semi-skilled and unskilled labour, as well as highly trained technical specialists and managerial staff. Vocational schools – now viewed as crucial to helping the economy and the industrialization process – became the topic of national debate in the early years of the Republic.[78]

Social Democrats, bourgeois feminists, socialist women, and organized housewives participated in this debate by deliberating how to prepare young female workers for their future roles as housewives and mothers through vocational schooling.[79] Women doctors similarly thought that the key task of vocational education was to prepare girls for domesticity, and sought out ways to accomplish this in their positions as school doctors. Their vision of domesticity, however, was based on their own middle-class ideals in which the vocational school would serve as a wholesome refuge from "the stresses of the workplace, the [perceived] unhealthy environment of the proletarian neighborhood, and the chaos of the working-class household." It provided working-class female students with middle-class values based around "regular work and a rationally-organized lifestyle."[80] Female physicians argued for their employment in these schools precisely because adolescent girls were developing their reproductive organs, constituted a population at risk, and ultimately needed health guidance regarding how best to prepare their bodies for housework and motherhood. Most of the discussion among women doctors, then, centred around the need for separate female doctors for female students in vocational schools, as well as a distinct physical education curriculum based upon girls' differing needs and maturity levels during puberty.

In general, women doctors agreed that it was acceptable for male and female students to be cared for by a male or female doctor in elementary school. Dr Heusler-Edenhuizen, a practising doctor in Berlin, did not see the necessity of starting a different physical education curriculum until the adolescent years, at which point the objective of male physical education became focused on potential performance and outward strength, whereas the priority for females was to strengthen them for activities "which nature has imposed on [their bodies]" – namely, childbearing and motherhood.[81] Dr Paula Heyman, a Jewish, socialist school doctor in Berlin, agreed that for students above the age of fourteen, boys should have a male doctor and girls should have a female doctor. These doctors would answer older students' health questions and teach sex education. Heyman viewed it as "inadvisable to assign these duties to a female doctor in boys' schools or to a male doctor in girls' schools," and she recognized the opposition that female doctors in male schools faced from parents, teachers, and school board members.[82] Heyman clearly had no interest in challenging her male colleagues in the higher schools. Although she sought to minimize exaggerated differences between male and female physicians, she advocated for separate school medical care based on sex. While she did little to help change the situation for her female colleagues by restricting female doctors' expertise to girls, Heyman likely drew less attention to herself and opened a new female space that she and other women in the profession could profoundly influence.

While female physicians acknowledged the necessity of cooperating with the teaching profession in promoting the health of the *Volk*, they fiercely defended their right to teach health to the nation's youth, especially in the upper classes. The combined theoretical and practical scientific skills certainly allowed teachers and doctors together to detect physical irregularities or disease in schoolchildren.[83] Gym teachers could send their complaining students to school doctors to confirm that no medical abnormalities existed, while doctors used an "expert eye" to spot threatening conditions while supervising gym courses – a method that Heusler-Edenhuizen considered to be superior to a basic medical exam.[84] It was physicians, however, who women doctors argued should ultimately be responsible for health education. Responding to pedagogical appeals for teachers to assume the task of health education, physicians like Josephine Höber asserted that doctors, with their medical training, were more qualified to teach health education, especially because it was a field that involved weaving nutrition, disease prevention, and the detection of infections into the lessons.[85]

The rationale behind providing female doctors for female students in the upper classes was to teach older students about health matters and to provide suitable sex education, especially since women physicians assumed the mothers of their students often failed to educate their children adequately in matters of sex, health, and hygiene at home. This was a primary reason why Heusler-Edenhuizen and Susanne Altstaedt believed these problems could be solved by staffing schools with doctors. Altstaedt, a school physician who took over the medical care of a few girls' vocational schools in Lübeck in 1924, viewed school doctors as the most appropriate professional group to teach children about the dangers of venereal disease and other issues they did not learn about at home. She thought doctors fit this role well because they understood the importance of tact and respected the appropriate boundaries of their patients when discussing sexual matters and thus would not harm the modesty of young girls.[86] Heusler-Edenhuizen praised the important educational capacities of schools, particularly in light of problems that occurred at home. She targeted "poor" and "mentally endangered children" as worthy of special treatment.[87] It was in instances like these that Heusler-Edenhuizen's class biases became tied to her eugenic leanings, as she conflated the intelligence of certain children with their class backgrounds. It was these types of "problem" children to whom teachers and doctors had to give the most attention. By intervening in the lives of working-class or mentally ill children, Heusler-Edenhuizen reveals how her reform efforts were tinged with class-biased eugenics that she also confused with a sense of social justice, as she aimed to minimize the risks these children posed to the rest of society. She claimed female physicians could care for disadvantaged and mentally inferior female bodies to prevent further risk to the German national body. In other words, she could aid her students and the German nation at large.

By criticizing the abilities of mothers to provide adequate sexual and health education for their own children, female physicians elevated the significance of school instruction and created a place for themselves within the educational system. Edith von Lölhöffel, a practising doctor in Charlottenburg and a contributor to various physical education organizations and courses in Berlin, pointed out the "great ignorance" that existed among mothers and housewives of all classes – "the educators responsible for childrearing" – about how essential physical exercise was to the health of their children. She suggested a number of exercises mothers and housewives could do with their children at home. She also praised a workshop held in May 1929 by the German College for Physical Exercise, in which housewives gathered for six days to participate in daily exercise and to hear affiliated lectures from doctors – a number of them by von Lölhöffel herself. Von Lölhöffel thus presented a desire to impart her knowledge about youth physical education to these mothers, but she also literally instructed them how to do so in lectures like "Physical Exercise for Infant and Small Children." Alice Profé gave a lecture entitled "Physical Exercise for School Aged Children." Two other women physicians from Berlin, Elisabeth Hoffa and Hedwig Bergmann, gave lectures on "Puberty" and "Physical Exercise and

Motherhood" respectively.[88] These women fashioned a role for themselves as parents to these parents and created a new way to participate in health education, and thereby the medical profession.

The BDÄ, which extensively discussed girls' physical education programs in its journal, addressed the failure of German mothers with regard to health education and advocated health parenting in the home – an example of the state's intrusion into the private sphere that became much more common under the Weimar welfare state. In 1925, the welfare office of Bautzen in Saxony asked the BDÄ to assist in producing a school leaflet to be distributed to mothers of school-aged children – an opportunity for female physicians to formulate welfare policy. This brochure, passed out to schoolchildren on the first day of school and intended for them to take home to their mothers, offered very basic guidance on how a child should sleep, bathe, eat, play, and even when he or she should go to the bathroom. Dr Lina Ramsauer, a practising doctor in Oldenburg who wrote the medical portion of the brochure, described how school doctors assisted mothers in educating and caring for youth. The mother was accountable for ensuring the mental and physical development of her child; the doctor only provided additional information in undertaking this task. Ramsauer recognized, however, that there were thousands of mothers in Germany who were either unable (based on their living or economic conditions) or unwilling to convey satisfactory advice and education to their children.[89] Having witnessed how these working-class mothers failed to provide basic care for their children, female physicians crafted a professional identity in which they assumed responsibility for the upbringing of other people's children and imposed middle-class values of motherhood on their working-class students' families. After all, the girls enrolled in vocational schools tended to come from working- and lower-middle-class families. Female doctors fashioned a rhetoric that elevated the significance of doctors in educating these vocational school students. Their professional journal accused working-class mothers of failing to fulfil their responsibilities as parents, and presented women doctors as uniquely positioned to interfere in people's domestic lives (at least discursively) and remedy this absence. This provides further evidence that the public–private dichotomy dissolved during the Weimar era. As Atina Grossmann notes, "sex reform journals, advice books, and pamphlets carried their interventions straight into the home and bedroom," as expert professionals gained insight into people's private lives under the rubric of social welfare, marriage counselling, and now school health education.[90] Through their rhetorical intervention into people's parenting principles, women doctors became a driving force behind the blurring of public–private boundaries in the Weimar welfare state.

Female physicians also claimed that issues of confidentiality and trust dictated that female doctors be employed in girls' vocational schools. Dr Ilse Szagunn asserted that it would be a "downright dereliction of duty" not to provide young girls, who were exposed to a variety of risks in their professional lives, education and words of warning, and "above all to give them the opportunity to turn to their female school doctor in full confidence with their needs." Protecting the privacy of female students about the taboo matters of sex and hygiene was reason enough for Szagunn to present the employment of female school doctors as "absolutely natural and self-evident."[91] Szagunn, who worked part-time from 1918 to 1931 as the nation's first woman vocational school doctor, took the same approach in school health care that she did in marriage counselling: young adolescent girls, she thought, trusted female school doctors with their intimate questions and problems, just as the female visitors to marriage counselling centres felt more confident speaking with female physicians there. Szagunn also recognized how work in school health care and marriage counselling overlapped, as she encouraged school doctors to teach the dangers of venereal disease and abortion, highlighted the meaning of health for a marriage, and pushed for premarital counselling. According to Szagunn, it was not just women doctors who advocated this view; her membership in a health delegation showed that the majority of men also supported the employment of female school doctors in girls' vocational schools.[92] Dr Josephine Höber, an advocate for school health reform and a practising Jewish physician in Kiel for over ten years before she immigrated, also confirmed that male authorities desired the cooperation of female doctors in evaluating adolescent girls during routine medical check-ups.[93]

Käte Gaebel, a representative for the BDF's women's professional office, defended the employment of female physicians in vocational schools because she feared that female students were not as honest with doctors of the opposite sex. She suggested that girls might withhold or exaggerate information in the presence of a male doctor, whereas they discussed the same information with a woman "without risk." Women in the upper classes, she claimed, had already opposed male doctors conducting their standard health exams.[94] For Höber, the "erotic atmosphere" of school health classes, which addressed embarrassing subjects for girls between the ages of twelve and eighteen, merited the need for female school doctors, who "[could] provide the most valuable and most comprehensive material" for girls experiencing menstruation, severe cramping, and other difficulties with the female genitalia during physical activity.[95] These presumptions that their working-class students were embarrassed or concerned with infringements upon their modesty might reflect doctors' class biases or ignorance more than their female students' actual inclinations. This was an era, after all, in which young women were inundated with information and witnessed charged debates about sex, health, and the body with political campaigns to abolish the statute that prohibited abortion and the use and marketing of birth control.[96] Nevertheless, by enticing female students with a trustworthy consultant and dependable source of information on taboo issues like menstruation, women doctors presented themselves as indispensable to the Weimar Republic's schools – one of the few medical spaces open to them, but one that they solidified through their writing, which emphasized their maternal abilities to help female students during a difficult time in their lives.

Expanding the Role of Women Doctors in Schools

Once employed in vocational schools, female doctors portrayed themselves as providing more than a feminine presence during school medical exams. They also linked birth control, eugenics, and childbearing to girls' physical education and the nation's future. In this sense, school health care generated an opportunity for female physicians to push professional boundaries, as they attempted to regulate not only their students' mothers, but also their students' bodies. Höber serves as one example of how female doctors engaged in elaborating these biopolitical discourses. She criticized the lack of available female doctors for school girls in Kiel, noting the demands for women to treat adolescent girls during their annual school medical exams. She suggested making regular tours through schools in order to round up students suspected of being sick and sending these "abject" children to school medical offices at the discretion of parents or teachers. In addition to her attempts to remove unhealthy students from schools and thus from having contact with healthier students, she also recommended recording their medical exam results in a health book that would accompany a child throughout his or her lifetime (as well as into the marriage counselling centre). The tracking of students' individual and family medical histories in this health book could then, in Höber's opinion, be used to determine who should and should not receive birth control. Through the compulsory recording of students' health conditions, she sought to prevent "never-ending misery" and maintain "the most desirable assets of people."[97] Höber hoped that encouraging the working classes to participate in a state-wide birth control program, especially if they demonstrated a tainted family history, would counteract the mass distribution of birth control among the other classes. Handing out birth control only to people with a history of disease or in a more class-structured way was a means to achieving this end. Through such proposals, Höber rationalized a plan of action and showed her disapproval of the current system in which birth control was distributed unscientifically and was generally available only to the educated, well-off classes. She presented herself as helping both her working-class students, who likely lacked access to birth control, and society at large, which would become burdened with supporting the larger number of working-class individuals. By suggesting that birth control be offered to students, Höber was attempting to control women's bodies in the name of the collective body and fashioned a way to expand her own duties as a school doctor. Höber's motivations, then, can be connected to a class-biased eugenics ideology, what she perceived to be the practical needs of her students, and her own desire for improved status in the medical profession.

It is clear from this example that birth control was among the topics women doctors discussed (or at least suggested discussing) with their students – a heavily debated matter in the Weimar period, especially because of eugenicists' overwhelming fears that the "inferior" working-class individuals were producing far more babies and at a much faster rate than Germany's "superior" middle- and upper-class individuals, thus causing a weaker nation overall. Historians have examined the blending of eugenic and social welfare–based health and family policies produced during the Weimar era, and have found that biopolitically informed welfare discourses in interwar Germany combined eugenics, national rebuilding, and working-class welfare initiatives in a unique, seamless fashion.[98] The Weimar Republic, following on the heels of a devastating war, centred its health agenda on rebuilding the nation, as it promoted vigorous, lasting marriages and seeing healthy young girls as among the most "fit" segments of the population.[99] Rationalized through biopolitics, this meant preparing girls to be "fit" mothers from a young age and educating them about proper hygiene through school physical education. This is perhaps also why middle- and upper-class doctors admonished working-class mothers for the lack of attention to their children's health. Women physicians' concerns about rebuilding and improving the national body clearly led them to make assumptions about which types of physical exercise best served women and to find it acceptable to advise mothers about how to take care of their schoolchildren in the 1925 school brochure discussed above.[100] Through writing this instructional pamphlet and holding workshops for mothers about proper childcare, they moved their work from the schoolhouses into the home.[101] While liberating for women doctors, this had the potential to demean their students and their students' mothers, especially because of the clear class divide between doctors and vocational school students. At the same time, by seeking scientific solutions to mothering, doctors believed they were doing what was in their students' best interests. This type of radical intervention in their students' lives meant they offered much more than routine medical exams and advice about physical exercise. Instead, they presented themselves as forging the fields of women's physical and sex education. The professional identities they created proved to be a careful balancing act between their class biases, sympathies, opportunism, and activism.

In numerous essays advocating equal physical education curriculum for young girls, women doctors fashioned a professional identity as physician-activists committed to educational reform. Their demands for the employment of women doctors in vocational schools demonstrate their concerns that girls have access to doctors who they thought would make them feel comfortable. Their writings were also a veiled critique of the systematic discrimination against girls' physical education and of their male colleagues predominantly employed in these schools. Profé pushed for the equalization of funding in sports, while other doctors advocated the issue of equal gym time for boys and girls. For instance, vocational schools in Görlitz required a gym hour for boys but lacked the funds to offer the same course for girls.[102] While not many girls participated in physical exercise in vocational schools, this was certainly not for their lack of desire.[103] Female physicians thought most girls lacked time, opportunities, and the funding to participate in sports and pushed for their equal access to all three.

The stakes of vocational education for the *Volksgesundheit* were growing. Pedagogues, women's organizations, and health authorities continued to raise concerns that many youth were "professionally underdeveloped" when they finished school, meaning that when they started working, they frequently collapsed from physical unpreparedness or were forced to do menial tasks or even to change careers. In the fall of 1925, the Association for School Health Care and the BDF, through the Dresden school doctor Maria Snell, advocated a systematic medical survey of students at vocational schools at their respective meetings. Around the same time, Szagunn reported to a meeting that the Berlin chapter of the BDÄ held in conjunction with the Association for Berlin Vocational School Students on the topic of "The Medical Care of Vocational School Students." Some students were so "mentally under-developed" or "physically inferior" that they ended up in remedial classes or a *Hilfsschule*, a school for children with learning disabilities.[104] Clearly, some inferior learners in the vocational schools proved to be an additional social and financial burden, thus leading many different organizations, including those in the health profession, to improve the systematic health monitoring of these vocational students.

With the higher stakes of physical education now intimately tied to the health of the nation and viewed therefore as a burden shared by the whole, one female physician described herself and her colleagues as especially apt to handle abnormalities. Lotte Landé, a municipal doctor in Frankfurt, treated children who were "intellectually abnormal," meaning that she and her colleagues dealt with problems such as a lack of appetite, late-developing speaking abilities, asocial behaviours, fidgetiness, bedwetting, or an aversion to certain foods. In her view, "female care physicians with a motherly conscious generally empathize[d] easier and could give more practical advice than many male colleagues" for these problem children. Landé found that mothers and children also conveyed "a very special trust" to her and her colleagues, thus alleviating the challenges of this type of work because they would more readily go see doctors in a time of need. This was especially beneficial, Landé stated, in cases of "considerable mental or intellectual disorders or severe environmental degradation" because a doctor could intervene immediately to prevent a more acute problem.[105] Landé highlighted maternal qualities such as trustworthiness, compassion, and reassurance, which she claimed made female physicians more equipped to deal with problem children and also made this work altogether easier for schools.

Through her work treating "abnormal schoolchildren," Landé recognized a connection between poverty, a higher risk of mental abnormalities, and increased societal burdens. For one, she and her colleagues made a judgment about a child's intelligence level, including whether defects existed and whether unfavourable social conditions contributed to a child's abnormalities, or if a combination of both factors existed.[106]

Landé sometimes linked the mental abilities of schoolchildren to social conditions like alcoholism and poverty, confirming that such environmental problems – also thought to be genetically transmittable at that time – had grave consequences for German youth. She thought such social adversity led to children's mental imperfections, which also resulted in larger social and financial burdens. For example, Landé and her colleagues sometimes had to remove abnormal children from unfavourable domestic circumstances and place them in a multi-week recovery program and often in remedial school, all of which created additional costs for society. Landé further insisted that school doctors had a duty to advise abnormal children against certain professions because they were not as fit for these jobs as their healthy peers. Landé was especially critical of poor people, who often ignored medical advice and did not take their children to proper doctors until they faced severe problems.[107] Landé's regular contact and experience with lower-class individuals likely led her to make such complaints, but her own upper-middle-class background and privilege meant she likely lacked an understanding of how day-to-day working-class struggles influenced their medical decisions. She was one of a number of women doctors who had daily contact with working-class students in vocational schools and their working class-mothers, who, historian Atina Grossmann claims, struggled to keep their families afloat in light of the economic crisis and massive unemployment. Female physicians were not screened from social problems like elite male doctors working for insurance practices (from which women were often excluded) or in lucrative practices in high-class neighbourhoods. Therefore, they were more apt to seek eugenic solutions for overburdened and desperate women.[108] Landé witnessed first-hand how "asocial" elements developed as a result of destitute situations, and thus she sought both to lessen the stresses and strains of large, impoverished families and to reduce the number of mental abnormalities in society. By removing problem children from their bad home environments, she recognized that she could help overburdened families. By discouraging "intellectually abnormal children" from pursuing certain professional paths, she attempted to alleviate the social and financial costs of expensive remedial schooling. Her genuine concerns for schoolchildren were mixed with a distorted notion of social improvement.

The medical monitoring of female youth not just in schools but also in sports organizations additionally helped filter out unhealthy elements of the population and led female physicians to create other female spaces.

Laura Turnau, a practising physician in Berlin and one of the founding members of the BDÄ, advocated that all new members of female sports clubs be subject to medical examinations and that upon acceptance to a club their membership be dependent on medical diagnosis.[109] In other words, Turnau proposed a system that supported "fit" individuals with good medical histories and sought to prevent the propagation of diseased individuals by ostracizing them from sports clubs, similar to what Höber had done in schools. In her suggestion that adolescent girls undergo medical examinations as a prerequisite for acceptance into sports clubs, Turnau anticipated a new niche for female physicians, who would be needed to perform these exams and would work as sports teachers in girls' clubs. Turnau sought to extend the duties of women doctors beyond schools; they would now supervise girls' leisure-time activities under the same rubric of girls' physical education. Similarly, an article in *Die Ärztin* broadened discussions about school physical education to also include women at work, dispensing health tips to women working in factories, in the professions, and at home about how to avoid physical harm in the workplace, and joined the predominantly male discussions of whether greater intellectual activity of the brain could harm the reproductive organs of women.[110] These types of articles show how female physicians used the discussion about appropriate physical exercise in schools to command an additional site of women's expertise in describing what was most harmful for young girls.

In their conversations about vocational education, female physicians advocated modifying gym curricula in schools, thus offering female students an equal yet different health curriculum catering to women's bodies and abilities. In this regard, they were no different than their counterparts working in women's physical education in other Western countries.[111] In the past, pedagogues and doctors believed that women could be physically and mentally educated in similar ways to men, albeit in a weaker form based on their weaker compositions.[112] Dr Anna Fischer-Dückelmann was one example of physicians who advised the same rigorous exercise for men and women at the beginning of the century.[113] Prior to the First World War, women were also restricted in the types of physical and mental activities they could participate in based on gendered expectations and social etiquette. For example, women were discouraged from certain mental activities, such as university studies, because they were deemed "unfit."[114] In addition, there were a limited number of physical activities, such as croquet and ice skating, deemed suitable for middle-class women; biking, a new sport many women enjoyed, was deemed "improper for respectable women."[115] By the Weimar era, the notion that women were different (not equal) to men had replaced earlier ideas about women's parity to men. Because the female organism had distinct functions, women doctors argued that female physical education be adjusted to fit this more current view.[116]

Changes specific to women's bodies during puberty led female physicians to advocate a unique gym program for women. Dr Elizabeth Hoffa, a Jewish pediatrician and part-time school doctor in Berlin, advocated that a daily gym hour, particularly during the crucial developmental years at the vocational schools, would be quite beneficial if it accommodated the female body. She even reported the improvement of bad posture and scoliosis and enhanced breathing after daily exercise in a Wilmersdorf elementary school was implemented.[117] Until the age of twelve, boys and girls followed relatively similar developmental patterns, but after this, girls' bodies matured much earlier and much quicker than boys', thus leading to higher rates of disease, especially scoliosis, among adolescent girls.[118] During puberty, the pelvis of females also grew wider to prepare girls for childbearing. However, because the stomach muscles were not yet strong enough to hoist the pelvis forward, the backbone often bent abnormally. Because the female body experienced these particular changes, Heusler-Edenhuizen and Clara Bender, a school doctor and practising physician in Breslau, thought female physical education should include exercises for strengthening the back, as well as running games and swimming to bolster the torso muscles. They thought it was important to incorporate breathing techniques into the curriculum because the heart and lungs were often not developed enough to keep pace with the demands of such precipitous body growth.[119] The strengthening of back, stomach, and chest muscles in women not only was important for supporting the pubescent maturation of their bodies, but it was also vital, according to Heusler-Edenhuizen, for making a woman stronger for "her specific reproductive activity, pregnancy and childbirth." Because a pregnant woman required strong stomach muscles to restrain the forward-falling child and to push during childbirth, strong back muscles to counterbalance her baby weight, and strong chest muscles to replace breathing from her stomach with that of the chest, Heusler-Edenhuizen called for these areas to be the focus of physical education programs.

Heusler-Edenhuizen and Bender confirmed that women who participated in proper physical education or sports during adolescence showed positive results during pregnancy, especially if a woman was doing exercise long before she became pregnant. Only a few exercises, such as riding, skiing, and certain bar exercises, were deemed unbeneficial for bearing children later, primarily because they created a pelvic floor that was too strong and too muscular. Women who had neglected doing exercise prior to pregnancy often had doctors prescribe them a corset to replace the lacking stomach and back muscles.[120] Some women were even starting to exercise during their pregnancies. Heusler-Edenhuizen, for example, remembered the case of a patient of hers with eight children who had one of the most fit bodies she had ever seen. When she questioned her about whether she had done some sort of exercise for her body to remain looking so good, the woman turned dark red and ashamedly admitted that she was a professional athlete and had competed shortly before and after pregnancy. Instead of chastising her, Heusler-Edenhuizen claimed that this woman assured her that proper physical education sufficiently strengthened women for pregnancy and even gave them greater joy in knowing that their bodies would not become deformed as a result of childbirth.[121] Heusler-Edenhuizen became, in other words, a true believer in the benefits of participating in exercise at an early age. Tailoring gym exercises to fit the new build of girls' bodies during adolescence and to prepare them for pregnancy was one way in which female physicians claimed they could redesign current school physical education programs. Furthermore, the construction and disciplining of female bodies for childbirth could be justified by concerns about Germany's future.[122]

Women physicians also wanted to accommodate girls' menstrual cycles in their reconsiderations of physical education curriculum. They perceived that menstruation was an embarrassing issue for adolescent girls, and therefore underscored that it was a normal, physical process that every girl underwent.[123] It was for this reason that Heusler-Edenhuizen believed there was no excuse for healthy women not to carry on with their normal work and physical activities. She thought only unusual, extravagant activities, such as carrying heavy loads or mountain climbing should be avoided. Schoolgirls should be exempt from jumping exercises, but in general, they could participate in most other sports and gym drills. Physical activity benefited girls' health because it stimulated blood flow; Heusler-Edenhuizen thus supported restrained exercise during menstruation.[124] Based on her experience as a school doctor in Breslau, Bender agreed that swimming, riding, jumping, and all vibration of the body should be forbidden during menstruation, but she viewed moderate physical movement as harmless, and in fact, beneficial in cases of blood loss or physical ailments.[125] Most doctors agreed that insisting that women hold off on any type of exercise was wrong and that the importance of limiting women's physical exercise while they were menstruating or pregnant tended to be exaggerated.

The worst type of behaviour for menstruating women, according to Profé, was sitting for hours because all the blood collected in the inner organs.[126] Heusler-Edenhuizen confirmed that pain often occurred from a lack of blood flow. She observed that teachers and students experienced stronger bleeding and pain during the exam preparation period in which they were usually sitting in front of their books all day without movement. She recommended that whenever women began to feel pain associated with menstruation, they should immediately ride a bike or power walk because this would help the pain go away.[127] In addition, Heusler-Edenhuizen helped convince young girls, who were timid about bathing during menstruation, that hygiene was still important and even more essential during this time because of the higher risk of infection.[128] How much to expect of a healthy girl during her period, however, really depended on how ill or indisposed she was – a designation that, unfortunately, most adolescent girls came to believe while they were menstruating. Heusler-Edenuhuizen claimed that having a female doctor on hand to ease a girl's embarrassment when asking for an excuse from gym class, to empathize with her feelings, or to give explanations in the way that only a mother could, really consoled a young girl during this time of crisis in her life. Moreover, such a special mother-daughter bond between doctors and their students counteracted the tension between parents and their children at this age.[129] Heusler-Edenhuizen highlighted her maternal abilities to empathize and provide comfort, even suggesting that her relationship with her students could supplant the familial bond. Many children found it daunting to discuss sexual issues with their parents, and many mothers did not find it necessary to have a talk about sexuality, even when their daughters began menstruating.[130] Their roles as mothers both prior to and during their medical careers likely led female physicians like Heusler-Edenhuizen to use maternal traits, such as tact, care, respect, and empathy when handling teenage girls who were confronting menstruation for the first time. Female doctors claimed a superior ability to act with discretion during this confusing and pressure-ridden time of adolescence. Dr Hoffa reported that young girls felt ashamed when asking for class exemptions, especially when boys were also present. In

elementary schools, male gym teachers generally showed little understanding of girls' medical excuses. Female teachers and doctors, on the
other hand, were more lenient when it came to exemptions; some even
found them essential.[131] In addition to portraying themselves as quite
valuable in terms of guiding young girls in matters of physical exercise
during menstruation, female doctors' maternal concerns coupled with
their medical bona fides may have also motivated them to intervene in
girls' physical education and to chastise their students' mothers.

In their conversations about schools, female physicians continuously tackled the question of whether girls should participate in gym
or sports activities while menstruating, indicating that this "feminine
matter" was something they thought belonged in school health curriculum. The content of women's physical education that female doctors
proposed already included specific exercises to fit women's bodies, and
it now focused on how the natural bodily cycles of women might affect
their physical abilities. This new curriculum concentrated on restricting and extending what was acceptable for the female body; the core of
it was about control. The curriculum and the concepts behind it were
novel; a separate physical education program for girls, especially one
that considered *their* needs had not previously been considered. Female
physicians asserted responsibility for this new curriculum, showing
their gendered contribution to physical education and their expanded
possibilities within the medical profession. They sought to define what
girls' physical education entailed and determined the outcomes this
had for their students' lives and for their own professional prospects.
In their efforts to influence and adjust the content of women's health
curriculum, they claimed to broaden the role of the female school doctor, who would become an educational activist for a new type of public
health – one that aimed to bring their perceptions of women's concerns
(like reproduction and menstruation) to the forefront.

Beyond advocating for changes in the content of women's health curriculum, female doctors sought to modify the way in which subjects like
sex education were taught. Various groups had advocated teaching sex
education since the beginning of the twentieth century, but after the First
World War, it became compulsory in vocational schools in certain cities,
such as Hamburg.[132] In her call for the reform of sexual education, Dr
Helene Börner, a practising gynecologist in Hamburg, highlighted the
failures of these courses in German vocational and higher schools. She
thought schools compressed too much information into too few lessons.
She also thought sex education was too sensational and was offered

much too late to students, and thus, it often failed to protect children. In addition, Börner criticized its overemphasis on the negatives of sexual life; while sex education intended to warn children, this often resulted in a backlash among youth, who often adopted defensive attitudes.[133] Female youth, for example, may have made claims they never wanted to marry – a risky consequence in light of the already low birth rate and the extreme gender gap after the First World War. Börner suggested an alternative sex education program that divided responsibilities among teachers, parents, and doctors, while all working together. Teachers would give children a basic background in biology, parents would be responsible for their upbringing and for instilling in them a sense of responsibility, and doctors would raise their awareness of venereal diseases and other health matters.[134]

Other women doctors had ideas about the environment in which sex education should be taught. Instead of holding large lectures, Dr Susanne Altstaedt and Dr Erna Janzen, who both taught in vocational schools, saw the value in teaching smaller classes. Altstaedt advised other school doctors against the large lecture format in favour of small lectures like the ones she held in various vocational schools in Lübeck. She taught twenty to thirty upper-class students for an hour and a half at a time. These small lectures did not require much more time, and in her opinion, the extra work was definitely worthwhile.[135] It was in these smaller settings, after all, that school doctors could develop intimate relationships with their students. These were the types of relationships female students needed in order to trust authority figures with personal information about taboo topics. For example, Janzen, previously a practising pediatrician in Eisenach who also taught at the vocational school there, preferred teaching smaller classes because of the personal relationships she could develop with her students; she urged health education to adopt this format.[136] When Altstaedt was teaching in a small setting, she was able to recognize the hopeful faces of young girls, leading her to automatically think of her own small daughter and how she would be where they were sitting within a few years.[137] Women school doctors, harking back to their own experiences as mothers, often thought of these schoolchildren as their own. Heusler-Edenhuizen and Szagunn even used the personal pronoun "my" when talking about their students.[138]

Szagunn's 1961 autobiographical essay for *Berliner Medizin*, in which she reflects on her part-time position as a school doctor at a Charlottenburg vocational school, is a particularly noteworthy example of how she characterizes her wide-ranging responsibilities in terms that combine the professional with the maternal. Until the vocational school fired her in compliance with the *Doppelverdiener* (double-earner) law, Szagunn oversaw three thousand female students, promoted health care for children, fought for child workers' rights, and taught women about sexual health.[139] Szagunn writes with evident pride about her work with working-class fourteen- to seventeen-year-olds, a generation of students who faced considerable social and economic obstacles: "Looking back, I always admired how they overcame all these difficulties and how the girls' approach – I always said 'my' girl in my mind – was healthy and brave in face of the duties of work and life."[140] Decades later, Szagunn presents herself as having served as a surrogate mother to her students, emphatically insisting that she silently laid claim to them as her own. Szagunn also frequently describes how, faced with her students' material suffering, she extended the scope of her responsibilities beyond routine medical exams and advice. She explains, for example, that following the 1929 stock market crash, she was moved by her students' suffering to lead a relief effort, distributing forty to fifty packages of groceries per month to needy students. Szagunn presents herself going above and beyond the normal duties of a part-time school doctor with anecdotes of collecting shoes, coats, and money, even finding a job for a student in especially dire need.[141] In this way, Szagunn collapses an archetype of maternal care into a professional identity in order to valorize her work and that of others like her. Szagunn, Altstaedt, and Heusler-Edenhuizen clearly related better to their students because they saw the work they did as an extension of their maternal duties. Szagunn, additionally, understood the impact that her being a mother had on her students. While she gave lessons at the women's vocational school, her younger son often played with other children in the Kindergarten affiliated with the school. Szagunn acknowledged that her students felt a deeper connection with her because in instances like this, she was more than just a teacher in their eyes. This, she claims, also accentuated her own teaching experience as well.[142]

Conclusions: Women Doctors as Educational Activists *and* Traditional Caretakers

Szagunn's reflections synthesized her maternal and professional roles as she proclaimed a significant non-medical influence over her students. Szagunn echoes the kinds of claims that women doctors made in their efforts to preserve and expand their place in the medical profession. Female physicians worked in schools for the same reasons that they were employed in other fields of Weimar public health and social welfare: these positions were some of the only jobs they could procure in the face of an overcrowded, male-dominated, and unreceptive medical profession. Female physicians maximized their marginalization, however. These positions offered them the flexibility to balance their domestic and professional lives as working mothers and allowed them to work primarily with women and children – something that both they and their male colleagues saw as suitable – thus enabling them to carve out and solidify a professional domain.

In these new spaces, women physicians conferred on the word "doctor" a whole new set of meanings. They tapped into a feminine niche by acknowledging their ability to serve the nation's female youth and showcasing their expertise. In their professional discourse, they made women's health education their calling, casting themselves as indispensable to this new subject by offering what they considered superior knowledge over their male colleagues. They saw schools as a particularly fruitful site for intervention where they could stress their gendered contributions to the profession and medical practice, and where they could make unique interventions to girls' physical education. They suggested, for example, that they were best suited to answer questions about what type of gymnastic activity girls required in preparation for motherhood or how much exercise they could perform while menstruating. In short, they offered something to adolescent girls that male doctors did not: professional training *and* personal experience. While male physicians pushed their female colleagues to the margins of the medical profession, schools became one of the few places where women doctors could get jobs in the Weimar era, but women doctors also laid claim to schools, underscoring their importance to the field of girls' health education. Through their maternalist and eugenics discourse, women doctors carved out a space and expanded their own professional opportunities as experts about and activists for adolescent women's health.

While female school doctors portrayed themselves as educational activists for their students, this was often at the expense of lower-class women. They issued advice to working-class students and working-class mothers based on their own middle-class values. Dr Edith von Lölhöffel's participation in workshops that taught mothers how to properly educate their children in health matters was a noteworthy example of this.[143] Lutz Sauerteig shows that pedagogues, feminists, and medical authorities had a history of educating working-class youth and their mothers about sexual behaviour on the basis of their own middle-class values.[144] As Dr Ilse Szagunn demonstrated in her position as a school doctor, she also offered practical aid and advice to the less fortunate during times of financial need. For these women, class alongside gender became crucial categories for understanding their position vis-à-vis others in Weimar society.[145]

They took the path of least resistance by rarely entering conversations about male physical education, unless it was in relation to female physical education.[146] Adopting a physical education curriculum centred around women's traditional roles as mothers and housewives was a means for them to avoid drawing further attention to their threatening presence in the field of medicine. This was a way for them to portray themselves as experts in a new field of women's health because they could use their own domestic knowledge and experience in their classrooms. Through their regulation of girls' bodies and their physical education program, women doctors demonstrated how they were able to push the limits of school health care. By raising awareness and expanding the boundaries of what women's health entailed (and where it could be practised), female doctors founded another space for themselves in medicine.

3 Fighting the Vices That Threatened Women and Children: Sex, Alcohol, and Disease

The social ills of prostitution, venereal disease, and alcohol particularly affected women and children in the Weimar period, thereby creating a site for women doctors to intervene. Women doctors began to address these problems precisely when alcohol and venereal disease started to affect marriage and familial relations and when youth became exposed to VD and prostitution. They became especially concerned when these vices encroached on the upper and middle classes, especially when middle-class men visited prostitutes, when middle-class women turned to prostitution out of economic desperation, or when the "civilized" classes began to drink, revealing their class biases; they especially sought to purge alcoholism – believed to be a heritable trait and therefore dangerous to the people's health – from the upper echelons of society.

Women doctors' work in the movements against alcoholism, venereal disease, and prostitution appealed to them for a number of reasons. For one, their interest in public welfare fields during the Weimar period marked an extension of similar types of activities they undertook during the Kaiserreich.[1] Their work in Weimar marriage counselling centres and school physical education reform efforts indicated women physicians' strong commitment towards public health. Similarly, their engagement with the Weimar social and political campaigns against prostitution, venereal disease, and alcoholism reaffirmed the importance of this type of social health care to their professional identities. Next, the anti-alcohol movement and anti-VD and prostitution campaign (practically one and the same), which both reached a height in the 1920s, developed and expanded along the same timeline and trajectory as female physicians entering and securing their foothold in medicine. Women's medical professionalization grew independently of these movements and was not necessarily correlated to them, but they certainly coexisted. Therefore, involvement in alcohol, prostitution, and VD was both easy and available for women doctors, and they were often building on the work and concerns of different strands within the women's movement. These growing fields offered new employment possibilities for female doctors (in VD clinics for example), but more importantly, they provided them with an abundance of opportunities to influence and shape discourse about new policy and legislation as it was being debated and produced.

Finally, female physicians were drawn to these movements precisely *because* of the harm they caused to women, children, and the home – already deemed the woman's domain by the early twentieth century. The destructiveness that VD and alcohol had on women and their families was well known and well publicized in the interwar period. Youth, with whom women doctors were already engaged through the new school health curriculum, became vulnerable to prostitution and alcohol as people migrated to cities. Wives and, as a result, marriages suffered from disgruntled, alcoholic husbands and infidelity, which occurred either during the First World War or immediately after and often brought disease into the home. Women's organizations began to recognize that the anti-VD campaign unjustly singled out women for being the carriers of disease and that VD clinics failed to provide them equal medical care. These reasons combined drew women physicians into either one or all of the movements. And yet, the primary focus around women and youth within the anti-alcohol and anti-VD movements that surfaced in *Die Ärztin* and in female doctors' efforts in related debates, conferences, meetings, or associations was also the by-product of the fact that they *were* involved and therefore centred the discussion towards their concerns and the interests of their readership.

Female physicians invoked distinct identities as women and as doctors as they sought to influence the discourse of these movements. This was enabling for a group that was attempting to carve out a niche for themselves in medicine. By focusing their rhetoric on the negative impact alcohol had on nursing mothers, for example, or on the treatment of women in VD counselling centres, these doctors located a means to influence contemporary dialogue about public health issues. Moreover, they worked to make their voices more discernible at professional events or at scientific and governmental gatherings or in respected journals, as they fashioned themselves as authoritative figures on how alcohol, VD, prostitution, youth, and women intersected.

Their participation in associations or in jobs – like the women doctors employed in VD clinics after 1927 – where they had not been able
or allowed in the past also showed the new possibilities available to
female physicians. Unsurprisingly, women physicians focused on the
way these problems manifested themselves in the private sphere. They
recognized the realm they could influence and did not stray from it,
thereby laying claim to a sphere they sought to vacate by becoming
professionals. Analogous to their work in other medical spaces, they
limited themselves to treating women and children, just as their male
colleagues had encouraged.

In addition to examining the types of work women doctors undertook within these movements, and how they infused this work with
maternalism, this chapter also argues that women doctors broadened
their medical roles by presenting themselves as political advocates for
women in the fight against state-regulated prostitution and in their
demands for equal treatment in VD counselling centres. The political
activism female doctors demonstrated differentiated their work in the
anti-VD campaign from their anti-alcohol endeavours, and aligned their
anti-VD work with the types of behaviour they displayed working in
marriage counselling centres and in school health reform. Their understanding of fundamental women's rights manifested in their demands
for equal treatment in VD clinics, in their fight against the double standard in the 1927 Law for Combating Venereal Disease, in their requests
for greater access to female physicians and birth control in marriage
counselling centres, and in their advocacy of equal attention and funding to women's physical education in vocational schools. In all of these
medical spaces, and especially in their anti-VD discourse, women physicians demonstrated an acute awareness of the injustices that women
faced. To a certain degree, they fell in line with the strong feminist and
abolitionist critiques of *Reglementierung* (regulated prostitution), as they
recognized the unfair treatment women received under this system.[2]
In school physical education, too, female doctors recognized that girls
were treated like second-class children compared with their male peers,
with fewer facilities, limited time to use those amenities available, or a
lack of gym curriculum altogether. Whether in schools or VD counselling centres, female doctors aspired to put an end to this second-class
treatment of women. The nature of their arguments was also similar in
these two fields. They called for women's equal access and treatment
in VD clinics and school physical education by pointing out women's
differences. This, they asserted, merited their students and patients a

separate yet equal health program in schools and VD clinics with doctors of their same sex. In marriage counselling centres, female physicians also recognized the basic rights of women because they argued that overburdened, poor women should have free access to contraception, and also that their inner-most secrets about marriage and motherhood deserved the ear of someone who could best understand them based on their similar life experiences. Supporting women's basic needs and rights in these different medical spaces confirmed female physicians as political beings.

Venereal Disease and Prostitution: Interwar and Interconnected Problems

Government officials, policymakers, and health-conscious organizations and individuals perceived alcoholism, venereal disease, and prostitution to be among the most widespread and interconnected social problems, alongside poverty and unemployment, that plagued the immediate post–First World War period. According to historian Paul Weindling, these problems emerged primarily because of industrialization and urbanization in the early twentieth century but were exacerbated in the postwar period. Industrialization – a relatively late phenomenon in Germany – conveyed the image of expanding cities that lacked adequate infrastructure of housing, education, sanitation, and medical care. Sickness and poverty proliferated, particularly among working-class populations. Disease spread rapidly, especially in overcrowded urban tenements. Industrial workers, often working between ten and twelve hours a day, six days a week "in hazardous conditions involving contact with noisy and dangerous machinery, poisonous fumes, and dusty, toxic substances" and the urban poor turned to prostitutes and alcohol to alleviate their squalid living conditions.[3] Extramarital affairs and alcoholism, especially among men, nurtured a marriage crisis with divorce rates at an all-time high.[4] Women were often left to take sole care of their already-struggling families, as their husbands drank away their meagre incomes and often returned home with a sexually transmitted disease. Alcohol only increased people's susceptibility to catching and transmitting a venereal disease because all cautions tended to be ignored.[5] Weimar-era economic circumstances forced desperate women to start working, sometimes as sex workers because of the perceived economic benefits. Even middle-class women and adolescent youth turned to prostitution out of desperation.[6]

Historian Bernd Widdig shows how fears of prostitution among the middle class "occupie[d] the public imagination" especially during periods of inflation.[7]

The First World War and its associated outcomes – increased alcohol consumption, prostitution, and the rise of women in the workforce – removed parents from the home and caused them to neglect their children, which resulted in a loosening of morals among youth. The Reichsministerium des Innern (Reich Ministry of the Interior; RMI), increasingly disturbed by the damaging consequences the First World War had on the supervision of youth and on adolescent health, especially on youth susceptible to prostitution and venereal disease, demanded that schools and organizations expand their efforts to educate youth about the dangers of sexual activity [8] The Deutsche Gesellschaft zur Bekämpfung der Geschlechtskrankheiten (German Society for Combating Venereal Disease, DGBG), founded in 1902, also recognized that the absence of parents, who either lacked authority or were ignorant of the risks of VD, necessitated government intervention to get local and state municipalities and teachers to participate in the "urgent teaching and warning of young people about the dangers of venereal disease."[9] The same anxieties about the health of the nation and its citizens that fuelled government intervention into marriage after the First World War also led to a massive expansion of new health and welfare policies under the catch-all rhetoric of *Bevölkerungspolitik* (population politics).[10] Society became increasingly medicalized as physicians now used their professional knowledge to serve the state; they were among the growing number of government personnel at all levels who were confronting the problems associated with urbanization, the rise of the working poor, and the rise of VD, prostitution, and alcoholism.[11]

With millions of soldiers returning home after being exposed to prostitution and venereal disease, new anxieties emerged about the dangers VD caused for the country.[12] Annette Timm discusses how soldiers have often "been recognized as conduits of venereal disease," but that the "unprecedented scale of military conscription" during the First World War led to increased military and government intervention in VD control. Already before the end of the war, in February 1918, the War Department attempted to curb the spread of VD, calling on soldiers to remain healthy and fit during such a vital time for Germany. Unfortunately, its efforts were ineffective, as cases of VD continued to infiltrate the army.[13] Coinciding with the return of millions of soldiers from the front, discussions for a new uniform national Law for Combating Venereal Disease began in the Reichstag later that month. An Emergency

Decree was issued on 11 December 1918 which stated that VD would include syphilis, gonorrhea, and chancroid; that people deemed likely to pass it on could be forcibly treated unless treatment was life-threatening; that whoever engaged in sexual activity knowing (or suspecting) that he or she had a venereal disease could be punished with up to three years' imprisonment or more; and that education about the mode of transmission and legal provisions for prosecution would accompany all treatment. The RMI also began its own efforts to reform VD control in 1919 by forming a special working committee on the VD epidemic because they were concerned about the lack of military intervention.[14]

In light of population losses during and after the war, "venereal discourse" came to dominate public debates because, as historian Julia Roos argues, "the perceived dramatic spread of STDs seemed to jeopardize Germany's prospects of regeneration."[15] VD became a metaphor for the moral decline of all society.[16] Most of the population had little knowledge about the possibilities of contracting VD or the consequences, and VD rates appeared to be on the rise.[17] An example from southwest Germany showed an increase in new cases of VD being treated in hospitals between the beginning of the war right up to war's end, and especially in the two years following the war when rates nearly doubled.[18] Venereal disease became such a serious concern that the RMI attempted to gather a reliable count of the number of Germans with VD. The Reichsgesundheitsamt (Reich Health Bureau; RGA) carried out the survey, which tracked all cases of medically treated venereal disease between 15 November and 14 December 1919 and showed that some 136,000 individuals were being treated for venereal disease. The RGA also noted that a portion of infected individuals either did not receive treatment at all or did not go to a licensed doctor, and therefore, this survey only included a portion of actual cases of VD.[19]

Gathering accurate statistics about the rates of VD was certainly difficult in the Weimar era. The press did not help alleviate growing worries about the alarming spread of venereal disease after a flood of infected men returned from war. Wilhelm Heinrich Dreuw, an anti-government campaigner and police doctor who specialized in VD, for example, convinced journalists and welfare associations that six million Germans were infected with VD in 1920.[20] Franz Bumm, head of the RGA, insisted that this was a clear overestimation, seeing as how this would account for 10 per cent of the total population in Germany. He instead estimated that over one million Germans had VD.[21] Venereal disease rates reported in the press, in fact, were often higher than the actual numbers that government data produced, sometimes resulting in complaints from the Health Bureau, but such stories still placed pressure on politicians.[22] As Timm has claimed, "the question of whether the VD crisis was exaggerated or not seems impossible to answer definitively" because patients generally wanted to keep the disease private and doctors were not required to report cases. However, fears of sexual degeneration and moral decline, as well as changing gender roles, certainly also shaped the crisis.[23] The creation of and prolonged debates over a national Law for Combating Venereal Disease throughout the 1920s undoubtedly stemmed from these anxieties – either real or imagined – about the impact of venereal disease on the *Volk*'s health. After almost a decade of political debates over its content and breadth, the Reichstag passed the law on 18 February 1927, and it took effect on 1 October 1927. Intended to replace the Emergency Decree of 1918, its provisions were very similar, and now only accredited German doctors were deemed acceptable to treat VD. Doctors were also required to distribute an official educational leaflet at the beginning of treatment.[24]

The RGA's attempt to extrapolate the number of individuals nationally infected with VD did, in fact, confirm the suspicion that VD was tied to geographic location and thus to prostitution. Unsurprisingly, those states with a strong industrial setting, or those with heavy sea traffic (Bremen, Hamburg, Lübeck) had a higher rate of venereal disease than those of a predominantly agricultural character, seeing as how prostitution was generally more prevalent in port cities. The relationship between venereal disease and prostitution was so close, in fact, that according to one women's journal, "one [could] see the spread of venereal disease as an indicator of the spread and use of prostitution." The journal also confirmed Bumm's contention that there were over a million people who needed treatment for venereal disease, adding that "its most dangerous source" – prostitution – had caused a "hundred thousand new infections."[25] Anita de Lemos, a female physician working for the police in Hamburg, was well aware of the blatant prostitution as well as the overwhelming presence and seduction of youth there. In her discussion of the conditions in Hamburg, she observed a dreadful environment in which solicitation by prostitutes occurred on the street openly, where working-class families and prostitutes lived together in completely unhygienic conditions, and where children witnessed all kinds of immoral acts.[26] De Lemos, a member of the privileged class of doctors, was clearly making her own moral judgments about the openness of prostitution in Hamburg, views that the working class – the background of the majority of German prostitutes – may not have shared.[27]

Weimar-era concerns about the growth of prostitution were also based on a combination of fact and fiction. Prostitution was in principle illegal in early twentieth-century Germany but was tolerated under a system of state police regulation known as *Reglementierung*.[28] Based on the French model of police-controlled prostitution, most German states introduced *Reglementierung* in the first half of the nineteenth century, and Germany's concerns about and regulation of prostitution did not occur in isolation of other European states during this time.[29] In order to avoid criminal prosecution, prostitutes had to register with the special division of the police – the *Sittenpolizei* (morals police) – created to supervise "moral" matters, including public indecency, sexual indiscretion, homosexuality, and prostitution. In an attempt to curb the spread of VD, police could arrest any women suspected of prostitution and subject her to a health exam. In many cities, registered prostitutes had to report for health exams as often as twice a week. Infected women were then hospitalized and underwent compulsory medical treatment. If they failed to do so or violated police regulations, they could be imprisoned for up to six weeks.[30]

Ascertaining the number of prostitutes in any given year was extremely difficult because only a small number of them registered with the police. In her observations of prostitution in Hamburg, Dr de Lemos calculated the number of women who were under police regulation to be about 2,400, but estimated that the actual existing number of prostitutes was eight to ten times as many as this.[31] Richard Evans argues that "the registered prostitutes formed an increasingly small proportion of the total number."[32] Julia Roos explains that experts estimated in most German cities there were five to ten unregulated or clandestine prostitutes for every woman registered with the *Sittenpolizei*. At the turn of the century, there were an estimated 100,000 to 200,000 prostitutes in Germany and by the beginning of the First World War, there were anywhere between 330,000 and 1.5 million prostitutes.[33] Moreover, prostitution rates sharply increased in certain major cities during the wartime and postwar period. The number of registered prostitutes in Berlin skyrocketed between 1913 (3,611) and 1925 (6,191). Clandestine prostitution also soared in cities like Hamburg and Frankfurt, especially during the severe inflation of 1921–2.[34] Even though prostitution rates did not rise in all major cities, starting in the late nineteenth century and continuing through the Weimar period, contemporaries viewed the problem of prostitution as both large-scale and endemic.[35]

Female Physicians and the Debate over *Reglementierung*

Debates about the new Law for Combating Venereal Disease, both while it was being drafted and after it was passed, afforded women doctors a plethora of scholarly opportunities to participate in the campaign against prostitution and venereal disease. They directed their conversations toward how the law most affected prostitutes – presumably the group that these women doctors thought they could potentially most influence. They attempted to frame the debate around prostitutes and their equal protection under the law, showing how they laid claim to a new area of medicine.

Women doctors had been active members in the campaign against venereal disease since their entry into the German medical world. Fridericia Gräfin von Geldern-Egmond, originally licensed in Switzerland in 1897 and then in Germany in 1902, was a member of the DGBG (founded in 1902) by 1903 and a participant at its First Congress in March of that year in Frankfurt, along with Elisabeth Winterhalter, who was on the organizational committee of the congress. Hope Bridges Adams-Lehmann, recognized as a German licensed physician in 1904 through a federal court decision some twenty-five years after she had passed the state medical exam in Leipzig, was, like von Geldern-Egmond, a specialist in women's health and an early member of the DGBG. Other early members included Agnes Hacker, Pauline Rosenthal, Jenny Springer, and Franziska Tiburtius.[36]

While the Reichstag was debating the Law for Combating Venereal Disease throughout the 1920s, the first generation of female physicians was finally gaining a strong presence in the medical profession. The portion of the law that attracted particular attention from female physicians involved the restrictions imposed on prostitutes under *Reglementierung*, which, in addition to subjecting prostitutes to regular hygienic controls, restricted their place of residence, freedom of movement, attire, and public behaviour. In the majority of German cities, registered prostitutes were confined to particular streets or houses approved by the morals police, also known as *Kasernierung* (quartering).[37]

German prostitutes' experiences and prostitution management during the Weimar era, including the debate over the regulation and treatment of prostitutes, have received a fair amount of recent attention. Some of these histories use prostitution as a lens through which to view sexuality and sexual politics, population policies, eugenic theories, and medical discourse within interwar and Nazi Germany.[38] Centring women doctor's discussions about prostitution and venereal disease shows how this group of women professionals reframed the conversation around prostitutes' equal rights within the 1927 law and VD counselling centres. By doing so, women doctors highlighted the ways they could influence and manage women, their health, and their bodies for the Weimar welfare state, thereby arrogating power within this women's medical space.

As the 1927 law was being debated in the Reichstag, women doctors weighed in on both sides of the debate about quartering prostitutes; they expressed the advantages and disadvantages of prostitutes being restricted to certain areas. Dr de Lemos's ideas articulated some of the reasons why doctors favoured quartering. She stressed that the housing of prostitutes on certain streets or in certain areas of the city protected them from the exploitation that they often faced in brothels. Moreover, they could inhabit their own apartments and the city would generally leave them to practise their trade within these designated areas. Quartering was also advantageous to society as a whole, she noted, because it attempted to eradicate all unregulated streetwalkers, making the streets cleaner and safer. It also allowed for the monitoring of hygienic conditions, which in addition to protecting women from abuse also protected the middle class – perceived as the primary group threatened by prostitution – from unsanitary conditions and disease.[39] De Lemos, then, saw quartering as a means to end the exploitation of women. She also viewed quartering as beneficial to the general welfare of society, and especially the threatened middle and upper classes, whom women doctors aimed to protect from the vices of the working class. In their discourse about quartering, female physicians like de Lemos put the interests of their patients *and* those of society in the foreground and often conflated the two. She saw how lower-class women prostitutes experienced police exploitation, but she also recognized how the community suffered from disease because of the unhygienic conditions associated with unregulated prostitution.

Police doctor de Lemos's rhetoric about quartering also stressed some of the disadvantages of the practice. Quartering as well as brothels, simply through their mere existence, induced curiosity and were seductive tourist spots for locals and foreigners. Rather than providing health protection for prostitutes and middle-class customers, she thought quartering was a ploy for health security and would only reassure hesitant men seeking a prostitute. This would thus augment the demand for prostitutes as well as increase the number of venereal diseases. She suggested that segregating prostitutes was senseless in the fight against VD because infected men would continue to infect healthy women unless a doctor examined every individual who entered the quartered zone – something she saw as "unfeasible."[40] Perhaps what was needed was the type of reformed state monitoring that Hildegard Canon, another female physician active in the fight against VD and prostitution, proposed much later in 1934 – a time in which it was, in fact, more viable. In Canon's proposition, this new form of quartering would make the state responsible for assigning women to certain houses, determining apartment prices, and supervising the health of prostitutes by establishing a station in each house to examine customers for infection.[41] Ultimately, women doctors like de Lemos favoured the abolition of quartering in the Law for Combating Venereal Disease, viewing it as unnecessary. She was not as critical as some of her colleagues because she still recognized some of the benefits state-controlled prostitution had on protecting the upper classes from prostitution and the unhygienic conditions associated with it.

The BDÄ adopted a more critical approach, which viewed *Reglementierung* as a repressive system that perpetuated a misogynistic sexual double standard – an assessment that also aligned with mainstream women's organizations.[42] One way the BDÄ highlighted this stance was by publishing an article by Anna Pappritz in 1925. Pappritz, a leader in Germany's branch of the International Abolitionist Federation (IAF) and longtime Bund Deutscher Frauenvereine (League of German Women's Associations; BDF) executive, strongly criticized state-regulated prostitution, which she thought singled out women as the only carriers of VD. German abolitionists opposed *Reglementierung* on the grounds that the system legally discriminated against the female sex by exclusively penalizing women for an act committed by both sexes. In 1902, the BDF officially adopted an abolitionist position.[43] Pappritz hoped the new law – still under debate – would help change this mindset and lead authorities to see that the reporting and treatment of men was also crucial to the fight against VD. This would add to the positive ethical strides the law had already made in breaking with the double standard. Pappritz also saw the efforts of female doctors in welfare offices, schools, VD counselling centres, and in police forces as essential to managing the terrible epidemic of venereal disease.[44] By drawing attention to the unfairness of *Reglementierung* and praising more recent efforts to hold men and women to similar sexual norms, the BDÄ – initially claiming to be an apolitical association when it was first founded – through its mouthpiece, *Die Ärztin*, revealed itself as becoming more political, siding with the abolitionist viewpoint that advocated for the equal treatment of men and women.[45]

Dr Meta Oelze-Rheinboldt is one example of a BDÄ member who adopted this political rhetoric in her critique of state-regulated prostitution in 1925. Oelze-Rheinboldt, a dermatologist in Leipzig, harshly noted Germany's failures in terms of drafting a uniform national law on prostitution and VD, and thus she thought Germany fell considerably behind other "civilized states." Attempts at reforming the current version of the law had, in her opinion, been unsuccessful and only resulted in more confusion in various states and cities. Because the current draft of the law was lacking any discussion of the "indisputable right of female patients to be examined by female doctors," Oelze-Rheinboldt considered it a "significant failure." She saw this as especially problematic because women were frequently suspected of having VD (albeit often falsely) under *Reglementierung* and counselling centres did not consistently employ female doctors, whom women most often sought for their examinations.[46] Oelze-Rheinboldt fashioned herself as an activist for women, underlining the bias in state-regulated prostitution, which viewed women as the main source of infection, and declared it absolutely necessary that the new law legally establish the right of a female patient to receive treatment from a female doctor. Dr Marie Kaufmann-Wolf, a specialist in dermatology, similarly insisted on fairness for men and women, who she thought should take joint responsibility for the same (sexual) offence committed. She admonished the idea that men could walk free at the cost of women, who were usually targeted as the supposed "source of infection" under state-regulated prostitution. Prostitutes, in fact, were not the source of all VD, and Kaufmann-Wolf found it ludicrous that the men who visited prostitutes multiple times and then repeatedly passed their diseases on were, in a sense, relieved of any sort of obligation. The anti-VD campaign could, in her view, never be described as successful or just if it never held men accountable, which was why she, like some of her colleagues, maintained that equal, anonymous reporting and treatment were needed for both sexes.[47]

By backing women's access to fair treatment, female physicians like Oelze-Rheinboldt and Kaufmann-Wolf framed the discourse about the 1927 law around equal protection under the law and presented themselves as pioneers for this cause. Directing the discussion toward women's medical rights was perhaps also somewhat opportunistic since women physicians would be the ones receiving jobs if these demands came to fruition. Female doctors promoted sameness in terms of the law and VD treatment, and yet they also understood that their differences as women, which they argued entitled them (and not men) to be tending to female patients, would benefit them professionally. Kaufmann-Wolf also encouraged other women to become involved in the anti-VD and abolitionist movements by drawing attention to women's instinctive desire to fight the double standard present in *Reglementierung*. She asserted that women should never tire of the fight against the double standard, which undermined the prestige and dignity of all women. She wanted women to stand together unanimously and to bury their political differences when demanding that men and women be subject to the same law. She declared there was an "instinctive feeling of awareness in us [women] to be the defenders of fundamental women's rights."[48] Kaufmann-Wolf, by using this type of essentialist language reminiscent of the German women's movement, showed that her gender influenced her opposition to the inequality women faced in state-regulated prostitution. She adopted political rhetoric, thereby expanding her medical role and responsibilities.

Various conferences also allowed Kaufmann-Wolf and Katharina Klingelhöfer, both of whom were part of the first generation of women doctors in Germany, to participate in discussions about the draft legislation. Klingelhöfer, an anti-VD activist, discussed the waiver of medical confidentiality and the classification of patients at a 1920 meeting, "Combating Venereal Disease, Prostitution and Criminality through Social Measures."[49] Kaufmann-Wolf gave a lecture entitled "Medical Perspective to the Law for Combating Venereal Disease" at a BDF Conference on the Question of the Forthcoming Legislation to Combat Venereal Diseases in October of the same year.[50] At this conference, which sought to bring together women from parliamentary, municipal, law enforcement, medical, and feminist circles to adopt a uniform opinion about the legislation and to discuss their further demands of the new law, Kaufmann-Wolf talked about the nature and consequences of syphilis and gonorrhea and evaluated the advantages and disadvantages of compulsory treatment for each disease. Embracing the goal of the conference – to demand a higher and equal sexual morality for men and women – she "spoke out of a strong, intuitive sentiment of women (*Frauenempfinden*)," demonstrating how women doctors (and women's organizations) chose to coalesce to fight VD.[51] They insisted on similar standards of sexual morality for men and women, especially in the new legislation, and they also claimed an instinctive ability to treat women in newly opened VD counselling centres. They fought for equivalent sexual mores and legal rights and subjected themselves to a paradigm of difference.

Once it passed, the 1927 law officially abolished *Reglementierung* and decriminalized prostitution in general. The conditions under which prostitutes worked and lived greatly improved. The police could no longer confine prostitutes to certain streets or houses. Prostitutes had protection against exploitative landlords and could now live in neighbourhoods of their choice, as well as with other prostitutes. They could dress however they liked and move freely throughout the city. There were no longer restrictions on their access to public transport or public areas, museums, theatres, or restaurants. Prostitutes no longer needed police permission if they wanted to travel, move, or leave their homes after dark. Women suspected of prostitution could not be arrested or penalized without a proper trial. There was also now a legal basis for requiring health exams of women suspected of prostitution: medical certificates required of people "urgently suspected" of being infected with VD. Women under medical supervision had the right to choose a private physician to be tested for VD, which, Julia Roos claims, many of them did despite the fact that they had to personally incur the cost to do so. Even though public solicitation was outlawed in towns with less than 15,000 residents or in places deemed offensive, such as near churches, schools, or areas where children congregated, open public prostitution ceased to be a criminal offence. Because the 1927 law granted prostitutes key civil rights, such as due process and freedom of movement, Roos has called it a triumph for bourgeois feminists, Social Democrats, and other opponents of *Reglementierung*.[52] Female physicians like those quoted above, who advocated for prostitutes' equal protection under the law, could be included in this group; their rhetoric, after all, pushed for more rights for prostitutes, which the law afforded them.

Whether the 1927 law was coercive or emancipatory for women remained unsettled after it went into effect.[53] Pappritz noted the "pleasing first signs of progress" in the fight against VD in *Die Ärztin*, and Dr Oelze-Rheinboldt reported the falling syphilis rates in the *Leipziger Neuesten Nachrichten* (*Latest News of Leipzig*).[54] Dr Eva Hensel, on the other hand, claimed that the enforcement of the law was "extraordinary inconsistent" and that the sought-after repeal of *Reglementierung* had not transpired.[55] While the law targeted and limited the working-class prostitutes they primarily worked with, for the few female doctors focused on prostitution and VD reform, the law served as an emancipatory means for them to enter conversations about these heavily debated topics. In addition, after the law went into effect, it took responsibility for managing prostitutes away from the morals police and gave it to welfare offices and health departments, thus creating a number of new jobs for middle-class women – another emancipatory effect of the new law.[56] Practically, this benefited female physicians in places like Hamburg, where the health authorities created positions for them to implement the law.

Hildegard Menzi and Anita de Lemos, both dermatologists, worked for the Tag- und Nachtdienst (Day and Night Service) for the Hamburg health authorities. Hamburg's prostitution problem was particularly severe due to the rapid industrialization of the city in the late nineteenth century; it was a port city and a hub for the shipping, manufacturing, and processing industries. The Hamburg health authorities were among a number of local government and bureaucratic agencies that historian Victoria Harris claims devoted significant energy to intervening in prostitution policy and managing prostitutes' behaviour.[57] While Menzi was active for only one year with the health office, de Lemos had been involved in venereal disease care for a long time. By 1921, she had already opened a specialty practice for skin and venereal diseases in Hamburg, the first female doctor to do so. From 1922 to 1927, she was the examination and trust doctor for the welfare office of the Hamburg police (Pflegeamt der Polizeibehörde).[58] Starting in 1924, she was the house doctor in a home for runaways (Durchgangsheim) for homeless girls for the Alstertwiete neighbourhood youth authority, and beginning in 1927, the police authorities commissioned her to examine young girls who had been apprehended by the police for the first time.[59] These "feminine activities of women doctors" appeared attractive to city authorities, who sought to fill these types of positions with female physicians only. Moreover, the nature of this type of work was such that women physicians could be replaced only by other women physicians, meaning that in order for one woman to get her vacation time approved, she had to find a female colleague to take over as her substitute. After all, female doctors were caring for female patients and male doctors for male patients, according to Menzi's descriptions of her activities.[60] Gender-specific views somewhat motivated the establishment of positions for women, and therefore, they were assigned to a field of activity that was connected with gender specific expectations. In this regard, the Hamburg health authorities followed a precedent that had existed since the end of the nineteenth century to employ female police doctors to perform the mandatory examination of prostitutes or suspicious women under *Reglementierung*. People like the Swiss trained Agnes Hacker, who by 1900 had a contract with the Berlin *Sittenpolizei*, and Natalie Ferchland, who took over Hacker's job in 1905 and worked on a part-time basis until 1929, were pioneers in the field and made the morality argument their focal point. Many men also viewed the potential shame young girls felt if not treated by female physicians as a serious problem during the first decades of the twentieth century.[61]

In discussions of the 1927 law, women doctors focused primarily on the equal treatment of women under the law and on the rights of prostitutes. They became advocates for women and their equality, which is one example of how they laid claim to a new area of medicine. Only on rare occasions did the new VD legislation lead to actual job opportunities. As Sabine Schleiermacher illustrates, and as the examples of doctors Menzi and de Lemos demonstrate, there were only a few cases in which female physicians' engagement in social welfare themes, including the fight against prostitution and venereal disease, actually led to an active political health career in political organizations, associations, or parties.[62] It was primarily through their writings about VD legislation that female physicians made their impact by becoming a political voice for underprivileged women. In newly opened VD counselling centres, they adopted similar rhetoric about women's fundamental rights and equality.

Venereal Disease Counselling Centres: A Space for Female Physicians

While government authorities were debating a new national Law for Combating Venereal Disease, state-sponsored, health-insurance-supported venereal disease centres began to appear throughout the Reich. These counselling centres were an element of Weimar population politics, a catch-all term that justified the expansion of health and welfare services and policies.[63] Female physicians, seeking to participate more broadly in Weimar health and welfare initiatives, used the issue of trust, already a rallying call for various women's organizations, to demand that women doctors be employed in new venereal disease counselling centres. In their view, if these centres wanted to gain the trust of their patients, one means of accomplishing this was to ensure that female doctors were always present to treat the rising number of female patients who visited the centres. No longer was it sufficient for the public to rely on the services of these clinics to help prevent the spread of venereal disease; it now became essential to employ a certain type of doctor who best catered to the needs of the patients. In this regard, VD counselling centres were reminiscent of Weimar marriage counselling centres, which sought to employ physicians who could develop trusting relationships with their patients.

The primary goal of counselling centres was to help supervise the growing number of VD patients. The first clinic opened as an experiment in Berlin-Lichtenberg in the early twentieth century but later moved to Beelitz because it failed to attract enough patients. The Reich Insurance Bureau set up a meeting of regional health agencies in 1913 to discuss the possibility of a national network of VD clinics that could survey patients when they moved between jurisdictions. No such network was ever established, but these discussions inspired the opening of the first permanent municipal centre for syphilitic patients on 1 January 1914 in Hamburg, as well as a Prussian War Ministry decree in July 1915 that mandated the examination and treatment of venereal disease for all discharged soldiers in military clinics.[64] The BDF also urged the treatment of all discharged soldiers – if necessary, by compulsion – and the reporting of their names to local insurance-supported counselling centres in a petition submitted to the *Bundesrat* (upper legislative house).[65] In November 1915, the German state insurance institutions convened again. Aware of their responsibility to organize an effective fight against VD, they decided to establish counselling centres for the monitoring of venereal disease in consultation with the medical profession and health insurance institutions. Although they had no disciplinary powers, they aspired to help control the spread of VD by raising public awareness and by improving access to medical advice and treatment. Educated medical specialists became the leaders of these clinics, which were modelled after lung care clinics, as they made advice, prevention, and control (not treatment and healing) their goals. Only in necessary cases did the clinics administer treatment for people suspected of syphilis, gonorrhea, or chancroid, and then kept patients under medical supervision after the conclusion of treatment. Most importantly, the clinics aimed to acquire and maintain the trust of infected patients under all circumstances.[66]

In the following years, more clinics opened, often with opposition from free-practising doctors, who saw this new system of VD counselling centres as threatening to their economic well-being and their ability to handle patients on a personalized basis.[67] Overcoming these restraints

and prejudices of the medical profession was one of the difficulties the
centres faced, but the needs of society as well as propaganda promoting the clinics proved to be beneficial in gaining the public's trust. In
August 1916, for example, the state insurance institution in Westphalia
had already opened three counselling centres, which quickly acquired
the trust of patients.[68] The state insurance institution in Westphalia
added two additional clinics in March 1918 and another four at the end
of 1918. Such expansion reflected both the massive number of people
seeking advice who suspected they might have VD (and many of them
did) and the increasing trust people put in these centres.[69] By 1920, there
were over sixteen clinics in Westphalia, the most of any province.[70] The
situation in the VD clinic in Berlin was similar. The counselling centre
there opened on 2 May 1917 and saw 3,550 visitors that year. In 1919,
8,567 people (7,230 men and 1,337 women) visited the clinic, rising to
10,321 people (8,586 men and 1,735 women) by 1920.[71] By the end of
1919, the German state insurance institutions had over 138 centres, with
100,361 visitors, one-third of whom came on their own accord.[72] There
were 185 centres in 1922, and although a number of these closed during
the inflation years, their number rose to 187 in 1926 and 264 in 1931.[73]
The population's growing trust in these establishments was unmistakable because they were visiting the clinics unceasingly and voluntarily.
The increasing number of centres reflects the reality that more people
were infected with VD, but also that people were more aware of clinics and were more willing to visit them to seek the advice of a medical
professional.

   Similar to how female doctors positioned themselves as ideal confidantes for female patients in marriage counselling centres, women physicians and women's organizations also maintained that women would
be drawn to the new VD counselling centres if they knew they would
be examined by a female doctor. Katharina Scheven, a leading member
of the Association for the Promotion of Morality (Verband zur Förder-
ung der Sittlichkeit), the German branch of the IAF, asked the RMI in
June 1919 to establish VD counselling centres specifically for female
patients in all large and mid-sized German cities. She also requested
that these clinics be placed under female leadership, which she thought
would attract more female patients. In her opinion, "female patients
would, in fact, utilize counselling centres if they were given the opportunity to confide in a woman doctor." After all, "a venereal disease is
often perceived as shameful," and "therefore, it [was] necessary to give
these patients any relief necessary to spare their feelings." She saw it as

especially crucial to protect the modesty of the large number of women and girls who contracted VD after they had illegitimate sex. Rather than continuously condemning them as "morally inferior," Scheven thought it was better to seek them out to prevent them from falling into prostitution.[74] Scheven promoted an interventionist method focused on prevention and reform in which young girls trusted VD centres and doctors enough to visit them and heed their advice. Allowing them to lapse into further moral degradation, she suggested, would only exacerbate the societal burden they had already caused. Scheven saw it as her maternalistic duty to help these lower-class "fallen women." In doing so, she also advocated middle-class morality, reflecting her own class background and biases. After all, VD counselling was a means to enforce middle-class morality, including sexual self-control.[75]

The BDÄ also championed the cause of endangered women and girls. Even more important than assisting girls with loose sexual behaviour, Dr Canon, for one, believed VD counselling centres needed female physicians to help inexperienced, frightened, and sexually abused young girls. According to patient statements, as well as Canon's communication with welfare workers, the aid women doctors could offer to these types of patients significantly facilitated the ultimate decision to let female physicians govern the examination and treatment of women at risk in VD clinics.[76] The BDÄ argued that only through the union of welfare and medical work, which emphasized care, education, counselling, and prevention for these individuals, could the fight against venereal disease be effective.[77] Arguments for this type of integrated welfare and medical care stemmed from the fact that several different agencies counselled the same families for related yet overlapping problems. The prime example was the family who sought marriage counselling because the couple was having marital problems; alcoholic care and VD counselling because the husband was a casualty of both; youth welfare and psychiatric care because the children lied, stole, and severely disrespected their parents; and financial aid because of the unemployment of one or both parents.[78] These interconnected problems were no longer only private matters; divorce, alcohol, VD, criminality, and unemployment were perils that weakened the nation. In terms of venereal disease, then, education and prevention became the key components of an effective anti-VD campaign. Women doctors – already the nation's educators in spaces like marriage counselling centres and schools – were ideally suited for these types of tasks, at least in terms of treating female patients in venereal disease clinics.

The BDF, as an advocate for women, recognized how valuable female physicians could be in propelling the anti-VD movement. In its plea to the Reich Ministry of the Interior in December 1927, the BDF also insisted on the employment of female doctors in VD counselling centres with the founding of the new law. The BDF highlighted the fact that female patients in various cities throughout Germany had already complained about the lack of availability of female physicians, and on behalf of the feelings and wishes of these patients, the organization now demanded same-sex treatment.[79] In addition to the fact that young women and girls felt shame visiting VD clinics, the examinations to test for VD were also quite intimate – another argument in favour of employing women doctors in these spaces. Dr Marie Kaufmann-Wolf noted the closeness with which female prostitutes – often unfairly singled out for VD testing under *Reglementierung* – were examined. Doctors would examine at least their faces, mouths, lips, arms, breasts, neck glands, and auxiliary glands, and usually a woman's anus, small and large labia, stomach and thigh skin, inguinal glands, ducts of the Bartholin's glands, urethra, vagina, and cervix.[80] Women doctors and feminist organizations, then, put some pressure on the government to account for the treatment of men as well as women, as it debated the provisions of the Law for Combating Venereal Disease throughout the 1920s.[81]

The government response showed little sensitivity to requests that a patient's sex be considered during VD reporting and examination. The president of the RGA, Franz Bumm, for one, dismissed the Association for the Promotion of Morality's claim that female patients felt more shame about revealing their cases of VD to doctors. He asserted that men felt just as much shame about their own venereal diseases and required an equal amount of courage to disclose personal information about their sexual affairs. In addition, he rejected the suggestion that women and girls had fewer anxieties about visiting VD counselling centres under female leadership, noting that such claims had no basis in reality. In fact, Bumm claimed that experience had shown that many women preferred to go to male doctors, who they thought would not judge them as harshly as their same-sex companions, and who they believed had more experience, expertise, and discretion. Bumm maintained that the formation of trusting relationships in VD counselling centres depended less on the gender of leaders and more on their performance, reliability, philanthropic spirit, and tact.[82] Female physicians like Canon responded to such allegations by noting than in her twenty-four years of practical experience, she found that even those women with less shame (because of their frequent sexual encounters) treated the opportunity to see a family doctor as a "blessing."[83]

The toil of female physicians and feminist organizations, in the end, was not completely overlooked. By the late 1920s, the government had become more supportive of the idea of employing female doctors in counselling centres to treat female patients; in certain states like Prussia, they were included in the guidelines for the 1927 law. The law also included provisions allowing for women to demand female doctors when they were available.[84] After the government recognized the necessity of same-sex treatment, it became standard practice, and women doctors had to be available even on Sundays and holidays and could not find male substitutes if they needed time off. When the new Nazi regime attempted to fire some female physicians working in VD counselling centres, Canon criticized the Nazis for attempting to destroy a system that had been in existence for almost thirty years, for impairing the fight against VD, and for standing as an obstacle to the effective enforcement of the still relatively new law. Even with a new totalitarian regime in place, Canon's perseverance in the fight against venereal disease and prostitution remained; she saw it as her duty to ensure the employment of women physicians in each counselling centre for women infected with VD.[85]

The founding of venereal disease clinics throughout the German Reich, like the creation of marriage counselling centres and the expansion of youth welfare, coincided with the entry of large numbers of women into the medical profession, and women doctors would come to fill this new public welfare niche. Like marriage counselling centres and the youth welfare movement, VD clinics were especially attractive to female physicians because of the structure and nature of the services they offered. Because the clinics functioned similarly to marriage counselling centres with office hours a couple of times a week, women physicians could adequately balance their professional and personal lives. Those women who desired families had time to stay at home with their children while also dedicating themselves to the welfare causes that were important to them. In addition, any woman doctor who worked in her own primary care practice or, as was often the case, with her husband, also had time to work a few hours on the side in a VD clinic. The goals of the clinics – educating patients about how to avoid spreading VD, acquiring the trust of the public and developing trusting relationships with patients, and in extreme cases, caring for patients afflicted with VD during treatment – also corresponded to the inherent qualities that women suggested they possessed from their work in the home as well as other fields in medicine. They fashioned themselves, in other words, as the dependable, nurturing, and experienced educators that these clinics and the Weimar state needed to attract the public, and especially women in the fight against VD.

Women's most important contribution to the anti-VD campaign, however, was the treatment they claimed to offer women. Doctors and feminist organizations alike never demanded the presence of female physicians for any other reason than to treat female patients. While this certainly helped the Weimar state's anti-VD movement, drawing otherwise embarrassed and reluctant women to VD clinics, and enabling women doctors to occupy new positions in medicine (particularly after the 1927 law made the availability of female doctors for female patients standard protocol), such language was also limiting. By confining their treatment to women, these doctors fulfilled the expectations of their male colleagues who maintained that women were needed in the profession only to treat other women and children. By also advocating this view (and following it in practice), women remained just where men wanted them – in subordinate, lower-paid, often part-time jobs, or in other words, in places where they could be kept under a watchful eye to prevent any threat they posed to an already vulnerable group of male physicians. Yet, without calling attention to the care and trust they could provide exclusively to women, neither female physicians nor the anti-VD campaign would have benefited. Dr Josephine Höber, for one, a member of the BDÄ's Committee for the Prevention of Venereal Disease, and her fellow members of the BDF's Committee for the Prevention of Venereal Disease, drew attention to the role of women: "only through the vigilance and active participation" of women and women's organizations (like the BDÄ) would the effective implementation of the 1927 law be possible.[86] This was true since the law asserted that in certain states, female physicians should be available for women. And although it is unknown whether more women visited venereal disease clinics after the implementation of the law, this law offered several new job opportunities for female physicians in addition to health officials, social workers, psychiatrists, and teachers.[87] Similar to the anti-VD campaign, the movement against alcoholism opened up a plethora of new opportunities for women and doctors, and women doctors, to exert their influence over how alcohol impacted marriage and family life.

Anti-Alcoholism and Its Appeal to Eugenicists, Women, and Doctors

The anti-alcohol movement became a space where eugenicists, women, and doctors could all make their specific interventions. Each group of individuals, many of whom overlapped, sought to arrogate some power through their participation. Often, they tied their efforts to improving the health and productivity of the nation, which alcoholism – a symptom of moral decline and degradation alongside VD and prostitution – threatened.[88]

The German anti-alcohol movement traced its origins to the 1880s, long before women doctors ever articulated their views about how alcoholism affected women and children. The German Anti-Alcoholism Association was founded in 1883, around the same time that the leading German anti-alcohol journal, *Auf der Wacht* (*On Guard*), began by publicizing the dangers of drinking.[89] The anti-alcohol crusade appealed to Christian moralists, who viewed it as an "evangelizing means of inculcating orderly behaviour in the masses." Led by university professors, they worked to replace Christian and moral reasoning with scientific and medical explanations for alcoholism. Members of the movement, which included psychiatrists, physicians, and medical students, continuously defined the causes and cures of alcoholism in both medical and biological terms. As Paul Weindling argues, eugenic ideas also played a strong role in the early anti-alcohol crusade: "Alcohol was perceived as a medical threat to heredity, and condemned as a cause of physical degeneration, moral depravity, crime, prostitution and a range of other pathological forms of behavior. Drunkenness resulted in seduction, VD, unwanted pregnancies and criminal abortion. Eradication of alcoholism was regarded as the means of raising productivity, enhancing emotional stability and curing a broad range of social ills."[90]

Alcoholism became further linked to a number of other social and heritable traits. "Social misery," Weindling writes, "was deemed to be the pathological product of alcohol on conception, of venereal diseases in causing sterility and congenital syphilis, and of female industrial labour resulting in the overstrain that brought on miscarriages, inability to breast feed and inherited malformations."[91] The professional community involved in the movement had become dissatisfied with solving society's problems through economic or political solutions, instead seeking biological explanations for alcoholism.

In addition to these eugenic ideas, eugenicists themselves also influenced the anti-alcohol campaign, which caused it to gain momentum by the turn of the century. Weindling discusses how the founder of the German eugenics movement, Alfred Ploetz, and other German eugenicists, Agnes Bluhm, Alfred Grotjahn, Wilhelm Schallmayer, and Ernst Rüdin, were active in the anti-alcohol crusade. They linked alcohol with hereditary illnesses and to the fitness of future generations, and championed eugenic solutions to the destructive effects alcohol produced.[92] Alcoholism – a "racial poison" according to Ploetz and Rüdin – could damage the nation's hereditary stock, but such social and racial arguments went far beyond the chief eugenicists.[93] By 1914, there were 41,000 members in 240 local abstinence or temperance groups. The national anti-alcohol league alone had 30,000 members. According to Weindling, these anti-alcohol organizations were the breeding ground for comprehensive programs of social and racial hygiene, adopting a scientific way to alleviate an inheritable disease thought to be connected to industrialization and urbanization.[94] Daniel Kevles also notes how both conservatives and progressives sought biological solutions to issues of crime, prostitution, and alcoholism – the problems of modern, industrial, urban society.[95] During the First World War, the military restricted alcohol consumption because it threatened its efficiency. In the immediate postwar years – a period marked by a decline in fertility – anti-alcoholism often became a measure of positive eugenics that could help improve the quality of future offspring and prevent "bad racial elements which cost immense sums to state and society."[96] Added medical expenditures to address the consequences of alcoholism were a concern for the suffering Weimar state. Anti-alcohol brochures during the Republic sometimes employed eugenics language. For example, the Committee for the Ban of Alcohol in Germany noted that Bavaria – the state with the highest overall alcohol consumption – had the largest number of infant and child deaths and "the most idiots born" there.[97] While claims like this were likely exaggerated to fuel the anti-alcohol cause, eugenicists' early influence on the anti-alcohol movement persisted.

Aside from eugenicists, the anti-alcohol movement, especially prohibition, became a women's concern that dominated several countries. The United States, Soviet Union, Hungary, Norway, and Finland all attempted prohibition during the war and interwar years. While Germany never implemented a policy of prohibition, reformers viewed the US as a good model and praised the anti-alcohol campaigns in other countries.[98] German anti-alcohol efforts focused instead on combating and treating alcoholism – deemed to be on the rise – rather than on limiting or banning the sale and use of alcohol.

The increase in alcohol consumption during the early Weimar Republic became particularly evident with the rising numbers of alcoholics who received treatment in hospitals, asylums, or in the newly opened municipal welfare clinics. One of the functions of welfare centres – where clinics were housed – was to identify patients for referral to a hospital, sanatorium, or asylum. The idea for these clinics grew prior to the war, but they opened mostly between 1919 and 1921. They identified alcoholic or individuals infected with VD and provided treatment for these two chronic diseases, offering a number of other services as well. By 1928, 828 such welfare offices existed.[99] Also, the welfare offices specifically for alcoholics showed a significant increase in admittances. In places like Nuremberg, the welfare office for alcoholics (Fürsorgestelle für Alkoholkranke) showed dramatic growth in the number of admittances. Some of these reported cases were also tied to criminal activity.[100] Hospitals and asylums in Bremen, Munich, and the Prussian states similarly described large increases in the number of admitted alcoholics.[101] In 1922, the Committee for Banning Alcohol in Germany (Ausschuß für das Alkoholverbot in Deutschland) estimated that nearly 50 per cent of mental illnesses, 84 per cent of sex crimes, 65 per cent of felonies, and 75 per cent of misdemeanours could be linked to alcohol.[102] Excessive drinking registered significant impacts on society's productivity because alcohol caused inefficient work habits, unemployment, and early death. Alcohol impaired judgment and morality, thus resulting in high rates of crime and mental illness.[103] Similar to how authorities, policymakers, and individuals in health-related fields perceived VD and prostitution to be a grave concern, they saw this rising alcoholism as problematic, especially because of its impact on marriage and family life. This is precisely why abstinence became a women's issue in the 1920s.

By 1933, sixteen different women's groups were engaged in the anti-alcohol campaign, a number that only grew after the Nazis came to power because it fit with their push towards a more "natural" way of living which they thought augmented military prowess.[104] While women were sometimes excluded from participating in the central decision-making organizations, their involvement in women's organizations could be empowering because they could utilize their positions within the home to make a difference in their husband's and children's lives.[105] However, the anti-alcoholism campaign was also burdensome for women, who were encouraged to make their homes more welcoming for alcohol-prone husbands, to prepare healthy meals and beverages, and to create an alcohol-free culture for their children.[106]

One of these groups, the Deutscher Frauenbund für alkoholfreie Kultur (German Women's League for an Alcohol-Free Culture), founded in 1900, was central to the role that women played in the effort to eliminate alcoholism in German society. On several occasions, it petitioned the Reich Ministry of the Interior for financial support, noting that anti-alcoholism required women's "altruistic, voluntary devotion" for this "specific female [task]."[107] The League also published organizational literature and brochures that showcased alcohol as a woman's matter, aiming to attract a coalition of women and mothers who recognized the dangers that alcohol posed to the *Volk* and who could empathize with the plight of the wives and children of alcoholics. In one advertisement, the League stressed alcohol's connections to domestic strife and illness.[108] Family life, after all, was destroyed when men spent the family income at the tavern, as women and children often went hungry. The use of important nutrients in the brewing and distillation of alcohol deprived women and children; thus, the League presented fighting alcohol as a "woman's business." It noted that the increase in immorality and venereal disease – for which alcohol bore the biggest blame – hit women the hardest because they were infected with VD once their drunk husbands came home after visiting a prostitute. Women also endured the burden of caring for "crippled" and "mentally deficient" children produced as a result of the father's alcoholism.[109] This eugenics language, characteristic of the German anti-alcohol movement, appeared in League advertisements that linked alcohol consumption to a number of other social problems including criminality and poverty.[110]

The Women's League for an Alcohol-Free Culture is one example of the panoply of organizations, government institutions, and individuals, both in Germany and elsewhere, that marketed the anti-alcohol campaign as a women's concern and subsequently reached out to women. Comprehensive alcoholic care and education, they claimed, required the types of skills that women had already developed in the home – those which some individuals thought men could not achieve.[111] Others recognized that women were sensitive and empathetic and were already accountable for the maintenance of family life and the moral upbringing of children in the domestic realm, where they could encourage anti-alcohol measures.[112] This sort of work, then, could be extended to the public sphere through household visits or participation in a community association, charitable organization, or an alcoholic welfare clinic. Caring for alcoholics also meant more than just caring for the individuals themselves; it emphasized attention to families, especially providing women and children with protection against abuse.[113] Even male doctors thought women were absolutely necessary for employment in alcoholic welfare centres because "feminine forces often [had] a particularly good instinct and [understood] it quite well to handle alcoholics or the wives of alcoholics."[114] This rhetoric suggested that women were involved in the fight against alcoholism because it affected the domestic sphere, but also because the instinctual social understanding they developed at home prepared them to serve as ideal advocates.

Just as women's organizations used discourse to suggest their leading role in the struggle against alcoholism, so too did doctors. For one, doctors had been medically trained and licensed, and alcoholism was, in fact, a *medical* problem.[115] Alcohol harmed the body, and thus it was the duty of doctors to be on hand for treatment and advice. Specifically, it was the duty of the doctor to give guidance about possible nerve or organ damage caused by alcohol. Doctors were needed for medical counsel in the selection of cases where alcoholism was the symptom of a serious disease like mental illness or epilepsy.[116] Therapy for alcoholism also demanded consistent intervention from doctors. As one medical counsellor explained, an alcoholic was in principle a sick person and therefore the object of medical custody and handling.[117]

Doctors, medical organizations, and medical journals used language to suggest that they were the most suitable individuals to spearhead the anti-alcohol movement, claiming they understood the health and social consequences of alcohol. The Freiburg Doctors' Association (Verein Freiburger Ärzte) believed that they "as doctors saw first and foremost the health damages caused by the abuse of alcohol," but that they were "also able to follow the disruptive moral and economic consequences, especially within the family."[118] Doctors in the *Aerztliches Vereinsblatt für Deutschland* (*Medical Association Journal for Germany*) subscribed to the view that physicians should not only be advisers at alcoholic welfare centres, but head them. After all, it was in their professional interests to do so.[119] Historically, lay practitioners had treated chronic diseases like alcoholism and VD through hypnosis, but the medical profession slowly joined politicians and police authorities throughout the first decades of the twentieth century to keep lay practitioners under control.[120] Moreover, in the postwar period, the overwhelming number of physicians (with male practitioners returning from war and women entering medicine at higher numbers than ever before), combined with the shortage of positions in the economic downturn, created an atmosphere of rigorous competition – another incentive to eliminate the rivalry stemming from lay practitioners in the anti-alcohol movement. Other medical journals – *Münchener Medizinische Wochenschrift* (*Munich Medical Weekly*) as well as *Deutsches Ärzteblatt* (*German Medical Journal*) – similarly advocated for doctors to take a leading role in the campaign against alcohol consumption, especially through anti-alcohol organizations. Dr Max Fischer suggested to his colleagues the advantages of joining a large association dedicated to the fight against alcohol, namely their public health presence through articles, events, or lectures. He thought every doctor should belong to an anti-alcohol organization, whether it advocated temperance or pressed for full abstinence. This type of involvement illustrated a fulfilment of their medical-ethical duties as the "natural trustees of the people's health."[121] The Freiburg Doctors' Association also agreed that as the "guardians of health," doctors could not let the misuse of alcohol continue to go unnoticed.[122] Using such authoritative labels, as well as rhetoric that emphasized their medical and social expertise, physicians sought to endorse their powerful position within the anti-alcohol campaign.

The Anti-Alcohol Campaign: A Fitting Place for Female Physicians

Both women and doctors suggested how suitable they were to take up the anti-alcohol campaign. Fittingly, female physicians fashioned themselves as the ideal candidates to become engaged in the anti-alcohol movement because they possessed both unique nurturing qualities as women as well as a strong scientific background, which meant they could provide support to alcoholics and their families and keep them all informed of genetic or medical problems. Women doctors were not working in the campaign against alcohol in extraordinary numbers, instead devoting much more of their time (and publications in *Die Ärztin*) to marriage counselling, school health care, the new Law for Combating Venereal Disease, and abortion.[123] The few physicians involved adopted maternalist rhetoric, focusing on the ways in which alcohol influenced women, children, and the family, thus limiting their professional expertise to domestic matters.

After founding their professional organization and journal, female doctors claimed early on that they could offer something special to the anti-alcohol crusade. Their male colleagues agreed. In its first year of publication, an article in *Die Ärztin*, "The Female Physician and the Alcohol Question," endorsed the medical profession as the best vocation for knowing how to prevent and address dangers like venereal disease and alcoholism that threatened the *Volk*. The author, physiologist Emil Abderhalden, specifically lauded women within this field: "much deeper than the doctor, often the female doctor grasps the enormous damages which venereal disease, alcoholism, and so on bring to the family and how they affect many generations."[124] Women physicians, according to Abderhalden, were the most suitable for this type of work because they personally felt the impact of alcohol on children and families; not only did female doctors see the troubles drunken men caused to their primarily women patients, but they may have even experienced such misfortune themselves. Women physicians treated desperate pregnant women all the time, observing their powerlessness to abstain from sex with their alcoholic husbands or to encourage their husbands to use contraception. Historian Atina Grossmann suggests that their sympathy for women led to female doctors' widespread support of legal and easily accessible contraception, abortion, and sterilization.[125] Women physicians' struggle against alcoholism was intimately linked to their other advocacy programs, such as their insistence that birth control be distributed in sex and marriage counselling centres, their demands for Paragraph 218 to be overturned, and even their calls for the sterilization of asocial elements of the working class.[126]

In addition to extolling the merits of women doctors working in the anti-alcohol movement, Abderhalden also questioned their lack of participation in anti-alcohol organizations. In total, only some 400 male doctors and 12 to 15 female doctors were involved in anti-alcoholism – shameful in comparison to his native Switzerland, a country with as many residents as the city of Berlin, which already had 150 male and female doctors working in the anti-alcohol campaign. In fact, although the alcohol problem had become more severe, he suggested that female medical students and doctors were no longer abstaining from alcohol and cooperating in the struggle against alcoholism as they had in the past.[127] According to Abderhalden, there were undoubtedly more women doctors who drank than those who were members of the Association of Abstaining Physicians (Verein abstinenter Ärzte), even though experience had shown that this organization boasted a considerable amount of power due to its large member base. Individual efforts in the crusade against alcohol, he claimed, had very little influence, which was why he recommended that each one of his colleagues – male and female – join the association. With more members, the Association of Abstaining Physicians would be better equipped to implement alcohol-free youth education, expand alcoholic welfare, create tasty, alcohol-free drinks, and support more extensive research on the effects of alcohol.[128]

Male voices like Abderhalden's likely held significant credence and were included in *Die Ärztin* because of the fervent cooperation he asked of women. While encouraging members to join organizations dedicated to the fight against alcohol, the BDÄ also condemned female colleagues who advocated alcohol for medicinal purposes. Dr Grete Schüler-Helbing, a long-established specialist in orthopedic rehabilitation in Berlin, published an article entitled "Woman and Alcohol," in which she recommended between a half litre and a litre of strong beer for sleep and wine, cognac, or liquor to cure a depressed mood or to give one temporary confidence. In this first ever public recommendation for the use of alcohol by a woman, Schüler-Helbing maintained that alcohol in small doses was not a poison but in fact was quite beneficial. The BDÄ responded to Schüler-Helbing by publishing a scathing criticism of her article in *Die Ärztin*, indicating the clear stance of the organization on matters of alcohol. Dr Else Liefmann, the co-chair and later the chair of the BDÄ's Committee to Combat Alcohol (Ausschuß zur Bekämpfung des Alkohols), found it "almost grotesque" that a female doctor could support the consumption of alcohol.[129] Up until Schüler-Helbing's endorsement, only men had defended alcohol consumption because, according to Liefmann, women were the ones who had suffered from alcohol abuse, as had their children and their orderly family lives. Liefmann disparaged Schüler-Helbing for neglecting the fact that her endorsement of drinking, even if it was only one glass of wine to help ease pain, could result in overindulgence or create a drinking habit. Liefmann further disapproved of Schüler-Helbing's recommendation to new mothers to consume only low dosages of alcohol. Schüler-Helbing was clearly unaware that alcohol passed to the milk of nursing mothers, which was by no means healthy for infants. Lastly, Liefmann admonished Schüler-Helbing for ignoring the links between alcohol consumption and venereal disease, and especially the vulnerability of adolescents to both.[130]

Through her critique, Liefmann revealed first and foremost a maternalist disposition characteristic of the few women doctors involved in anti-alcoholism. By mentioning the destruction alcohol and venereal disease had on youth, Liefmann demonstrated that alcoholism became an issue for her especially when youth were concerned. Helping youth avoid the enticement of alcohol was the type of work that Liefmann and other female physicians sought to achieve within the anti-alcohol crusade, indicated by the fact that alcohol-free youth education became a primary objective of the anti-alcohol organizations they joined.[131] Liefmann also showcased her expertise on the ways alcohol affected nursing mothers and infants, thus exhibiting the way she and others claimed to influence the anti-alcohol movement.

Similarly, Dr Agnes Bluhm – one of the early eugenicists involved in the anti-alcohol movement – spoke on the influences of alcohol consumption on expectant and nursing mothers at the Second German Congress for Alcohol-Free Youth Education, held 21–25 May 1922 in Berlin. At the Congress, fifty youth associations with approximately 2.5 million members presented a resolution that called for sharp anti-alcohol provisions.[132] A large number of young people spoke at this event, but Bluhm's lecture highlighted her belief that alcohol-free youth education had to begin in the womb, at the moment a woman became conscious of her pregnancy. Thus, she said it was necessary to dispense advice to expectant mothers, who Bluhm stressed should abstain from any alcohol consumption because mothers transferred a large percentage of the alcohol they drank to their offspring in the womb. Nursing mothers also passed alcohol to infants through their milk, leading Bluhm to call for these mothers to avoid all alcoholic beverages.[133] Bluhm, like Leifmann, focused her attention within the anti-alcohol campaign on helping women and children. Although Bluhm was engaged with other academics in the anti-alcohol movement, primarily in Zurich, she displayed her most prominent participation in congresses like this one (focused on youth) and focused her work in anti-alcoholism to women's issues, such as breastfeeding. In this way, Liefmann, Bluhm, and other women physicians remained tied to a medical track in which they evoked their female identity to make claims about their ability to serve women and children.

Beyond their maternal tendencies, the efforts of Liefmann, Bluhm, and their colleagues within the anti-alcohol movement also exhibited their class-biased eugenic leanings. In addition to supporting a campaign that eugenicists had pioneered since its very founding, some female doctors were also quite explicit in their views that alcoholism was a destructive heritable trait that needed to be eliminated from the population. *Die Ärztin* reported in 1932 that the controversy over whether alcohol could damage one's genetic make-up had been resolved through the work of Agnes Bluhm. In a 1930 experimental study on alcohol and offspring, Bluhm had determined that alcohol was capable of causing genetic changes – knowledge that she did not think was required to justify a fervent battle against alcoholism. In her opinion, the severe social and moral costs of alcohol misuse were enough to fully rationalize a strong movement against alcohol consumption.[134] Bluhm defended the fight against alcoholism in light of the overwhelming amount of social (and what some considered moral) problems – poverty, crime, venereal disease, prostitution, abuse, and overpopulation among the poor – that could be associated with it.[135] Such widespread alcoholism could cause damage to a group that Bluhm called "civilized people," a matter of concern because of the overwhelming number of "inferior" elements who eugenicists believed were taking over the struggle for existence.[136] Bluhm was certainly trying to protect particular members of the population – namely, the upper classes – from the harms of alcohol that were spreading among the underclasses and social deviants.

Liefmann also understood that there were "weaklings" (*Schwache*) among the *Volk* – something she, in fact, had criticized Schüler-Helbing for neglecting. By promoting the use of alcohol, Schüler-Helbing had ignored "a social hygienic sense of responsibility" and tempted these "weaklings," only compounding the problems of impoverished or diseased individuals (already considered part of this "weakling" category).[137] Liefmann proclaimed to understand the consequences alcohol had on destitute individuals and supported a eugenic view that prevented the further spread of alcoholism among these "weaklings."

Like their colleagues in the youth welfare movement, certain female physicians also pinpointed alcohol as the root of other social ills. Helenefriederike Stelzner, a school doctor and practising physician in Berlin who grappled with school health care from what she called a "sociomedical-psychiatric" view, concluded in a 1929 study that in families of female welfare pupils, more than 50 per cent of their fathers were alcoholics.[138] Her study joined others by male physicians that confirmed the relationship between alcoholic parents and youth welfare or youth criminality.[139] Hertha Riese, the medical leader of the Bund für Mutterschutz's sexual counselling centre in Frankfurt, also noted a connection between alcoholic parents and the destitution of children. She found that of all advice seekers from the sexual counselling centre, alcoholic women had the highest average number of children, with 5.4 live births, and the highest average number of abortions with 1.6 (out of an average of 7 pregnancies for each of these women). Furthermore, Riese reported that the health conditions of those children conceived under intoxication were even worse than those in socially damaged families. Lastly, she stated that the mortality rate of the children of drinkers surpassed that of all other groups.[140] The research of Stelzner and Riese within anti-alcoholism not only displayed female doctors' continued attention to alcohol's impact on children, but it also illustrated that they were no strangers to the idea – present throughout the larger anti-alcohol movement – that alcoholism only compounded other social problems considered to be heritable (like poverty and crime) and was becoming a greater burden on society, and thus needed to be eradicated.

Because women doctors treated many lower-class women and children in their other work spaces – municipal marriage counselling centres and vocational schools – they learned first-hand that alcoholism only exacerbated the suffering these individuals often faced. Many of these women and children were already susceptible to conditions like criminality, poverty, venereal disease, and overpopulation, and alcohol consumption only augmented their difficulties. It was precisely these alcohol-caused social (and genetic) problems that affected their patients and students, as well as the mental disorders believed to emerge as a direct result of alcoholism, that led these female physicians to take up the anti-alcohol cause and to side with a eugenically founded movement that called for alcohol's elimination from the gene pool. Women doctors like Bluhm, Liefmann, Stelzner, and Riese especially wanted to protect the upper classes from the perils of alcohol, and worked to prevent the further destruction of alcoholism among the lower classes. More to the point, in the few articles that *Die Ärztin* did incorporate regarding the work female physicians were doing in the anti-alcohol movement, the topics primarily revolved around youth or women, reflecting the areas in which its reader base was both interested and involved.

Conclusions

Alcoholism, prostitution, and venereal disease affected women, children, and the home, which was the reason women doctors initially intervened, but female physicians also used maternal rhetoric to underline the upheaval these vices and diseases caused to women's lives and domestic spaces and to carve out a professional domain. They centred their concerns in the anti-alcohol campaign around how alcohol affected the families of alcoholic men and nursing mothers. They directed their efforts in the anti-VD movement at fighting the injustices against women in state-regulated prostitution and at demanding equal access and treatment for women in VD counselling centres. They promised to offer women seeking VD treatment a trustworthy confidante.

Perhaps one of the most remarkable things about female physicians' commitment to these fields was the way in which, in addition to heralding their specialty in women's health, they also presented themselves as political advocates for women. Dr Kaufmann-Wolf, for one, claimed that her natural, womanly instincts motivated and enabled women's participation in the fight against state-regulated prostitution and VD.[141] Her colleagues, too, advocated that discrimination against women in VD counselling centres be overturned by employing a strategy that focused on women's inherent differences, which they thought granted them the basic right to be examined by doctors of their same sex. The tactics of women doctors in the anti-VD campaign combined the notion that the female body was different, and thus merited special treatment, with the suggestion that all bodies (male or female) be considered equal under the law. Their language about bodies and an innate womanliness opened up a new discursive space for them to make political demands. No longer were these doctors debating venereal disease as a purely medical topic; VD became a political space for them as well, as conversations now turned towards fundamental rights and equality.

Simultaneous with their calls for the equal treatment of female bodies, female physicians participated in the management and regulation of women's bodies and sexual behaviour characteristic of an expanded Weimar welfare state. This control of individual bodies in the name of the national body (or what the Germans called the *Volkskörper*) – biopolitics – was characteristic of Weimar Germany.[142] The passage of the 1927 law particularly amplified the power of the medical profession to control their patients, especially because authority was now in the hands of practitioners and health departments rather than the morals police.[143] While this made them more vital to the Weimar state, it also meant that their professional (read: class) privilege lent them the ability to advance in their medical and political careers at the expense of lower-class women, who were susceptible to prostitution and therefore VD and primarily targeted by this new law.

Female physicians were not alone in their belief that VD, prostitution, and alcoholism plagued the lower classes. Of particular concern, however, were the fears among some female doctors that venereal disease and prostitution were spreading to parts of the so-called "respectable society" due to the economic circumstances of the time.

Dr Oelze-Rheinboldt, for example, became concerned that the "staggering infections" of VD in the masses were now drifting into all classes.[144] Dr de Lemos asserted that middle-class women now turned to prostitution to support themselves during a time of badly paid female work.[145] Partaking in these campaigns also meant attempting to prevent the spread of veneral diseases to the upper classes and adding to the further degeneration of German society.

Female physicians had already become political advocates for themselves with the formation of a professional organization and accompanying journal and through their various efforts to include more women and enhance their status within the medical profession. In addition, they claimed to be political activists for their primarily female and youth patients, focusing on political issues such as gaining women access to birth control in marriage counselling centres, equalizing school health care programs for young girls, fighting the double standard in the 1927 law, and calling for equal treatment for women in VD counselling centres. After 1933, the female medical profession would take a much more political stance.

4 Building the *Volksgemeinschaft* and Supporting Racial Hygiene in the Bund Deutscher Mädel and Reichsmütterdienst

In a 1937 article in *Die Ärztin*, Emmi Drexel, a school doctor in Berlin, lauded the opportunities that National Socialism offered to her and her colleagues. She said they would be able to contribute to national education, publicize racial political requirements, and indoctrinate hesitant mothers to support Nazi ideas about health. While she appreciated that the Weimar Republic was certainly committed to promoting large families and a distinct German nationalism, she praised National Socialism for making the "spiritual recovery of the *Volk*" a national goal and one of the most important duties of German doctors like herself.[1] Drexel exemplified the number of women who gained new health and population policy positions under the Nazi umbrella of ideals like the *Volksgesundheit* (people's health). The Nazi Party offered supporters like Drexel a myriad of opportunities for employment, education, funding, and to both create and feel a part of Hitler's *Volksgemeinschaft* or people's community.[2]

The Nationalsozialistische Deutsche Arbeiterpartei (National Socialist German Workers' Party; NSDAP) had already received especially strong support from traditional professionals, such as lawyers and civil servants, who became disillusioned with the Weimar Republic as the crises of overcrowding, inflation, status loss, and organizational competition within their various occupations grew. Doctors were no exception to this rule and in fact were among some of the strongest supporters of the Nazi Party before 1933.[3] More than half of women physicians also became affiliated with Nazism.[4] Many female doctors like Drexel saw the appeal of Nazism, as it presented them a number of new opportunities. In fact, this chapter demonstrates that Drexel and other non-Jewish female physicians who continued their professional work under Nazism were resourceful as they recognized the ways in which they could best serve the regime. Despite their expulsion from the elite health insurance practices, they continued their work for women and children in the Bund Deutscher Mädel (League of German Girls; BDM), teaching and enlightening young girls, and for the Reichsmütterdienst (Reich Mothers' Service; RMD), educating mothers. Women doctors also claimed to be valuable to the regime's racial hygiene agenda because of the authority they commanded with their women patients, particularly their abilities to promote pro-natalism by awakening women's inner desires for children.[5]

This chapter explains the allure of National Socialism for non-Jewish female physicians. About one-third of female physicians, either by choice or coercion, left Germany or were forced out of the profession and purged from the BDÄ after 1933.[6] This chapter highlights the activities of those female doctors who continued their professional activity in Nazi Germany. Despite the regime change, I argue that women doctors continued to perform similar types of work that they did in the Weimar Republic, championing themselves as experts in women's and children's health through their employment in the BDM and the RMD. They maintained that they could create and enhance the *Volksgemeinschaft* by preparing young girls in the BDM to be the healthy, responsible members of the future generation and by moulding mothers in the RMD to be more health conscious. While they continued to promote women's and children's health, their rhetoric took on a far different meaning than it had during the democratic Weimar era because it emphasized the goals of the party and the state alongside the needs of their patients. Medicine became tailored to fulfilling the ideological goals of the Nazi state, which consciously used women doctors to indoctrinate women and children to its exclusionary, racial health policies. In addition to carving a niche for themselves in Nazi medicine by proclaiming a particular "feminine" expertise for the health of approximately one-half of the *Volksgemeinschaft*, female physicians also participated in racial hygiene training at Alt-Rehse, the doctors' training school for racial hygiene matters during the Third Reich. Women doctors, who reported favourably about their experiences at the racial hygiene educational camp at Alt-Rehse, then translated this training into practical application either in the BDM or onto the pages of *Die Ärztin*, where they discussed the special role they would play in achieving the racial hygiene goals of the Nazi state.[7]

Female physicians who remained involved with the BDÄ upheld the aims of a repressive dictatorship. In emphasizing the unique "doctor-mother" roles they could play, they situated their professional work within the paradigm of the feminine-doctor duties of the new state, which included protecting mothers and their children and educating and indoctrinating German women to be responsible comrades.[8] On the one hand, this can be viewed as an honest attempt to make room for themselves in an overcrowded, unreceptive, and, at times, hostile profession. Even if their rhetoric proved somewhat hollow after the Second World War started, when women were needed in the medical profession, it is well documented that in the early 1930s, the Nazis sought to keep women out of universities and certain professions and initially upheld laws that discriminated against married women doctors whose husbands already had adequate income. And yet on the other hand, this raises questions about women doctors' complicity, as they fought so determinedly to work for the National Socialist state. Historians Johanna Bleker and Christine Eckelmann contend that creating this concept of the "doctor-mother" in the new state was a defence strategy of female doctors, who were battling an antagonistic medical profession.[9] While this was certainly true, these female physicians were opportunists. They recognized openings in women's and children's health available to them under the Nazi state, and they were well prepared to assume these jobs because their work in the Weimar era had groomed them for similar activities in the Nazi period.

Coordination of the BDÄ

In the first few weeks after Hitler came to power, there was no immediate sign of change for the BDÄ or the lives of women doctors. In 1933, the organization had over 900 members, which was nearly one-fourth of all practising female physicians in the Reich (4,367 women out of a total of 51,067 physicians in Germany).[10] Of these, 572 identified themselves as "non-Aryan."[11] Whether "non-Aryan" in this case equated to "Jewish" is unclear, but what is clear is that the number of Jewish female physicians was not insignificant, especially in cities; they made up perhaps as high as one-third of female physicians in the BDÄ.[12]

When Hitler took power, he initiated a *Gleichschaltung* or coordination of all social and political institutions in Germany to bring them under Nazi control. This process was carried out in the spring and summer of 1933 and affected all political parties, state governments, bureaucracies, trade unions, and organizations, including the BDÄ. Many of the changes that happened during the *Gleichschaltung* and much early persecution of Jews in the Nazi regime happened through announcement;

the BDÄ's early reports in May and June of 1933 follow this trend. *Die Ärztin* first reported on changes within the organization in May 1933. In light of the political changes, individual local chapters requested a board meeting, which took place 2 April 1933. At this meeting, the board and editorial management resigned and provisional leaders were announced to replace them. The coordination of the BDÄ was completed two weeks later.[13] Bleker and Eckelmann view this initial action as one of obedience that allowed the BDÄ to continue its existence.[14] The board and editorial leadership quickly adhered to Nazi policies, but so too did individual chapters of the BDÄ. Hertha Nathorff, a Jewish doctor who was then working in a family and marriage counselling centre in Berlin, reflected on the transition taking place under Nazism in her diary. On 2 February 1933, she noted the first derogatory comments about Jews during her office hours, and on 16 April 1933, she reported on what happened when she attended a regular chapter meeting of the BDÄ. Although attending these meetings was a familiar practice to Nathorff, on this particular day she perceived a "strange atmosphere" and did not recognize many of the unfamiliar faces. After a man explained that the *Gleichschaltung* – an alien word to Nathorff and her colleagues – was required of the BDÄ, all Jewish doctors were asked to leave the meeting. Nathorff then described how all-Jewish and so-called half-Jewish doctors, and some "German" doctors silently stood and left the room, "pale, shocked to the core." She expressed how "agitated, sad, and broken-hearted" she was, as well as the shame she felt for her "German" colleagues.[15] Nathorff appears to be both confused and disturbed by the announcement at this meeting, and reacted accordingly, not knowing what to do at the time and then later reflecting on it in her journal, where she shows genuine emotion about what it felt like to be asked to leave. Her municipal counselling centre would later be closed down and she would eventually emigrate to New York.

The coordination progressed quite rapidly thereafter. Information, once again, came through announcement in the journal, namely in a June 1933 article that the new editors likely published in order to summarize the multiple "Events" that had happened over the last couple of months. In a 10 May 1933 meeting of the BDÄ, Dr Gerhard Wagner, already the Reich Physicians' Leader (*Reichsärzteführer*), appointed Dr Lea Thimm the provisional leader of the association. In addition, Thimm would take over the editorial staff of the *Die Ärztin*, which reported that these steps were necessary in light of the "threatening danger" of the association, whose existence now depended on the government.[16]

Already, the rhetoric of a newly Nazified editorial leadership was apparent. Moreover, the individual local chapters were required to make the following changes:

1. All local leaders of Jewish descent had to resign, but their membership and cooperation were not affected as long as they were "objectively scientifically acceptable" and did not allude to "organizational and ideological questions."
2. All local leaders of non-Jewish descent had to agree to the *Gleich-schaltung* "without conflict," and if they did not, they would have to temporarily step down from office until their desire for cooperation had been observed.
3. Local leaders not affected by measures 1 and 2 should send in a short report about the atmosphere of the local chapters and indicate the ratio of Jewish to German colleagues.

The subsequent member meeting in Hamburg was also cancelled because of the short amount of time Thimm had to prepare for it, but she assured members that she would arrange a new meeting time and place as soon as the necessary contacts and cooperation with various local chapters was under way.[17] Thimm was likely scrambling to keep pace with the rapid changes taking place.

Although there were some early indications (above) of allowing Jews to remain members of the BDÄ, the organization became officially closed to German-Jewish members at the end of June. After this, the organization abandoned its former non-alignment. In its founding, the BDÄ had proclaimed political neutrality and the majority of members avoided politics, at least in theory.[18] In the BDÄ's affiliation with the International Medical Women's Association, there were to be no political questions addressed at their annual congresses, as indicated in an early summons. Rather, these congresses were simply a time to exchange experiences in the field of social hygiene.[19] The BDÄ had been founded with a social hygiene agenda in mind; the original duties of the association included the "handling of social-hygiene questions from the standpoint of a doctor as a woman."[20] This implied control over social and health policy decisions, which female doctors clearly abided by through their involvement in marriage counselling, girls' physical education reform, and the campaigns against alcohol, venereal disease, and prostitution. By demanding that the state take control over people's fitness for marriage, the BDÄ was certainly fulfilling the social hygiene objectives it sought to embody. After 1933, however, the organization abandoned the social hygiene responsibilities in the statutes and the new leadership deleted the clauses about political and religious neutrality from the 1924 bylaws.[21] And although Nathorff recalled that some "German" colleagues walked out with her and her Jewish colleagues in April 1933, only one non-Jewish German doctor publicly quit the BDÄ.[22]

In June 1933, the editorial staff of *Die Ärztin* reported that the "coordination can be labelled as a sweeping success." By that time, twenty-one of the twenty-six local chapters had "declared their full willingness to work further under the changed political circumstances and in accordance with the spirit of the new age."[23] Two chapter leaders even resigned without having yet received notification of the new regulations. With the exception of three local chapters, all had complied by sending information about the attitudes of their members. These letters reflected "a fresh and hopeful spirit," and the editors declared that the overall depression that had been weighing on Germany since the beginning of the year "appeared to give way to new life and new hope" in the BDÄ.[24] Although these early editorial reports suggest a successful *Gleichschaltung* of the organization, I use them judiciously because the BDÄ was rapidly changing its political stance and becoming more and more Nazified.

The reports do allow a glimpse into how individual members were adapting to the political transition. The editors showcased Dr Maria Monheim's report from the Munich chapter of the BDÄ. The editors, quicker to become politicized, viewed her report as exemplary of the spirited attitude of the BDÄ. However, she exhibited some uncertainty about and distance from the new regime and attempted to highlight the ways the change might benefit the nationalist sentiments of members. She claimed reluctance to participate in politics in the past due to her feminine disposition and the overall apolitical attitude of the BDÄ. Monheim asserted that she and her colleagues were "always neutral" unless they were occupied "with questions that corresponded to our feminine-medical interest or to which we as women had something particular to say." She recognized how members might benefit from the regime's recognition of the BDÄ, expressing hope that women would now be able to work with the state to craft policy. She described a "strong sense of community" among members of the BDÄ resulting from their shared material plight, suggesting that she recognized how difficult it was for women to achieve status in the medical profession.

Monheim defended the obvious "national" feelings of her chapter's members as well as their ability to socially adjust their medical activity and professional ethical views in light of the regime change. Rather than exhibiting extreme nationalism, she initially appeared detached from the new regime and also apologetic about the anti-Semitism of her chapter, emphasizing the nature of Bavarians as "more down to earth, closer to nature," and therefore, as also "more race-conscious," which led to the successful purge of Jews from her local chapter, leaving only three or four remaining out of forty members.[25]

Monheim's changing disposition was emblematic of many non-Jewish German members of the BDÄ in 1933. She had been educated under the old system, distinguished as part of the first generation of practising female physicians in Germany. After attending medical school in Munich, she received her licence in 1912 and then embarked upon her long career as an assistant and subsequently a practising physician. Like many of her peers, she worked in a pregnancy clinic and then eventually as a gynecologist. And she, along with many colleagues, joined the BDÄ in 1927, but remained apolitical and admittedly only pursued interests that involved women and children and the family.[26]

It was not until 1933 with the coordination of the BDÄ that Monheim slowly began to articulate her political voice, often with the encouragement of higher-ups in the organization. While she had initially been hesitant to join a political party, she attested to her hope that she and other women could become participating members of the state. And even though she still sought to protect the interests and opinions of her chapter's members, cautious to reveal too much about the atmosphere of the group in her report, she assured Thimm and the other editors of the Munich chapter's willingness to serve the *Volk* and "to do their duty with the use of all force."[27] Monheim was clearly an opportunist, which is likely why she was willing to adopt the regime's racial policies despite her own feelings about purging Jewish members of her chapter or the tensions this may have caused. She encouraged the BDÄ as a whole to abandon its political neutrality and discard any reservations about Hitler, who had since acknowledged all their previous concerns about the position of women and mothers in the new state. Monheim assured the BDÄ that while Nazism purportedly restricted women to reproductive roles, the new regime offered women doctors an unprecedented opportunity to cooperate in the promising work of reorganizing the care of women, mothers, and the family.[28] Monheim became even more politicized after 1933, first by proposing that certain colleagues serve on the BDÄ's board (among them herself) and then by becoming a member of the National Socialist Women's Organization (NS-Frauenschaft).

Monheim was not alone in her support of Nazism. Ilse Szagunn, who had also been a part of the first generation of women physicians in Germany and seasoned in clinical and educational medicine, experienced few professional changes with the rise of National Socialism. Under the new regime, she continued her advocacy for children's medicine and pregnancy care, a bulwark of population politics and racial hygiene.[29] Szagunn typified women doctors who blurred social hygiene and racial hygiene – categories that were not wholly defined at the time and that were not necessarily mutually exclusive. Szagunn defined social hygiene broadly, and her life's work demonstrates that she fused her professional ambitions with social needs by promoting marriage and large families and making the welfare of the German *Volk* a primary concern in her public health efforts.[30] Her early interest in social hygiene was inspired by her work with Adolf Gottstein, a practising physician and one of the founders of social hygiene as a discipline. She first worked as a part-time school doctor at the girl's vocational school in Charlottenburg, where she was responsible for 3,000 students.[31] She saw the state's "preservation and support of motherhood" as fundamental, and she thought health curriculum should include sex education, professional health advising, and marriage counselling, and noted that some of her own landmark work included teaching women that they had a greater societal responsibility when it came to sex.[32]

Although she was fired from her job as a vocational school doctor in 1932 because of the *Doppelverdiener* (double-earner) law, Szagunn continued her work, at last on a voluntary basis, in the Friedenau marriage counselling centre well into the Nazi regime.[33] While numerous marriage and sex counselling centres closed during the Nazi period or had to shut down for financial reasons, Szagunn's clinic continued to exist, as Protestant marriage counsellors found opportunity in cooperating with the new state. Szagunn's spiritual counselling, which complied with Nazi ideology, promoted the preservation of marriage to visitors and underscored for them the importance of sexual duty to the German nation. She even insisted that Protestant marriage counsellors familiarize themselves with Nazi laws concerning racially or confessionally mixed marriages.[34] Szagunn posed no threat to the regime, and her earlier ideas about marriage and family mirrored Nazi politics, making it easier for her and her clinic to exist in the Nazi state. After 1933, Nazi

policy demanded that conservative marriage counselling centres provide advice on the sterilization of people labelled "inferior."[35]

Szagunn, unlike Monheim, had been quite political before 1933. Her
activism can be traced to her first semester of medical school, where she
founded the Berlin chapter of the German Academic Women's League
(Deutsch-Akademischer Frauenbund), an anti-Semitic organization
with very nationalist overtones that sought to educate women about
their responsibilities to their country. Women even had to be of German heritage and speak the German language to join, which ultimately
excluded about 40 per cent of the medical students at the time because
they were of Russian descent.[36] This anti-Semitic women's group had
enough university branches to form a national organization, the German Association of Academic Women's Organizations (Deutscher Verband Akademischer Frauenvereine), in 1914. In an effort to cultivate
Deutschtum (Germanness) among the female student population, the
organization banned Jews.[37] Szagunn's nationalist and anti-Semitic
leanings likely hardened from her participation in this organization
and would make it easier for her to embrace Nazism later. At the time,
her work with this organization was instrumental in creating a more
hospitable medical school environment to a group of female students
immediately after they were first admitted. Szagunn campaigned for
the establishment of female student housing and fought the ongoing injustices against women medical students. Szagunn carried this
political disposition into her career. She served as the Charlottenburg
district health deputy for the German People's Party (Deutsche Volkspartei; DVP) from 1925 to 1928, as well as the Berlin central health
deputy for the DVP – a centre-right party from which the Nazis would
eventually gain many of their supporters. As a member of the Prussian Health Council (Preußischer Landesgesundheitsrat) from 1921 to
1933, Szagunn was a member of the Committee for School Health Care
(Ausschuß für Schulgesundheitspflege) and the Committee for Population Politics and Racial Hygiene (Ausschuß für Bevölkerungspolitik
und Rassenhygiene). Through these committees, she participated in a
discussion about eugenics-based abortion and sterilization laws, which
would have, as she claimed, served the *Volkswohlfahrt* (welfare of the
people). Moreover, she embraced the eugenic leanings of the Health
Council, which made the eugenic education of youth a priority and supported the voluntary exchange of marriage health certificates. While
the Health Council condemned the death of unworthy lives and doctors who conducted voluntary sterilization for research, it promoted

housing developments for "genetically healthy families as a positive population measure."[38] Szagunn was well immersed in so-called positive eugenics before 1933.

When the Health Council dissolved in 1933, Szagunn made a smooth transition to the Nazi political sphere. Her earlier experience in an organization that purged Jews likely made the *Gleichschaltung* of the BDÄ familiar and a bit more seamless. Szagunn's work prior to 1933 in social hygiene and eugenics spheres likely made her both attractive to the Nazi regime and prepared to take on a number of important leadership roles. In 1940, she worked for the Office for People's Health (Amt für Volksgesundheit), an NSDAP-authorized bureau, covering the situation of stillbirths in Germany.[39] She also received a special order from the Ministry of Labour (Reichsarbeitsministerium) in 1941 to ascertain the state of working mothers who breastfed.[40] In addition, she assumed editorial responsibilities of *Die Ärztin* after the death of Dr Edith von Lölhöffel from 1941 until its termination in 1944 – a position the Office for People's Health approved her for. And it was no secret that by then, *Die Ärztin*, once the mouthpiece of the BDÄ, had pro-Nazi inclinations.[41] In reflecting on these political experiences later in life, Szagunn expressed gratitude for the numerous chances she had to sit on committees and especially to voice the opinions of women's organizations against measures, such as Paragraph 218, to influential national committees.[42] In allying with the regime, Szagunn drew from her past nationalist, eugenic, and anti-Semitic experiences, but also still had a desire to prioritize women, as she had done in medical school and in her jobs as a marriage counsellor and school doctor.

Szagunn was exceptional compared with other BDÄ doctors precisely because she acknowledged her political leanings and openly discussed professional cooperation with the Nazi regime. However, most non-Jewish German female doctors in the BDÄ continued their work under Nazism, attracted to the new regime's promises to allow them to continue their personal and professional advocacy, crafting comprehensive social programs for women and children. By participating in Nazi programs like the BDM and RMD and endorsing Nazi policies through their work in these programs, women doctors in the BDÄ, in effect, became political actors, even if they did not openly admit it.

Overall, from all official accounts, the coordination of the BDÄ appeared to transpire quickly and easily and was unexceptional in transforming itself into a politically and racially homogeneous professional group.[43] After the announcement of successful coordination in June 1933, the local chapter's managerial board assembled in Berlin on 24–5 June to express their concerns about the continued existence of the organization, but Thimm attempted to allay these fears, taking over the board. Monheim proposed that Thimm become the leader of the BDÄ, but it was not until the 28 January 1934 member meeting that she was officially voted into office. At this meeting, she spoke assuredly about the continued existence of the BDÄ and opportunities for women's employment under the Nazi state.[44] She then named her new co–board members, who were also aligned with the goals of the new regime.[45] Doctors like Laura Turnau, a founding member of the BDÄ and board member, who was also Jewish, had already stepped down from her position as the career adviser the previous year.[46] Of the eight board members serving when Hitler came to power, four were eliminated on the basis of their Jewish background, including Lizzie Hoffa, Erna Ball, Gertrud Bry, and the managerial editor Käte Wassertrüdinger.[47]

Although *Die Ärztin* reported matter-of-factly about the successful coordination of the BDÄ, the journal itself had already been purged of all Jewish and left-leaning influences, and thus, we get no official information from the BDÄ about how much tension the *Gleichschaltung* may have actually caused. It is likely that Jewish members of the organization, especially those who were founding members and had been serving on the board, felt furious or upset (as Nathorff expressed), but unfortunately, accounts of their transition out of the BDÄ and perhaps out of Germany do not exist outside of Nathorff's. What is likely a more telling example of how many non-Jewish German doctors felt is the shame that Nathorff alluded to in her diary. Even Monheim's initial detachment from the new regime and defensive statements about the purge of Jews in the Munich chapter provides a more accurate picture of how certain non-Jewish doctors justified their actions because of their ambition and opportunism. After all, even someone like Monheim, who was originally diffident about the transition, got promoted to a leadership position, alongside Thimm and Szagunn once the competition had vanished. Atina Grossmann has also argued that some women gained opportunities through new spheres of activity and influence, and I would argue that doctors like Monheim and Szagunn recognized how they could move up the hierarchy, but also how the new spheres of opportunity revolved around helping women and children – work they were already pursuing. As Grossmann also states, younger women doctors were attracted to Nazism because they did not have to suffer through professional struggle and could easily fill the positions of their former Jewish colleagues. Women doctors could argue that they were more necessary overall because of the shortage caused by the purge of all Jewish male and female doctors.[48]

At the regional level, the organization also became ostensibly Nazified where it had not already been. For example, Dr Erna Orlopp-Pleick, a member of the party as well as the Nazi Physicians' League, became the BDÄ's area director in Köningsberg in East Prussia by the fall of 1933.[49] Between 1933 and 1935, the Nazi state enacted further measures against German-Jewish doctors by eliminating them from civil service positions, dismissing them from state and city hospitals, barring them from the health insurance practices, and revoking their licences if they were classified as Jewish.[50] In total, Johanna Bleker has estimated that some 600 female doctors were affected.[51]

By the fall of 1933, the BDÄ became a subgroup of the newly created Nazi association for women, the Deutsches Frauenwerk (German Women's Front). The organization continued to fight for female doctors' privileges over the next few years. The new leader, Thimm, who had been a party member with a clean record since 1926, quarrelled with *Reichsärzteführer* Wagner over the right of women to study medicine and the impending suspension of female panel physicians as early as 1934. While the Nazi regulation of physicians and their organizations was still ongoing, Thimm brazenly appointed women colleagues with no Nazi affiliation whatsoever. For instance, Elisabeth Geilen was appointed the BDÄ's executive secretary in December 1936. As Michael Kater has shown, during those first years under the headstrong Thimm, the BDÄ provided "the organizational underpinning for the battles of principle these women physicians were waging against their Nazi male cohorts."[52]

All of this changed in 1936. On 1 April of that year, a law went into effect that stated that the Reichsärzteführung (Reich Physicians' Leadership) would regulate all medical organizations and that all medical associations with professional or economic interests could continue to work only with the approval of the Reichsärztekammer (Reich Physicians' Chamber; RÄK).[53] In the fall of 1936, the Nationalsozialistischer Deutscher Ärztebund (National Socialist German Physicians' League; NSDÄB) officially took over the ideological leadership of doctors and held its first training course for female physicians at its new racial hygiene training centre in Alt-Rehse. These first training courses were in no way affiliated with the BDÄ; rather, the NSDÄB summoned the first 130 voluntary BDM physicians to attend. This was the beginning of the NSDÄB's ideological and political takeover of the BDÄ, which up until that point, Thimm and other party comrades had administered somewhat independently. Thimm was silenced at the end of 1936 alongside other outspoken intellectual Nazi "feminists." This type of marginalization of women in the political sphere was the norm through all phases of the Nazi regime, according to Claudia Koonz. The Nazi Party and state, she argues, consistently prevented women from influencing policies that affected their own lives and relegated them to the private sphere or leadership positions within their own organizations.[54] Wagner dissolved the organization a few weeks later "on the characteristic pretext that the 'seclusion of the female doctor' would have led to the establishment of a special university for women."[55] In January 1937, *Die Ärztin* reported that as of 15 December 1936, the BDÄ had disbanded.[56] Von Lölhöffel had taken over the journal in February 1936 and she would be followed by Szagunn; the journal, with its Nazi proclivities, continued to publish until 1944 and became an official organ of the RÄK in 1942.

The only semblance of another organization for female physicians appeared in September 1938 when the *Reichsärzteführer*, Gerhard Wagner, anticipating the impending war and need for women doctors, as one of his last acts as Reich Physicians' Leader, founded a "Female Physicians Department" within the RÄK. This department claimed to represent the interests of women physicians and adopted political stances for them. Dr Ursula Kuhlo, who had been a party member since February 1932, became the leader of this department.[57] Kuhlo, who had been petitioning Wagner for a new independent women physicians' group since 1937, joined thirteen men in her new position on the RÄK and, heavily outnumbered, eventually acquiesced to male physicians' views until the end of the war, thereby ending any autonomy or self-expression of female physicians.[58]

Working for the Bund Deutscher Mädels

With the *Gleichschaltung* completed within a year of Hitler's rise to power, women physicians laid claim to new spaces within the regime to continue their professional advocacy. One of these spaces was the League of German Girls (BDM), the female branch of the Hitler Youth. Within this organization, female physicians employed maternalist language to argue that they could be the ideal Nazi image of a woman and could offer more to the new state than their male colleagues because they claimed to no longer be *only* medical authorities, but also trust-worthy confidantes and role models to young girls. Female physicians continued to adhere to traditional understandings of gender roles, especially by championing marriage and motherhood for the members of the BDM. The ability of female physicians to serve as role models for their patients, to influence them on relevant national policies, such as alcohol consumption, and to develop personal relationships with them such that women felt comfortable enough to discuss intimate issues, had already led the Weimar state to value their work in spaces like schools and marriage counselling centres. But under Nazism, women doctors could continue this legacy while also upholding the goal of the state: to build a healthy *Volksgemeinschaft* within organizations like the BDM. Doctors could help girls in the BDM to feel like insiders and to enjoy a sense of belonging beyond family – something that Thomas Kühne claims had previously been the privilege of men.[59] By constructing the *Volksgemeinschaft* in the BDM, female physicians also participated in Hitler's larger *Volksgemeinschaft*, as they empowered themselves and entered the medical community and the public sphere.

Women doctors had initially marketed themselves to Nazis, espe-cially the medical leadership, by emphasizing the ways in which they could assist the regime in achieving its health and population goals. Because the construction and preservation of the *Volksgemein-schaft* was one of the main tenets of Nazism, women physicians like Dr Gertrudis Becker-Schäfer were not remiss to mention the social value of the work that she and her colleagues undertook for the *Volk*.[60] Becker-Schäfer, a practising physician in Wuppertal, advocated that female doctors, who came into daily contact with members of the *Volk*, were among the "most able" individuals to fulfil this task. In fact, she claimed they were much more capable of realizing the Nazi world view than their male peers. Becker-Schäfer criticized the "mechaniza-tion" of the medical profession, which stemmed from male doctors' growing specializations to earn more money. She argued that through their "mechanization," male physicians neglected treating patients in totality. Women doctors were not as interested in material rewards and valued developing close human relationships with their patients. Indeed, female physicians like her showcased their abilities to serve as a "doctor-mother" or *Volksärztin* (people's doctor) under Nazism, thereby extending the same holistic approach to medicine they had employed when they stressed their suitability to work in Weimar mar-riage counselling centres.[61]

To help execute the aims of population policy under National Socialism, women doctors emphasized their unique abilities to develop personal relationships with patients and to awaken and educate women's motherly instincts. According to Becker-Schäfer, in an early propaganda piece for the new state, female physicians could fortify "the heroism of motherhood" in all German women, similar to how men learned their military obligations to the state. Becker-Schäfer and her colleagues were both role models and confidantes for their women and youth patients, who identified and trusted them because they saw in them same-sex companions and, most importantly, women who were also married and mothers. It was this married woman doctor who was also a mother that Becker-Schäfer upheld as the ideal model and the most natural leader for other women.[62] Women doctors, in other words, could lead the way to the *Volksgemeinschaft* through example. They would be the individuals caring for working women, mothers, and youth while Germany continued on its path to physical and spiritual recovery. Dr Monheim also thought women physicians were especially capable of fulfilling the specific feminine-medical duties that accompanied National Socialism. She argued that women's instinctual nature and empathetic attitude led them to make the right decisions during very difficult times.[63]

The BDM, founded in 1930 as an extension of the Hitler Youth, was the only female youth organization in Nazi Germany. It did not gain a mass following until after Hitler came to power and it grew rapidly throughout the mid-1930s until membership became compulsory in 1936 for eligible girls between the ages of ten and eighteen. Eligibility requirements included German ethnicity, German citizenship, and physical and mental fitness. Just like the Hitler Youth, the BDM divided members into separate sections based on age. The Jungmädelbund (Young Girl's League; JM), formed in 1933, included girls between the ages of ten and fourteen, the Bund Deutscher Mädel consisted of girls between the ages of fourteen and eighteen, and Glaube und Schönheit ("Faith and Beauty"), added in 1938, embraced young women between the ages of seventeen and twenty-one on a voluntary basis.[64] The main activities of the JM and the BDM – a several-hour time commitment each week – entailed camping trips and other short weekend excursions, hikes, sports, outdoor training and field exercises, community service, political activities, such as participation at festivals and public rallies, summer camps, and social evenings that included singing and arts and crafts. This training was intended to educate girls in National Socialist ideology and to prepare them for their future tasks within the

Volksgemeinschaft, namely as wives, mothers, and homemakers. "Faith and Beauty" focused primarily on grooming young women for marriage, motherhood, and domestic life, with a strong emphasis placed on home economics so women could properly run a household and care for their children. It also devoted attention to education, job training, and helping young women meet their future career goals. Physical training and ideological schooling remained significant components of "Faith and Beauty," which required only two to three weekly hours of service from young women, who were often already busy working. "Faith and Beauty" served as a type of liminal organization for older adolescents between the BDM and NS-Frauenschaft, whose ranks women graduated into at the age of twenty-one.[65] The BDM was essentially training girls for lifelong membership in the party and its women's groups.[66]

Both physical training and health education were especially important for the young girls in the BDM. Hygiene and proper dress codes were of equal importance. National guidelines, in fact, dictated that two-thirds of the time in group meetings be dedicated to "physical activity and exercise" with the remaining one-third on "worldview [ideological] training."[67] With its focus on the body, the BDM rendered this once private issue public, thereby connecting physical fitness, health, and dress with the interests of the nation. Physical training and health also aimed to indoctrinate German youth to National Socialist racial-biological ideals. This could be seen in the form, regulation, and discipline of BDM sporting or dancing activities, which did not allow any expression of individualized or spontaneous movement, but instead sought to produce fit girls who would develop into healthy women, give birth to strong children, and ultimately preserve the heredity of the *Volk*. The creation of an achievement badge to reward physical prowess and training manuals for the JM and the BDM reflected the notion that sport emphasized building camaraderie among a generation of healthy girls who would become the nation's future mothers. Nazi ideology, in other words, was implicit in BDM physical training. Health education, too, focused on fulfilling Nazi goals to create a pure and fit race. BDM leaders stressed proper nutrition, comfortable clothing, sufficient sleep, adequate housing, good skin and dental care, and an overall way of life that balanced physical exercise with leisure and relaxation. BDM girls from urban areas also spent time in the countryside in order to gain an appreciation for the German homeland.[68]

Given the BDM's emphasis on physical exercise and health education, it is not surprising that female physicians became heavily involved in the organization. When it became clear that the BDM was the only female-only organization focused on girls' health, women doctors laid claim to this new space to implement their ideas about the health monitoring and care of its members. The BDM was only ever of marginal interest to *Die Ärztin*, which published sporadically on the work of BDM doctors after 1933. A wave of articles appeared in 1933–4 to coincide with these new positions opening to women. When this new field first opened to women doctors, there was an attempt to address the numerous questions and problems concerning the medical care of girls in the BDM at a workshop of all the upper-district (*Obergau*) female doctors in 1934 in Berlin. At this workshop, they discussed the extent to which individual female physicians were actually providing medical care, where they were lacking, and what type of medical care had proven to be the most necessary and appropriate, and they sought to standardize their medical work and create common target goals. Most, who were already involved in the BDM, were bursting with questions, problems, and work suggestions; it was good, then, that the conversation had begun.[69] In 1937, the BDM started employing women physicians on a full-time basis, and as the regional network of the Hitler Youth expanded during the war, the number of BDM physicians (as they came to be known) expanded as well. There were 1,300 female physicians working full time or in voluntary or advisory roles in the BDM by 1939 and 1,500 by 1941.[70] By May 1941, there were enough physicians employed in the BDM to merit a special issue in *Die Ärztin* on the health-care management of girls in the BDM, namely the objectives and work of leading BDM doctors. Working for the BDM became one of the most popular and gratifying professional opportunities for women physicians, and presumably may have been used as a springboard for future careers.

The BDÄ already considered it "one of the most important duties to enforce the health monitoring of German female youth," evidenced also by the work they did in school health reform in the Weimar period.[71] The work of BDM physicians paralleled their work in schools and, in fact, built on school medical exams and served to supplement the work of vocational school doctors. Some school doctors worked simultaneously as BDM doctors, as Dr Anneliese Panhuizen explained at the Meeting of Hitler Youth Physicians in 1937. In Frankfurt, where she worked, they had three female school doctors who also worked for the BDM. The cooperation between school doctors and BDM physicians could be very useful, especially with regard to the regularly scheduled school medical examinations. These occurred when children were admitted to school and then again when they were ten, which coincided with the year they were admitted to the BDM. School doctors, then, through these exams provided validation for BDM suitability, according to Panhuizen, and BDM doctors and school doctors could work together to compile a list and communicate about the girls who were permanently or temporarily "unfit" for membership.[72]

BDM doctors determined the health condition of individual *Mädels* (girls) through regular medical examinations that covered the heart, lungs, blood pressure, pulse, cardiovascular functions, mouth and throat organs, teeth, stomach, reflexes, and the condition of a girl's skin, posture, feet, and nutrition. In addition, BDM physicians searched for infections like angina, scarlet fever, rheumatoid arthritis, and any susceptibility to colds among parents and siblings in their medical histories. Most importantly, they checked for hereditary diseases, which, if found, would disqualify girls from membership. They recorded the physical activity of girls, along with height, weight, chest measurement, sight, and hearing. Finally, these exams assessed racial features to determine which girls would be admitted to the organization. After a little practice, female doctors were supposed to be able to quickly judge from a girl's skull, face shape, hair, skin, and eye colour if it was even worthwhile to perform an exam.[73] These health exams, which sought to record and isolate the physical and mental problems of young girls, reflected the goals of the BDM to incorporate National Socialist ideas about racial biology and the *Volksgemeinschaft* into its physical training and health education programs. By forbidding girls who were seen as physically, mentally, or racially unfit, or genetically diseased, from joining, the BDM created an exclusionary community of Germany's healthiest individuals. The female physicians performing these exams were implementing the dogma of the BDM, which ultimately mirrored that of the Nazi state to create an exclusive people's community.

Dr Lore Heidepriem-Friedel demonstrates one example of BDM doctors who became an empowered member of the larger medical community by embracing the eugenicist ideals of the regime and by adopting the *Volksgemeinschaft* concept as she attempted to create a micro-*Volksgemeinschaft* within the BDM.[74] She claimed that it was ideal to have only healthy, fresh girls in the BDM and that the BDM should refer to itself as "an elite of German female youth" who later became healthy women, physically and mentally. Heidepriem-Friedel recognized, however, that creating this elite group was not always realistic because the BDM included youth from "all walks of life," and thus, the political organization, surveying, and education of youth should be their most urgent goal. This was totally new and comprehensive medical work for women physicians and included "the sampling of [the female youth's] health condition, the indoctrination of the healthy, and the eradication of contagious patients or the morally inferior."[75] Heidepriem-Friedel suggested that in order to carry out this work, the BDM physicians must receive access to the files of the Hereditary Health Courts, set up after the passage of the Law for the Prevention of Genetically Diseased Offspring (14 July 1933) to determine whether individuals should be forcibly sterilized so that they could "weed out" hereditary diseased children, insofar as they were a danger to others. In her opinion, "we [BDM physicians] must be empowered to exclude girls who are physically ill or morally unfit from the BDM."[76] Because BDM doctors ultimately helped the state form an exclusionary community within the BDM, Heidepriem-Friedel believed the state should also empower doctors with the tools and authority to do so.

In this instance, Heidepriem-Friedel demonstrates some rather complicated motivations for her work. Her rhetoric reveals a seasoned eugenicist who might have truly believed in the Nazi regime's plan to weed out the hereditarily ill. More likely, she was an opportunist who recognized how she could assist the Nazi regime in fulfilling its radical eugenics policies. The passage of the Law for the Prevention of Genetically Diseased Offspring especially provided some women physicians who worked in hospitals, clinics, and organizations like the BDM the opportunity to carry out the task of weeding out the physically and mentally "unfit" and incentivizing the "fit."[77] She recognized how she could benefit not only herself with a wider breadth of medical access and knowledge, but also her patients with improved health. Heidepriem-Friedel may have been conflicted about both helping some girls while weeding out others, but this was emblematic of the larger Nazi medical strategy, as they normalized the seemingly contradictory. Heidepriem-Friedel most likely was some combination of all of the above – an avid eugenicist, an opportunist, and an advocate for her patients.

BDM doctors recorded the results of regular medical exams on health cards, which maintained consistency in all local chapters throughout the Reich. Although it is unclear how often doctors referred to these health cards, the cards noted the necessary measures to improve health (e.g., medical and dental treatment and recovery relocation), as well as to what extent individual girls could participate in their required service to the BDM, particularly physical exercise. BDM physicians then gave these summary findings to BDM-*Führerin* (BDM leaders) – selected girls within each section of the BDM (JM, BDM, and "Glaube und Schönheit") who completed a preparatory regimen and six-month probationary period before being appointed to the position, which they then worked on a voluntary basis.[78] BDM leaders were responsible for preserving the medical confidentiality of BDM members and for ensuring that the necessary medical measures were enacted. The close contact and cooperation between BDM physicians and BDM leaders was essential for the successful completion of these examinations. The leaders, according to Dr Auguste Hoffmann, the Berlin regional BDM physician and a medical consultant for the organization, had to trust the physicians, to listen to their advice, and to subordinate themselves unconditionally to their medical expertise on questions of health.[79] Dr Heidepriem-Friedel even went so far as to suggest that BDM doctors should do their best to influence these leaders.[80] Hoffmann claimed that the effective execution of medical care depended on BDM leaders knowing when to consult BDM physicians and putting an enormous amount of confidence in them and their authority.[81]

Dr Josephine Bilz, a BDM subdistrict (*Untergau*) leader and an employee for the Reich Youth Leadership health office, commented on this delicate relationship between BDM physicians and BDM leaders in the special issue that *Die Ärztin* published on BDM physicians in 1941.[82] She referred to the "special trusting relationship" that developed between physician and leader, but Bilz also highlighted the emotional guidance and companionship that physicians provided to young BDM leaders. These leaders, who were the same age as the girls in their squads or platoons, often confided in physicians throughout their maturation process. BDM leaders had the double burden of being responsible for other adolescent girls while experiencing the physical and emotional changes of puberty themselves and thus often sought out doctors for support. As Bilz recalled, the leaders would often plead to see doctors to discuss a concern about the physical or emotional well-being of one of their girls, but this was only a ploy to talk to doctors about some deeper need or conflict. Although leaders did not claim to be looking for a maternal friend or teacher, this was precisely what BDM doctors offered them. Hoffmann, Bilz, and other physicians like them presented themselves as medical experts as well as caring companions to these young leaders during adolescence, claiming their maternal abilities allowed them to grasp girls' deepest emotional issues without asking too many embarrassing questions. Bilz asserted that BDM physicians "instinctively sensed" the problems of the young leaders and guided them through any hardships with very few words.[83] BDM physicians, then, employed the rhetoric of motherhood and femininity to make a case that they were indispensable to the effective education and preparation of German female youth on all questions of physical and mental health, and portrayed themselves as intimate advisers or mentors to BDM leaders throughout maturity.

In addition to offering support and companionship to BDM leaders, BDM physicians cared for the *Mädels*. Besides performing routine medical exams, BDM physicians supervised the hygiene of members, indoctrinated young girls to Nazi ideas of racial hygiene, built camaraderie among the various age groups, educated girls in matters of biology, sickness, and health, and prepared them for motherhood. At the first workshop for BDM physicians throughout the Reich, held in Potsdam in November 1934, Hoffmann ranked the educational tasks as "one of the most important duties of female physicians in the BDM," alongside administering fitness exams and providing medical support for members.[84] Because BDM doctors interacted with girls during a critical developmental phase, physicians had a fundamental responsibility to counsel girls on biological questions and to teach them to maintain a clean and healthy personal lifestyle. Children often already received this type of health instruction in schools, but after the Nazi takeover of power, the boundaries of health care greatly expanded. This meant the Nazi leadership, even in wartime, supported educating girls on the basics of personal physical care, dental care, healthy nutrition, its position on alcohol and smoking, morality, and the management of a healthy family, *Volk*, and race – and the BDM echoed this message.[85] Schools, especially elementary schools, were supposed to provide German youth with this basic education, and the BDM would then supplement school lessons.[86] Later, during the war, BDM doctors would direct the first aid services of members after air raids and were tasked with caring for schoolchildren.[87]

Doctors like Erika Geisler, however, a BDM subdistrict (*Untergau*) leader and a department head for the Reich Youth Leadership health office, cited the deficiencies of school health lessons and praised the guidance and support the BDM offered girls until the age of twenty-one – throughout their crucial developmental phase.[88] While Geisler may have simply sought to draw attention to the work that she and her colleagues did, there was certainly some truth to the fact that the adolescent years were imperative because of the biological and psychological changes young girls underwent, and also because of the potential pressures they faced from their peers – both of which school doctors had already identified in the Weimar period. BDM physicians, then, performed an important service by guiding girls through adolescence. BDM doctors claimed that they could maintain a strong influence over the girls, especially as they struggled to find a community of accepting peers and exemplary adults. Dr Ursula Kuhlo, a BDM regional leader and an office assistant in the Reich Youth Leadership health office, in fact, argued that the BDM was more significant than the family during this time, and that the words of its leaders often meant more than parental instruction.[89] BDM physicians like Kuhlo declared their profound educational influence over *Mädels*, even if they did not always disclose the concrete success of such efforts. Even if she exaggerated physicians' authority over girls in the BDM, Kuhlo demonstrated how BDM physicians laid claim to this female space and self-mobilized an archetype of maternal care, all in the name of the Nazi state.

Seemingly, the impact that BDM physicians had on *Mädels* would be minimal, considering they saw them about twice a week. Kuhlo expressed concerns about the effectiveness that she and her colleagues could have on shaping BDM members' lifestyles. She believed that the childhood home or workplace – where girls spent the majority of their time – were the most influential. While Kuhlo recognized the important role of parents and household routines in educating girls about healthy lifestyles, she also acknowledged their failure. According to her, few parents and educational institutions devoted attention to matters like owning a toothbrush and using it twice a day. The support that homes and schools offered with regard to these basic requirements of personal hygiene, Kuhlo claimed, left much to be desired. She observed a lack of basic health knowledge among *Mädels*, especially those from the countryside, and blamed mothers for their negligence in teaching the easy, practical goals of health education to their children. Kuhlo maintained that it was the responsibility of BDM doctors to intervene when mothers failed to advise and aid their daughters during adolescence.[90] BDM physicians, then, claimed to compensate not only for the deficient education girls received in schools, but also for the shortcomings of their mothers as well. Some of the same class biases against Weimar vocational school students and their mothers clearly carried over to the Nazi period and translated into an urban-rural divide between BDM physicians and certain BDM members from more rural settings.

It was often during the regularly scheduled BDM mother evenings (*Mütterabende*) that the failures of mothers were exposed. These evenings, in which BDM physicians and leaders worked to establish and deepen their relationships with the parents of the girls entrusted to them, glaringly demonstrated just how little assistance mothers provided their daughters and how often they lacked an understanding of their daughters' needs, according to Kuhlo. As Kuhlo reported, during these evenings, BDM doctors begged mothers to get involved.[91] Dr Grete Deicke-Busch, a BDM district leader and regional doctor in Düsseldorf, described how physicians made themselves available to mothers during these evenings to answer their health education questions. BDM physicians also shared information about the health lifestyles and moral attitudes required of girls in the BDM – information that mothers were both interested in and thankful for. Deicke-Busch also noted that in her district, they often asked married female doctors who were mothers themselves to participate in these evenings. She found that it was difficult, if not impossible, for physicians to speak in front of mothers without the expertise that emerged from their personal experiences as well as their medical training.[92] The tendencies of female physicians to remain tied to their traditional maternal roles that existed in the Weimar period persisted in the Nazi era, as they continued to promote marriage and motherhood as attributes that enhanced their medical expertise.

During these mother evenings, BDM physicians, who were also ideally married mothers, and therefore trustworthy professional and personal references, educated mothers about the health activities of their daughters. Doctors also provided mothers the tools to help their daughters when they came to them with health or sexual questions. This was especially important after 1939 because of the strains the war put on family education with the absence of fathers and the employment of mothers. Deicke-Busch encouraged mothers to learn to develop open, honest relationships with their daughters at a young age so their daughters would be more apt to turn to them for problems they faced during adolescence. BDM physicians also instructed mothers to maintain positive educational influences in the home at all times. In the case of alcohol and smoking, for example, Deicke-Busch encouraged mothers to stop any teasing or pressure their daughters received from older siblings. The BDM already taught girls to reject alcohol and cigarettes, but if parents did not echo this message at home, the work carried out within the BDM would be futile.[93] To reinforce this, the RMD launched its own anti-alcohol and anti-smoking initiative.[94] BDM physicians could also significantly influence mothers in terms of proper nutrition as well as the best types of recreational and physical activities for their children. In general, BDM physicians professed to be educating mothers about motherhood – something that Deicke-Busch admitted she was consciously and unconsciously doing.[95] Teaching motherhood was also the primary goal of the RMD.

If BDM physicians created trusting relationship with mothers, they could ultimately do their own jobs more effectively. But effective work meant much more than enlisting mothers as allies in promoting health education; it also involved successfully achieving the overall educational goals of the Nazi state.[96] Because female doctors gained the confidence of mothers through events like the mother evenings, they proclaimed to exert strong influence over *Mädels* and thus could indoctrinate them to National Socialist ideology. As one *Jüngmadel*, Ursula Mahlendorf, reported, this indoctrination was certainly effective: "For us, the cohort born between about 1925 and 1930 and socialized from age ten on by the Hitler Youth, being German and being National Socialist became indistinguishable."[97] Hitler and the Nazi state would ultimately reap the benefits if a relationship developed between BDM physicians and mothers.

The state benefited because BDM doctors indoctrinated girls to Nazi ideology such as the *Volksgemeinschaft*. The health fitness admission examinations, which prohibited membership in the BDM altogether if one was deemed "unfit" due to a "serious disease, physical malformation, or asocial element" trained ten-year-old girls in Nazi exclusionary policies; such negative medical results may also have had more serious consequences than exclusion from the BDM for these children. The BDM implemented similar segregation policies in the case that a *Mädel* became "temporarily unfit" to participate in BDM activity or service because of an "acute disease" or if a girl was deemed "limitedly fit."[98] In addition, BDM doctors indoctrinated girls through health training. *Jungmädels* learned from a very early age to take pride in keeping their bodies clean, wearing matching uniforms (usually a blue skirt and white blouse), and rejecting vices like alcohol and smoking, but most importantly, they also ascertained that these were requirements of national pride. On their first overnight trips and then through later camping trips or travel, BDM doctors schooled *Jungmädels* and then *Mädels* about healthy clothing and proper nutrition. Mahlendorf recalled the pride she felt in washing her uniform frequently and taking daily sponge baths, so much so that she annoyed her mother by consuming scarce cleaning supplies.[99] Girls in the BDM gained an appreciation for the joys of physical exercise through afternoon sports, and they discovered the importance of developing a connection with nature through summer camping – both of which were fundamental facets of National Socialist dogma.[100] The BDM clearly incorporated the Nazi ideology of *Blut und Boden* (blood and soil), which celebrated the relationship of people to the land, into its activities. For example, during the *Pflicthjahr*, or the year of obligatory service for girls seventeen or older in the home or on the farm, girls also acquired an appreciation for nature through strenuous rural labour [101] "Glaube und Schönheit" members learned that beauty was something that was always connected to health and racial purity by studying art from different periods of history and by performing weekly community work in areas like "Healthy Girl, Healthy *Volk*," which instructed girls about the relationship between personal health and lifestyle and racial and population policy decisions.[102] In fact, Deicke-Busch ranked the proper training of girls in racial hygiene and Nazi ideology with the medical monitoring of *Mädels* as one of the most important responsibilities of BDM physicians.[103]

Some physicians, such as Erika Geisler, recognized that "the Führer gradually grew into the youth" through these types of BDM programs, but also that such activities taught girls that their health and service in the BDM were vital for the community and the state.[104] Geisler proved to be right, as one *Jüngmadel* noted how Nazi ideas of *Blut und Boden* and racial ideology grew within her; she took solitary hikes in the woods, where she noted the beauty of the landscape and acquired a sense of racial superiority, stating that she "believed that [she] belonged to an elite," and at one point she berated herself for being mistaken for looking like a Pole and spent hours in front of the mirror trying to determine if she was the ideal Aryan type.[105] Melita Maschmann, a dedicated BDM leader, was fascinated by the *Volksgemeinschaft*, and stated that she "want[ed] to help create the National Community in which people would live together as one big family."[106] Drs Deicke-Busch and Kuhlo recognized that binding girls to the *Volksgemeinschaft* and to the German landscape or German culture were goals of both BDM physicians and the Nazi party, and these goals were certainly being realized.[107]

So too were feelings of comradeship, and BDM doctors were a keystone to fostering feelings of inclusivity and equality.[108] Dr Deicke-Busch maintained that the tight bonds of BDM members were necessary to the goals the organization set out to achieve, which included encouraging girls to care for their own health, physically toughening them through sports, and helping them detect social ills early in order to prevent any harm they might cause.[109] Singing German songs or viewing German art, moreover, built patriotism in *Mädels*, which the Nazis desired. Dr Kuhlo recognized that it was not until girls joined "Faith and Beauty" and pursued more individualized interests that the dominant principle of camaraderie began to wane. She thought participation in large celebrations like rallies or parades allowed young girls to remain connected to the larger youth community, which was a key part of Hitler's Reich.[110] Several girls who joined the BDM reported positively on experiencing such camaraderie, especially through their participation in team competitions and singing patriotic songs.[111]

Crucial to the success of creating this camaraderie were the behaviour, dress, and participation of BDM doctors. Externally, BDM physicians wore the same clothing as *Mädels* when they participated in a BDM function, abided by the same laws of the organization, and participated – so far as possible – in everyday service activities, sports, competitions, travel, and camping trips.[112] They had to carefully balance their youthful comradeship with the girls as well as their sense of authority. In other words, BDM doctors had what Dr Josephine Bilz called a "contradictory duty" of being in the centre of the youth movement and yet standing aside from it in order to allow the girls' process of maturity to occur on its own.[113] Some BDM physicians sought to enlist certain types of female doctors, who were better suited for this balancing act. BDM doctor Auguste Hoffmann, for one, urged finding younger colleagues to do this type of work, presumably because they would have more in common with BDM members, who ranged from ten to twenty-one years old.[114] Furthermore, Dr Ursula Kuhlo insisted that married doctors with children provided the best help on camping trips, demonstrating once again that women doctors defended marriage and motherhood as qualities that made them more able to connect with young girls.[115] BDM doctors ultimately understood that their participation led to stronger relationships with the *Mädels*. By wearing their uniform, experiencing their travels, singing their songs, and joining them in other activities, BDM physicians asserted that they gained the trust of girls in a way that they likely would not have had they remained outside of the community.[116] Wearing the uniform, alone, was an indication that doctors were "in" and were considered full-fledged members of the *Volksgemeinschaft*.[117] The physicians, in addition to becoming members of a macro-*Volksgemeinschaft* in Germany through their work, were becoming members of this micro-*Volksgemeinschaft* as they simultaneously created it among girls within the BDM. Consequently, BDM doctors like Deicke-Busch, Kuhlo, Bilz, Geisler, and Hoffmann, insisted that they could do their jobs more effectively and could perhaps even, through this close contact, awaken a desire within *Mädels* to become doctors themselves – a fundamental step to building the future medical profession.[118]

Besides directing girls toward the medical profession, BDM doctors also worked to prepare young girls for motherhood, thus instilling in them another basic element of Nazi ideology. First, BDM physicians made it clear that they understood it to be their responsibility to physically and mentally educate girls for motherhood. Deicke-Busch was not shy about admitting that she was rearing the future "leaders of German families" and therefore ensuring the growth of the next generation of healthy women, on which the German state depended.[119] Second, in schooling *Mädels* about the moral position of the BDM, doctors like Kuhlo connected a good moral attitude to proper motherhood.[120] And finally, in making motherhood the objective of health education, BDM doctors Hoffmann and Geisler discouraged girls from overexertion in their professional lives, sports, or BDM service, fearing that any damages, especially to the genitalia, would prevent *Mädels* from becoming mothers.[121] Accordingly, Kuhlo aimed to avoid any excess of physical or mental activity when designing the BDM service plan, and Heidepriem-Friedel agreed that preventing the overexertion of youth was one of their major tasks.[122] By centring the BDM program on grooming girls for motherhood – morally, mentally, and physically – women physicians sustained the same principles they had as school doctors in the Weimar period. As professionals, who were no longer fighting to solidify their place in medicine, they continued to promote a domestic lifestyle and maternity as the epitome of women's existence. Thus maternalism, as historians Seth Koven and Sonya Michel point out, worked on two levels – championing private domesticity while legitimizing women's public professional roles, especially their own.[123]

Working for the Reichsmütterdienst

In addition to encouraging motherhood through BDM curriculum, female doctors helped educate mothers through the RMD. Raising the status of racially valuable mothers was a primary concern of the Nazi regime. The party was devoted to elevating the status of Aryan mothers through well-known initiatives like the *Mutterkreuz* (Mother's Cross), which rewarded prolific mothers with preferential treatment, such as requiring members of the Hitler Youth to salute them in public. Racially valuable women who had three children under the age of ten received honour cards entitling them to preferential treatment while shopping. Large families received rent, water, and electricity rebates, as well as free theatre tickets, while young married couples received interest-free loans.[124] Hitler proclaimed that mothers were the most important of all citizens, and they enjoyed recognition – even celebrity status – that took concrete form, for example, with more baby-care stations and expanded health care services.[125] As Wendy Lower states, the German mother was the heroine of the German race.[126]

The party established the RMD early in 1934 as part of the Deutsches Frauenwerk (German Women's Front), a political organization that sought to ideologically enlist women. Analogous to BDM mother evenings, which coached the mothers of BDM members in proper motherhood techniques, the RMD taught motherhood through *Mütterschulung* (mothers' training). According to the *Mütterschulung* guidelines, this program aimed to physically and mentally train competent mothers, who recognized the important obligations of motherhood for the German *Volk* and the German state.[127] Mothers' training occurred either in newly opened mother schools in cities, in four- to six-week mothers' training courses, or during mothers' free time. In rural areas, the RMD held rotating courses and established *Heimmütterschulen* (home mother schools), where women could take abridged courses in the home and then advise and assist their neighbours since medical personnel were often unavailable.[128]

Similar to the BDM, the *Mütterschulung* curriculum indoctrinated mothers to National Socialist ideology and schooled them in their duties to the new state, which included ensuring the future *Volk* through the education and care of genetically healthy children. Moreover, mothers learned how to manage the household through courses in cooking, sewing, accounting, and shopping. They learned about pregnancy, birth, infant and childcare, how to raise physically and mentally healthy children, and how to handle difficult children. In courses on health and nursing, mothers gained knowledge about the health maintenance of the family, children's diseases, infectious diseases, and household nursing. There was also some discussion that a film about breast milk collection would be included in the curriculum.[129] There was a religious and moral educational component to mothers' training that taught women about marriage and religion, children and religion, and religious morals in the household.[130] The RMD offered classes for pregnant women to educate them in childcare and domestic science, which had been attended by over 1.7 million women by 1939, and offered a service which provided second-hand cots, prams, and children's clothing.[131]

The *Mütterschulung*'s teachers consisted of people educated in a number of different disciplines, including female caregivers, trade teachers, agricultural household teachers, youth leaders, nurses, and naturally, female doctors, who were primarily employed to educate mothers in health-related matters.[132] Female physicians like Erika Geisler viewed the work that she and her colleagues performed for the RMD as closing a noticeable gap in the health education that parents gave to their children.[133] In other words, female doctors sought to step in when parents were lacking, ignorant, or negligent. Similar to how school doctors taught the scientific art of mothering to their vocational students' negligent parents, doctors working for the RMD, like their colleagues in the BDM, also aspired to scientifically teach motherhood to failing mothers.

The RMD, as a whole, also worked to close the gap between the group of women who strongly supported National Socialism and those who were merely neutral. Rather than simply educating and training women in Nazi ideology, the RMD aimed to indoctrinate women to become active followers of Hitler. It was for this reason that Dr Erna Röpke, departmental leader of the RMD, explained that the organization was part of the Deutsches Frauenwerk and not the NS-Frauenschaft. Even though both were divisions within the National Socialist community, the NS-Frauenschaft included already loyal Nazi believers, whereas the Deutsches Frauenwerk amassed the women who did not belong to any Nazi organizations and ideologically guided them. The RMD, then, "posed a political task" for all those involved, and Röpke noted that doctors, teachers, and the like had to realize that they had a "political mission" to achieve.[134] This overtly political attitude in *Die Ärztin* was much different than the political neutrality the journal once exhibited. Medical journals and medicine in general became infused with Nazi ideology after 1933, as the individualized interest of patients most certainly came second to the racial political goals of National Socialism.

In order to accomplish this political mission, those women doctors and any other women who worked for the RMD had to be supporters of National Socialism. Moreover, Nazi ideology had to be consciously woven into all mothers' training courses, whether they were about health, household management, home design, or child and infant care. *Mütterschulung*, in other words, taught each German woman that the work she did as a mother influenced the entire *Volk*. For example, courses schooled mothers how to sacrifice for the good of the nation without protest, especially during rebuilding periods. In cooking courses, women learned the relationship between the small family household and the larger household of the German *Volk*. Household management courses instructed women to buy German products when shopping. Sewing courses taught mothers how to mend and alter clothing, how to make children's apparel, and how to produce something new out of something old.[135] Women learned how to create a comfortable home with limited resources – situations they encountered during the Depression and the Second World War. In home design courses, women learned how important it was to maintain the home as a place of rest since life was so hectic. Historian Claudia Koonz has suggested that examples like this demonstrate that German women maintained the home as a site of normalcy for their husbands and sons, many of whom were Nazis, and therefore they too must be counted as culpable for the regime's crimes.[136] On the one hand, *Mütterschulung* provided a scientific guide to mothering that aimed to help women deal with the practical problems they encountered in their daily lives. On the other hand, *Mütterschulung* fit well with Nazi ideology such as sacrificing for the *Volk*, especially during economic hardship and war.

The BDÄ insisted that the RMD, although it technically fell under the bureaucracy of the National Socialist state, should be given free reign to implement its maternal training and its medical assistance and protection for fit mothers.[137] This argument revealed just how critical female doctors thought this work was for the German state – so significant, in fact, that it should not be beholden to routine bureaucratic measures. The BDÄ also recognized that the most efficient way to teach motherhood was to have women educate women and, more importantly, to have mothers train mothers.[138] Dr Röpke, for one, understood that a man could never achieve the goals of *Mütterschulung*, and explained that the RMD would only invite male doctors to give lectures during their social evenings if they truly understood how to speak to women. She instead insisted that married female physicians were the most desirable candidates for this type of work.[139] Röpke insisted that these women could often still lead *Mütterschulung* courses alongside their responsibilities in their own practices and in their homes as mothers. If for some reason, a woman doctor could not complete an entire course, the RMD asked them to at least make themselves available on the last evening for questions, especially for those courses dealing with racial or genetic care. If anyone other than a doctor led the course, physicians had to be on hand to advise teachers and to ensure that they followed the required teaching method of open discussion, rather than lecturing, during the course.[140]

Röpke, after speaking with many leaders of *Mütterschulung* courses, remarked that they derived just as much enjoyment and satisfaction out of teaching the courses as the mothers did taking them. After all, according to Röpke, doctors had the opportunity, through their teaching, to practically implement their many years of experience. They were also able to contribute to the education of the *Volk* in an unprecedented way.[141] Overall, the *Mütterschulung* courses allowed mothers to develop "a bond of genuine camaraderie" with female physicians – their "understanding sisters" with whom they shared a common womanly duty: motherhood.[142]

Those female doctors working for the RMD, then, employed the same maternal rhetoric as BDM doctors. This language likely stemmed from their predecessors, who worked as marriage counsellors and school doctors during the Weimar Republic. And just as marriage counselling centres and schools were new work spaces for women doctors during the 1920s, the BDM and the RMD maintained the same function in the 1930s. Now, however, the benefits were twofold: female physicians found space for their medical and educational voices as well as a way to implement their practical experience as mothers under a strict totalitarian regime; additionally, the Nazi state could rely on some women doctors to indoctrinate women and children to become supporters of the regime. The Weimar state, although it may have recognized the value in using female doctors in particular welfare initiatives, did not as obviously employ them for larger objectives, thus signifying a point of demarcation between the two regimes. The BDÄ and women's organizations were generally the only institutions in the Weimar era that realized that women doctors could draw women into marriage counselling centres or attract them to the anti-alcohol and anti-VD campaigns. Only in the case of the 1927 anti-VD law did the state acknowledge the benefit of employing women doctors in VD counselling centres by making this policy. The Nazi state, on the other hand, consciously recognized how valuable physicians in the BDM and the RMD were, and could be, to train women and girls in its ideology. The Nazis' view of women in society as helpers and healers, alongside their belief in the separation of the sexes, implied that there was a need for women to be employed in medicine to cater to the needs of women and girls. Medicine also had a new ideological element to it. No longer were doctors assisting only their individual patients; they were also helping the goals of the party and state.

Working in Racial Hygiene at Alt-Rehse

One of the primary ways in which the Nazi state came to depend on female physicians was through women's racial hygiene indoctrination. Women doctors already attempted to sell themselves to Nazi medical leadership as the "people's doctor" who could offer women someone trustworthy to identify with. For example, Agnes Bluhm, a leading racial hygienist and physician, stated that "no profession [was] more qualified than the medical profession" to fulfil the regime's racial hygiene goals. She believed that females in the profession were at least as important if not more essential than her male colleagues to the Nazi racial hygiene agenda because "the woman doctor lent a more willing ear than the male doctor."[143] In her 1936 book, *The Racial Hygiene Duties of the Female Doctor*, Bluhm expanded on these beliefs, claiming that those doctors who had the deepest trust of their patients – oftentimes women – also had the chance to offer their patients the most effective education, especially in terms of racial hygiene.[144] This is a vivid example of how women doctors self-mobilized for the Nazi state. The Nazi medical leadership also recognized that because women physicians were influential examples to their patients, they could guarantee the enforcement of racial hygiene objectives. Female doctors could be the archetypes of Nazi health and population policies, which were infused with racial hygiene, among their women and youth patients.[145] Therefore, it seemed practical for the medical leadership to appropriately train female physicians in the principles of racial hygiene at the educational training camp for doctors at Alt-Rehse.

The *Ärzteführerschule* (leadership school for physicians) was a specialized ideological training centre for young physicians, midwives, and civil servants in the health sector. It was located in the small village of Alt-Rehse at the Tollensesee in Mecklenburg in Northern Germany. The NSDÄB, under the leadership of Dr Gerhard Wagner, planned and built the training centre, which opened on 1 June 1935. Hans Haedenkamp, the architect commissioned to design the *Ärzteführerschule*, broke ground on the property on 2 August 1934. Not only did he rehabilitate and reconstruct existing buildings, but he also built the school and dormitories and revitalized the village as well as the street between the train station and Alt-Rehse.[146]

The facility Haedenkamp planned purposefully included the landscape surrounding it. He constructed dormitories with views of the lake and arranged them among old trees. He intentionally placed the communal house at the highest and most beautiful place in the park with balcony views of the Tollensesee. By situating the leadership school in the surrounding landscape, Haedenkamp evoked the National Socialist ideology *Blut und Boden*, which championed nature, natural therapies, and rural living. This was also true for *Reichsärzteführer* Wagner, an avid supporter of naturopathy as well as an advocate for the construction of Alt-Rehse. Dr Hans Deuschl, the leader of the school, stated that because National Socialist doctors were "pioneers for new biological principles in medicine and natural science, which are most closely rooted with the blood and soil of [their] Fatherland," they chose to establish the educational site in the calm of beautiful landscape rather than in a bustling city.[147] To a great extent, female physicians' accounts of their experiences at Alt-Rehse recalled the natural beauty of the surroundings and how this made them feel more connected to the goals they set out to achieve there.

Starting in June 1935, the Reich medical leadership invited medical professionals to the training centre for short courses of between two and four weeks. These courses ran year-round. The program included topics related to Nazi ideology and its application to medicine and public health. The participants heard lectures about racial medicine, euthanasia, and public health from many famous German politicians and physicians and combined this intellectual component with physical training, sports, harvesting for the local population, and the construction of roads. All participants wore a common uniform and individuals from different parts of the country roomed together in order to create camaraderie. This reflected the atmosphere that Wagner thought should govern Alt-Rehse, which he outlined in a speech on the day the school opened. He asserted that doctors had to learn to subordinate themselves if they wanted to become leaders. They had to endure stalwart self-discipline in the school in order to later become the educators of the *Volk*. A "soldierly spirit of simplicity, obedience, and selfless devotion to duty" should dominate Alt-Rehse, as participants learned to cooperate as comrades in their service to the *Volksgesundheit*.[148] Nazi ideals of militarism clearly played a role in how these doctors were now trained. Under Hitler's totalitarian state, doctors became the army of individuals, not to defend the country from its invading enemies, but to protect the health of the *Volk*, and Alt-Rehse was their training ground.

When the training centre first opened, the medical leadership invited only National Socialist doctors in leadership positions to attend, but then opened the school to physicians at the beginning of their careers and to other professional groups who had connections to health management – namely, midwives. In 1936, for example, the school held two courses for young doctors as well as one for midwives alongside other courses for especially qualified medical practitioners and assistants. The courses for younger physicians were free and counted toward their medical internship.[149] The first National Socialist training course for female doctors at Alt-Rehse took place 16–24 September 1936. The medical leadership invited approximately 130 women physicians – most of whom were BDM doctors – from all regions of the Reich to participate. Overall, the participants reported that the course proved successful in every respect – the hospitality in the dormitories, the beauty of the landscape, and the good camaraderie among participants. *Die Ärztin* reported that all of this created the friendliest possible setting for their first experience at a large medical and ideological-political training week for female doctors.[150]

Die Ärztin viewed women physicians' participation in the training course as especially significant because for the first time, German medical authorities officially recognized the professional leadership of women. By inviting them to Alt-Rehse, according to the journal, the medical leadership acknowledged that women physicians were necessary and important members of the *Volksgemeinschaft*. This invitation also confirmed that medical authorities had accepted that women doctors required a deeper knowledge of politics and ideology (like any other professional group) to best provide for the *Volksgemeinschaft*.[151] In other words, despite all efforts to limit women's participation in the medical profession – for example, through health insurance practice and university admission regulations – the editors of the journal observed that women working in medicine finally received a stamp of approval from the profession's leaders. Even *Die Ärztin* admitted that the invitation to Alt-Rehse represented a reversal of policy, and while certain regulations against women would likely provisionally continue, they could be considered defunct. No longer, the journal predicted, would the regime attempt to gradually eradicate female doctors through economic restraint.[152]

Women physicians were hardly at the centre of the Nazi medical leadership's concerns, but the editors of the journal clearly made it seem as if they were of utmost importance. The editors likely bolstered the status of female physicians where they could, especially in light of the fact that the journal was intended not for the general public, but rather for their peers, who were still a relatively new and vulnerable readership. *Die Ärztin*'s reports about Alt-Rehse were certainly infused with propaganda, which is why I use the reports judiciously. Unfortunately, all other records and written material that capture the experiences of women doctors at Alt-Rehse were destroyed at the end of the war. The accounts of female physicians who spent time at Alt-Rehse emphasize the picturesque setting of the school, the camaraderie that developed among participants, and the structural and educational content of the training centre, which reveal more about how *Die Ärztin* chose to characterize these female physicians and the school, rather than about the physicians' experiences themselves.

In their reports about the first training course for female physicians, participants expressed how uneasy they felt upon arriving at Alt-Rehse, but how the "idyllic Mecklenburg landscape on the Tollensesee" quickly calmed all feelings of nervousness.[153] Dr Heidepriem, a head doctor (*Hauptärztin*) for the BDM, who attended the first training course, described the "tense expectations" that she and other participants felt after exiting the bus that brought them to Alt-Rehse. After receiving some food and being assigned a dorm room, usually with seven strangers, Heidepriem remarked that everything felt very unusual that first night and that sleep did not come easily.[154] Another account in *Die Ärztin* confirmed that participants felt "somewhat worried" as they were distributed into rooms with seven unknown people – something they had never experienced before.[155] Dr Gertrud Bambach's memory of the second women doctors' training course at Alt-Rehse, which took place 23–30 September 1937, also described the chaos upon their arrival at an unfamiliar train station. The participants stood together "with uncomfortable reticence" until they were pushed towards a van where they were ordered to load their suitcases, not knowing if they would ever see them again. There was no time for reflection, however, as they quickly loaded a bus and were on their way to Alt-Rehse.[156]

Despite the nervousness female physicians experienced after arriving at Alt-Rehse, or the uncomfortable feelings of sharing a room with strangers, their memories always testified to how the beauty of Alt-Rehse and the comradeship developed in the dormitories reassured them. After an uncomfortable, sleepless first night, a cruel, deafening bell roused them at 6:00 a.m. for the beginning of the day's athletic activities, regardless of the weather. This did not seem to matter to

Heidepriem, however, who noted that the morning mist and sun conjured an image of a fairy-tale landscape.[157] Bambach also observed how even in the chilly, dewy morning fog, the doctors became distracted from the activities they were doing when the sun slowly emerged over the horizon and illuminated the flags flapping in the morning wind. Such beauty encouraged them to give thanks for their experience at Alt-Rehse, according to Bambach. Even if every German doctor knew what Alt-Rehse looked like from the accounts in *Deutsches Ärzteblatt* (*German Medical Journal*), Bambach insisted that even the most perfect pictures and the most animated accounts could not come close to depicting the genuine beauty of the landscape. She thought "one had to see it with his or her own eyes and experience it with his or her own heart." Bambach described how the Tollensesee twinkled throughout the day and how the dormitories were isolated in the middle of a meadow. Even in total darkness, participants, especially those from the large city who rarely witnessed such natural beauty, could enjoy the "magical sight of a moonlit landscape." Their previous worries and the quotidian thoughts that accompanied them to Alt-Rehse "sank in the still of the night."[158]

Bambach, Heidepriem, and other women physicians claimed to feel a connection towards the beauty of the land, thus suppressing all their initial apprehensions. The participants gained a new appreciation for their Völkisch roots, more natural ways of living, and "blood and soil" – key components of both Nazi racial ideology and the *Lebensreform* movement that preceded it.[159] *Die Ärztin* reported that participants understood, for example, how the buildings and setting of Alt-Rehse consciously fit the harmony of the landscape.[160] Their experiences, therefore, allowed them to grasp how individuals could remain in touch with their Völkisch past in the face of modern urbanization and industrialization. Female physicians also reported a "spiritual revival" living and working in such a beautiful natural setting.[161]

The camaraderie that female physicians experienced at Alt-Rehse erased all of their preliminary feelings of uneasiness. What was initially an awkward situation – sleeping in a room full of strangers – quickly became the foundation of enduring friendships, according to the published reports. It was in these dorm rooms, Bambach declared, "where one did not talk about comradeship, but experienced it." To her and the other participants, "Alt-Rehse [was] more than a course, more also than just a community of female doctors." It was the beginning of an unspoken bond.[162] Heidepriem, who barely slept the first night because of the strangeness of the living situation, later attested that this style of living together was what contributed to the best camaraderie among the women – something that they hardly thought possible.[163] By the end of the course, participants reported wanting to stay longer because of the friendships they made in the dorms.[164]

Comradeship also developed outside of the dorms – through the collective march to the community house, the lining up of participants, the singing of songs, and the hoisting of flags. All of these pre-dawn activities were reminiscent of the annual Nuremberg Nazi Party Rallies. The service uniform that Alt-Rehse participants were required to wear also created a sense of unity among disparate individuals. Although there was some grumbling about not being able to wear fashionable clothing at the beginning of the first training course, one participant recounted how the matching uniforms contributed to the "unique camaraderie between 127 participants who were largely unknown to one another until now." The uniform abolished all class, age, or regional differences, and instead "quickly produced one community" – one that would endure well beyond their time in Alt-Rehse.[165] The uniform was the visible symbol of comradeship, and it stood for "recognition, prestige, and belonging"; through wearing it, these doctors were creating the *Volksgemeinschaft*.[166]

It was generally in the evenings, after the more serious activities of the day had finished, or in their free time between lectures and excursions, that participants developed the strongest sense of companionship. Heidepriem described how during their long evenings of getting to know one another, there were no strict rules and Dr Deuschl even loosened the smoking ban and allowed the young women to break curfew. These nights were full of laughter, happiness, and comfort, and in her mind they proved to be just as important at consolidating camaraderie as the excursions or more academic activities.[167] Bambach's accounts of the time "in between lectures" when they discussed their motivations, or when they sang, played sports, or collected nuts for the animals, were also some of her most memorable.[168] The same held true for Dr Elisabeth Baecker-Vowinckel, a participant at the eighth training course for female physicians, held 5–15 July 1939. She described the "spirit of comradeship" created through sailboat rides, swimming, singing, playing music, playing sports, and especially during the farewell party, when many of the doctors expressed their desire to remain at Alt-Rehse.[169] To Baecker-Vowinckel, the fact that they all felt so happy and united on this last night proved that the goals of the Nazi movement and its medical leadership had brought them closer together. She recounts, "We all put 'you' over 'I'. We did not see personal gain, but rather we only had the common higher goal in mind. It was a big family that came together in song, proud to be allowed to work for greater Germany."[170] Although these women physicians all claimed to prioritize communal interests over their own, just the opposite was taking place within the organization, as personal gain and opportunity in the medical profession and the Nazi system were likely motives for these women to attend the training camp in the first place; the training camp provided a chance for the regime to recognize them and to gain new ideological skills that would help them move through the ranks, especially as their Jewish colleagues needed replacing.

Die Ärztin highlighted recollections like this, true or not, to show that Alt-Rehse fostered feelings of solidarity that could easily be directed toward the larger Nazi regime once doctors left the training school. Participating in a march to the communal house was analogous to marching on the grounds in Nuremberg, revealing how Alt-Rehse indoctrinated participants to the ideological rituals of National Socialism. Most importantly, women doctors could convey these learned ideological practices to girls in the BDM. Because they had supposedly experienced feelings of camaraderie themselves at Alt-Rehse, they could be much more effective BDM physicians. They understood how to create comradeship among adolescent girls by singing songs and wearing matching uniforms, and they also recognized that these traditions helped absorb them into the larger Nazi state as well. However, these testimonies of the participants supposed experiences at Alt-Rehse are also shockingly infantilizing characterizations of highly accomplished professional women. The reports gush about the landscape and highlight the doctors' apprehensiveness about making friends, their misgivings about clothing, and how well they slept – all seemingly trivial matters. The editors of Die Ärztin painted an image of these doctors as overcoming their fears and creating a community at Alt-Rehse. Perhaps this was a way to assuage any fears that their readers had about joining the community of women practising medicine, and about participating in Alt-Rehse courses during an otherwise tumultuous time for doctors and German citizens overall. But such infantilizing language only reinforced the subordinate status of female physicians, who seemingly concerned themselves with inconsequential matters. The consequence of this for an organization and journal attempting to gain professional status and ground was likely the opposite of that intended.

In terms of the curriculum at Alt-Rehse, indoctrination to racial hygiene and *Blut und Boden* ideologies was quite blatant. In this sense, I agree with Anja Peters, who characterizes the school's structure and course content as promoting Völkisch, racial ideology.[171] The curriculum consisted of lectures from representatives from the genetic biological institute, the Hitler Youth, the BDM, the racial-political office of the NSDAP, and the offices for people's health and public welfare. These lectures covered everything from the Nuremberg racial laws and the education and protection of youth in associations like the Hitler Youth and the BDM, to the connected problems of abortion, venereal disease, nicotine, and alcohol. In addition, either the *Reichsärzteführer* – Wagner and then his successor Dr Leonardo Conti – or a representative from his office made the journey to Alt-Rehse to emphasize how important it was for doctors to ensure the health management of the *Volk*. These speakers, in particular, stressed the critical role doctors played in treating the large segment of the population who became unfit for work by the age of forty due to physical or mental stress. The treatment and recovery of the *Volk*, and the prevention of future disease, were the means by which doctors could serve the party and state.[172]

In the female physicians' accounts of their time at Alt-Rehse, which were biased because no journals could speak negatively about the regime, the doctors generally reacted quite positively to the lecturers. Heidepriem thought the speakers were "excellent" and considered it to be "extraordinarily gratifying" to hear several different people state that the cooperation of women doctors was both desired and necessary. She was also pleased with the fact that the medical leadership now made the education of female physicians a priority.[173] *Die Ärztin* reported that participants at the first training course understood that the lectures "served the greater goals ... of health management in the Third Reich." Women doctors may have spent only a short amount of time at Alt-Rehse, but these lectures clearly had an impact on them, as many experienced powerful motivation for the work they did in the BDM afterwards.[174] The women physicians at this first training course acknowledged the success Nazism had achieved in implementing its racial hygiene goals, and by the end they realized how the regime relied on them to preserve the legacy of the National Socialist *Kämpfertum* (struggle).[175]

The indoctrination that took place at Alt-Rehse, whether it was more indirect, through the promotion of comradeship or appreciation of the land, or more transparent, through lectures like "Influences of

Inheritance and Environment," prepared doctors for the types of work they were simultaneously doing in the BDM and RMD, and for work they might be asked to do during the Second World War. Anja Peters argues that "it is reasonable to believe that a substantial proportion of these young physicians later became active in different extermination programs and genocide actions during the war years."[176] Although there were not many female physicians directly involved in extermination and genocide, there were a few cases of women doctors openly participating in Nazi racial hygiene in authoritative positions. Dr Bahr, for one, an employee of the NSDAP's racial political office, checked for Jewish ancestors in the pedigrees of ordinary citizens. For those she found with Jewish lineage, there were disastrous consequences. Dr Herta Oberheuser, one of the most infamous of these women doctors involved in carrying out genocide, was a pediatrician who joined the Nazi Party at the age of twenty-six and eventually became employed on the medical staff at Ravensbrück, a concentration camp exclusively for women. She participated in cruel experiments and helped bring about the death of many victims. She was one of the most ambitious female professionals and also one of the most ideologically perverted. As Michael Kater writes, "To the extent that she may initially have been a victim of the politics of the Third Reich, she ended up bearing a major share of responsibility for its crimes."[177] Oberheuser was truly exceptional in how candidly she carried out the principles female doctors learned at Alt-Rehse.

The majority of female physicians brought the ideological training they received at Alt-Rehse back to their jobs in the BDM or the RMD, or conveyed it on the pages of *Die Ärztin*. Just as the medical leadership divided doctors at Alt-Rehse into three groups based on ability – experienced, intermediate, and physically handicapped – they, too, categorized their own BDM members into superior and inferior groups.[178] Not only was membership in the BDM open only to those *Mädels* deemed physically and mentally fit based on the successful completion of a medical exam, but there were also racial prerequisites to join the organization. Doctors could easily exclude girls from the BDM and even from the initial medical exam if they considered them racially inferior just by looking at them.[179] In addition, women doctors may have transferred what they learned at Alt-Rehse about championing motherhood back to their jobs within the RMD. For example, the medical leadership rewarded Alt-Rehse participants with the most children with a photo album as a special honour. Similarly, female doctors working in the RMD educated women about the incentives of being fit mothers with numerous children.[180] In both cases, mothers with large families were rewarded in a form of positive eugenics. This also coincided nicely with the government's policy of publicly honouring worthy German mothers by awarding them the *Mutterkreuz* if they had four or more children.[181]

Even if women doctors brought the principles learned at Alt-Rehse back home with them, the evidence suggests that Alt-Rehse functioned only as a teaching and preparatory site for introducing the ideology that would eventually lead to euthanasia, selections, special actions, mass sterilization, and medical experiments. It was a place for instilling theory, not for undertaking practice.[182] The editors of *Die Ärztin* presented female physicians as being pleased with their participation at the training courses at Alt-Rehse, and especially the medical leadership's acknowledgment that they played a crucial role in the promotion of the regime's ideology. These doctors already recognized the critical responsibility that women had in ensuring a healthy, future *Volk*. Women physicians also knew that they offered something unique to the Nazi state by instructing young girls and mothers about their important racial hygiene duties.[183] Now, by participating in racial hygiene training at Alt-Rehse, they portrayed themselves as fitting into the ideological medical goals of the Third Reich, and thereby the *Volksgemeinschaft*.

Conclusions: The Face of the BDÄ under Nazism

It is fair to say that the *Gleichschaltung* of the BDÄ was a success. The organization eliminated all Jews and political opponents, and Nazi sympathizers took over its leadership roles. The new editorial leadership certainly created the impression that this was an easier transition than was likely the case for many confused and disturbed doctors. The association, which was previously unaffiliated with a political party, assumed a rigid political, ideological stance – one that supported the Nazi goals of racial hygiene, and one that sought to indoctrinate women and children to become believers of Nazi ideals about health, nature, comradeship, racial biology, and proper motherhood. Atina Grossmann argues that the BDÄ easily succumbed to the pressures of Nazi coordination because the trusted language of motherhood, eugenics, and social hygiene from the Weimar Republic remained the same in the Nazi period; she claims only its meaning changed. The BDÄ did not always understand this altered language, but simply heard the familiar "motherhood-eugenics" discourse and adopted the new regime's politics.[184] While female physicians were, in fact, already familiar with class-biased eugenics because of their work in marriage counselling centres, schools, and the movement against alcoholism in the Weimar era, which allowed them to more easily accept the race-based eugenics of the Nazis, they were perhaps not as submissive as Grossmann suggests.

I instead see the BDÄ members who continued to work within the confines of Nazism as opportunistic, as they were active proponents of the services they could offer to the party and state. While the state recognized how it could employ women physicians to enlist other women and children to its causes, female doctors also identified the ways they could benefit the regime. For example, they fashioned themselves as trusted advisers for girls in the BDM and as role models for mothers in the RMD. Moreover, this type of work was a natural extension of both their activities in the home as well as the professional projects they undertook during the Weimar period. The Weimar state had already entrusted women physicians to train women to be proper mothers and to educate youth to be healthy, and this was a task women doctors succeeded at because women confided in them to a greater extent than men. Nazi medical authorities similarly recognized how appealing it was to employ women doctors, especially if they were mothers, in the BDM and RMD. Female doctors were no longer being outcast and marginalized to supplementary positions in women's and children's health that were part-time, that did not pay very well, and that were undesirable during the Weimar era. They were now working under a state and within state organizations that upheld women's and children's health, and therefore the work they specialized in was essential to Germany's future. By situating their activities within existing frameworks, members of the BDÄ adopted Nazi ideology.

This is not to say that all women physicians accepted and promoted Nazism. As Gisela Bock has pointed out, women under Nazism could become victims, perpetrators, bystanders, and followers, and sometimes fell under more than one category at different times or even concurrently.[185] For Jewish doctors, who were approximately one-third of women doctors in the BDÄ before 1933, Nazism meant loss of citizenship, emigration for the fortunate, and death for those unable to escape the so-called Final Solution.[186] The other two-thirds, the non-Jewish German female physicians, had careers that spanned the Weimar Republic and the Nazi regime. Many of these women claimed their value to both the Weimar and the Nazi regimes by placing themselves at the centre of women's and children's medicine. The Nazis created a very different version of the welfare state than that created in the Weimar Republic, though it was still focused on protecting women and children, meaning that women doctors could still appropriate the rhetoric of the state in order to articulate their professional identities. Under the German dictatorship, however, the welfare state supported women and children only insofar as the ideological aims of the regime could also be maintained, which was quite distinct from the social welfare provisions of the first German democracy. The same could be said about protecting women and children during total war as well.

5 Advocating Healthy Infant Nutrition Practices through Breast Milk Collection: Maternal Guardians on the Home Front

As the Nazis blatantly mobilized for war, a few female physicians carved out another novel professional space; they presented themselves as model caregivers for Germany's mothers and infants through the collection of breast milk. Breast milk collection facilities (*Frauenmilchsammelstellen*; FMS), which had existed in Germany since 1919, were intended to collect milk from women who produced a surplus and to redistribute it to sick, weak, or premature infants, or to women who did not produce a sufficient amount. With war looming, higher rates of infant mortality for bottle-fed children, and constant fears about a healthy *Volksgemeinschaft* (people's community) always in the background, the women doctors involved claimed that their experiences as mothers made them particularly suited to help a large number of vulnerable and sick infants through breast milk collection. They legitimized their work based on certain characteristics – nurturance, care, and empathy. By claiming that these "feminine" characteristics and experiences made them more capable of promoting nursing and breast milk donation among mothers, they offered something unique that their male colleagues did not because they understood the female experience of breastfeeding. Maternalism proved to be the means for female doctors to portray themselves as the leaders on the home front; the unique womanly act of breastfeeding, which many of them had done at home in their capacity as mothers, could now be translated into this new workspace and become vital for the nation. This was a strategic way for women doctors – whether intended or not – to gain new opportunities while the medical profession and the Nazi regime tried to sideline them throughout the early 1930s.

War changed much about science and medicine in German society – where scientific resources were filtered, how guidelines intended to secure the health and "racial purity" of Germans were compromised, and who could participate in scientific and medical endeavours. Michael Kater has noted how the outbreak of war changed the position of women in medicine, stating that "after the war started, and because Jewish doctors were rejected, married women doctors were called back to clinics, and the number of those unemployed decreased steadily from 1939 to 1942."[1] Although they were primarily working on the home front, war did not exist as a separate entity from everyday civilian life and certainly touched the lives of women doctors who often had close contact with the nation's female and youth civilians.[2] Female doctors recognized how the war exacerbated the central value the regime placed on women and youth because model mothers who would raise healthy children (who would become the nation's future soldiers) were increasingly vital to the war effort.[3] Some of these physicians also identified how a total war mentality could be spread to a mundane site of everyday life – breast milk collection – which they laboured to make even more central to the regime.[4]

Breast milk collection had started twenty years earlier, but with the build-up and eventual outbreak of war, female physicians (and the regime itself) took greater interest in this field. Female physicians linked breast milk collection to wartime nutrition, as they highlighted ways to maximize Germany's natural resources (which included breast milk) and its labour supply in a time of total war. The few women doctors involved in collection efforts emphasized the maternal expertise they could offer to women, whose bodies and labour were essential to the Nazi wartime state. They claimed they could exploit a unique natural resource during wartime – one that was unique to women and that they were uniquely positioned to help exploit. They drew regional and national attention and funding to breast milk collection, and by doing so, the number of facilities expanded as did women physicians' roles within them. The more important breast milk collection became to Nazi wartime efforts, the more vital women doctors working in this field became to the regime.

By underscoring their importance to wartime nutrition plans like breast milk collection, some female physicians were able to raise their own status in the profession as they became experts in this new field. This is especially true of Dr Marie-Elise Kayser, who founded the first breast milk collection facility in Magdeburg, made the promotion of breast milk collection her life's work, and became an expert for those within Germany and outside of it interested in opening their own facilities.

Although her early efforts can be seen as an innocuous attempt to help sick and weak infants in the aftermath of the First World War, the claims she made about the benefits of breast milk collection in the buildup to war and her attempts to gain the support of the Nazi regime show her as a pivotal actor under Nazism.[5] Adelheid von Saldern has argued "that the war was not merely a masculine venture."[6] Similarly, Nicole Kramer demonstrates that women were not merely objects of the Nazi government, but rather sought to shape and reshape their wartime roles within it.[7] This was certainly the case for Kayser. She understood that the more attention and funding that breast milk collection received from the Nazi regime (which took over its supervision and regulation in 1936), the wider the network of facilities, the more infants would benefit, and the more her own work and that of her colleagues would profit. In their breast milk collection efforts, doctors like Kayser certainly participated in a system that Wendy Lower states "granted [women] new benefits, opportunities and raised status."[8] In Kayser's case, that elevated status came in the form of both regional, national, and international recognition for breast milk collection, as well as a solidified place in medicine for herself and her colleagues.

In addition to gaining professional opportunities, Kayser and her colleagues advocated for nursing women's rights in the workplace at a time when this was largely unheard of. They did this, however, by making claims that they knew what was best for other women and their bodies. Moreover, after 1939 they were largely doing it in the name of the Nazi agenda, as they advocated that other women's bodies (and their resources) be used for the war effort. While this allowed women doctors to participate in and influence the new field of breast milk collection, they were making professional gains on the backs – or the breasts – of other women.[9]

Early Breast Milk Collection Efforts

Breast milk collection preceded Nazism. In the early twentieth century, in an attempt to improve infant welfare, reformers established "milk kitchens," which offered working-class mothers sterilized cow's milk at subsidized prices. Despite their positive reception, reformers then turned their efforts toward the opening of infant welfare centres, which at first provided mothers with sterilized milk and free advice, but then focused on educating mothers and tracking infant development.[10] The systematic collection of surplus breast milk had started in Vienna in

1909.[11] Because of the increasing need for wet nurses and the uncertainty of feeding vulnerable infants, doctors Ernst Mayerhofer and Ernst Pibram started collecting breast milk on a small scale in two children's clinics. They established a Centre for Breast Milk Care, which was unknown to Kayser when she set up her first facility, but it served as a precedent to later ones. In Vienna, the breast milk did not come from private donors, but exclusively from the birthing and women's clinic. In addition, surplus milk was used only by institutions and was not dispensed to private households. Mayerhofer's and Pibram's attempts did not last and were quickly forgotten.[12]

Kayser, who was among the first generation of female physicians, became aware of the importance of breast milk around the same time that Mayerhofer and Pibram began collecting surplus milk. Born in 1885 in Görlitz, Kayser started her medical study in Berlin and eventually enrolled in medical school in Jena. While in medical school, she studied for a semester in Rome, where she lived in her brother's house and witnessed an Italian wet nurse save her severely ill niece from dying. For the first time, Kayser clearly realized the immense importance of breast milk.[13] She passed the state medical exam in Jena in April 1911, and the next month, she began working as a medical intern on the obstetric ward at the university women's hospital in Jena, as well as in the department of internal medicine at the city hospital in Magdeburg. That summer, Kayser became the first female to receive her medical degree in Jena. The following year, she received her medical licence and became the first female physician in Jena. Thereafter, she briefly worked as a pediatrician in the university children's hospital in Heidelberg and then at the city children's hospital in Magdeburg.

Kayser opened her own pediatric practice in 1915, where she experienced the importance of breast milk and saw the daily difficulties of feeding infants. Witnessing the painful years of hunger and how this affected premature babies and sick, weak infants who lacked sufficient food, she sought out ways to improve their chance of survival. During the war, she saw that facilities were set up to collect valuable materials for the general population; the same, she thought, could be done with surplus breast milk, which she had often watched thrown out or fed to dogs.[14] In a medical news article for Saxony-Anhalt, one doctor reported that breast milk was even used as milk for coffee.[15] Kayser claimed that "probably no time was as advantageous for this idea [of breast milk collection] as the war years, which sharpened the sense of responsibility for all salvageable items."[16] Women's malnutrition during the war also

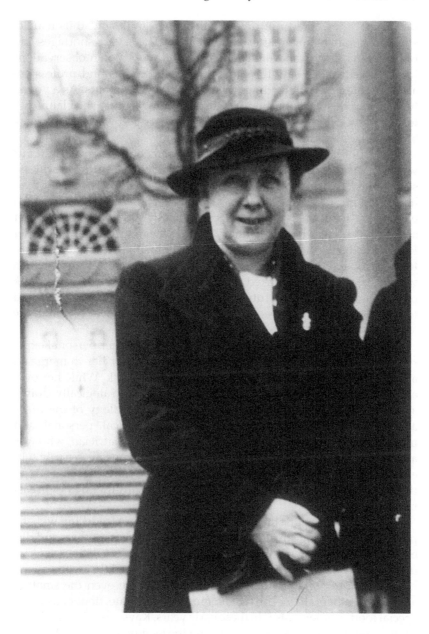

5.1 Dr Marie-Elise Kayser (1885–1950). Stadtarchiv Erfurt Photo Archive.

meant that they could not produce their own milk, and thus usually stopped nursing shortly after giving birth.[17] The severe shortages and hunger caused by war were coupled with Kayser's own observations in her practice. She saw the difficulties both parents and professionals encountered when feeding premature and new infants. As a young female specialist starting her own practice in wartime, she claims her teachers' shocking words often rang in her ears: "'If we had had more breast milk, the child would have been saved!'"[18]

In addition to witnessing the practical needs of mothers and infants who faced shortages, hunger, and lack of nutrients during war, Kayser claimed that her own experiences of "womanhood and motherhood" led her to the idea of breast milk collection.[19] Kayser conceived of the idea for a breast milk collection facility a few weeks after her son, Ruprecht, was born in January 1919: "One night a few weeks after Ruprecht's birth, the idea suddenly came to me that you must do this. It was probably because once again, I was swimming in milk which was overflowing. This stirred a decision to conserve the surplus milk of nursing women in the future based on the Weckschen method and to make it available for needy children. And I could never get rid of the idea."[20]

Her reflections on this moment demonstrate how her personal experiences as a mother provided convenient rhetoric for her to merge an archetype of maternal care into her professional work. While her own experiences were certainly sincere, she may have strategically drawn attention to them because it suited the gender ideology of the times and legitimized her work in this field. Her practical, personal, and maternal concerns overlapped: "As a practising pediatrician, who was at the same time a mother of a small child, it was for me necessarily self-evident to try to make this surplus useful in the right places."[21] After that, she became, as she claimed, "obsessed" with the idea of breast milk collection.[22]

Kayser opened the first breast milk facility in 1919 in Magdeburg with the purpose of collecting surplus breast milk from nursing mothers and directing it to those who medically needed it – namely *"ernährungsgestörte"* (nutritionally disturbed) children. A local ad requested that women who had ample nutrients for their own children donate even the smallest amount for others. To incentivize women to participate, donors received special food supplements.[23] In these early years, Kayser worked tirelessly to encourage women to donate milk, and the facility collected 1,973 litres of breast milk within its first four years of existence.[24] However, despite her efforts and her strong disagreement to any opposition this first facility elicited, it closed as a result of postwar economic inflation.[25]

Nevertheless, the idea of collecting and redistributing surplus breast milk lived on. In 1925, Kayser and her husband, Konrad Kayser, relocated to Erfurt, where he became the director of the state women's clinic. In 1927, the two of them established a breast milk collection facility in connection with the clinic where he worked. In Erfurt, Marie-Elise Kayser devised the scientific method and operation for breast milk collection that would serve as a model and educational training ground for other facilities, not just in Germany but abroad. A doctor in the Soviet Union, Marie Marezkaja, wrote to Kayser in 1930 to tell her they were replicating the Erfurt model of breast milk collection there.[26] Thereafter during the 1930s and 1940s, almost fifty breast milk collection facilities opened in German territory, following the Erfurt example.

The Establishment and Operation of Breast Milk Collection Facilities

Kayser was a strong advocate for breast milk collection facilities from their inception until her death and became an expert on the establishment and operation of these facilities. At the Erfurt facility, she founded a school so that interested parties could come and familiarize themselves with the work and create new facilities based on the Erfurt model. Along with two nurses, Kayser trained and familiarized doctors and midwives in the daily operation and examination methods. Erfurt, thus, became the centre of a national and eventually an international network of breast milk collection facilities. Kayser wrote prolifically about the establishment and operation of facilities, publishing countless articles on the topic and delivering numerous lectures to medical organizations, women's groups, and even schools.[27] In 1940, she published a book, *Breast Milk Collection Facilities: A Guide for their Establishment and Operation*, summarizing much of her doctrine about breast milk collection.[28]

It became clear from Kayser's initial pleas to mothers in all circles of the population that her feelings about helping humanity as a whole were particularly strong. She sought to find the greatest possible circle of private donors who would be willing to collect their milk in their own homes and then donate it to a facility for free or for a small fee in order to save as many nutritionally disturbed or vulnerable infants as possible.[29] Two of Kayser's peers, doctors Irma Feldweg and Friedrich Eckardt, who looked to Kayser when starting their own facilities in Pforzheim and Plauen respectively, claimed that this was a "truly social feeling of communal work," created without profiting anyone. In fact, breast milk should benefit children from all circles of the population.[30] While middle- and upper-class doctors would do the collecting, the initial donors (who were compensated) and recipients of breast milk appeared to come from all classes. This shifted once the Nazis came to power, as the regime required women to be medically examined before donating their breast milk, and presumably only members of the *Volk* were the recipients of breast milk.

Kayser's systematic method of collecting surplus breast milk placed special value on the strong medical monitoring of the entire operation in order to meet all health and hygiene requirements. When authorities later inspected the facility, it was often considered to be an exemplary model of health.[31] Kayser pleaded with mothers all throughout Germany to collect their excess milk within their own homes for donation to newly opened breast milk collection facilities. She demanded that the purity and integrity of the milk be regularly checked – an idea that was completely groundbreaking in Germany.[32] Breast milk stations, which emerged around the same time in the US, also strictly enforced hygienic procedures and monitored mothers.[33] The new German facilities would consist of a kitchen for the examination and preparation of milk, an office, an examination room for milk donors and their children, a lab, and a freezer or cool room for the storage of milk. While Kayser recognized the capability of a breast milk collection facility to thrive as a private, commercial enterprise, she rejected this idea as being inconsistent with the communal values of breast milk collection.[34] Because breast milk collection was relatively unknown, an affiliation with a state, city, or other similar public institution would ensure its survival.

In addition to the ideological basis behind breast milk collection as a communal enterprise, Kayser recognized numerous practical reasons for connecting collection facilities with city or state institutions such as a women's clinic or a children's hospital. For one, these types of institutions contained a large number of potential donors in the form of newly parturient mothers, thus streamlining the process for finding, educating, and examining them. These establishments also contained a plethora of women who had general nursing needs, either because of illness, complications during birth, or premature birth. Cooperation with a clinic or hospital, then, would offer the breast milk collection facility the opportunity to draw from a large pool of potential donors and link them up with women, who, for one reason or another, could not sufficiently nurse. Moreover, a collection facility with an affiliation could operate at a considerably lower cost than if it operated alone because in addition to providing the necessary room and inventory, a woman's clinic or children's hospital also had extra assistants on hand to help with the collection itself.[35]

The nature of the collection process was essential to the goals of the breast milk collection facility, according to Kayser. She recommended that the collectors be friendly, sociable people who also understood the worries of housewives. For this reason, she advocated that the work be carried out by women, stating that when the Erfurt facility was forced to employ a man as a collector, it learned that this came with disadvantages.[36] In her book, Kayser adopted maternalist rhetoric that she and female physicians would use to push for a feminine presence and authority in breast milk collection. She implied that only women could empathize with the needs of housewives because of their potential shared experiences. With this in mind, Kayser suggested that women's organizations could also offer assistance once facilities grew so large that one collector was no longer sufficient. Women's organizations could collect the surplus milk from people's homes in different parts of the city and bring it to so-called lower collection facilities, which could be housed in schools, factories, hotels, or – as the Magdeburg facility found to be quite convenient because of its ready-to-use refrigerator storage – in a dairy. Bottles were collected daily, but on Sundays, women or, in many cases, men and older children took to bringing the surplus milk into the facilities themselves.[37]

Breast milk collection facilities compensated the donors less if they had to send couriers to pick up the milk in order to offset the cost of transportation. Collection by foot was only possible, of course, in smaller cities and in the immediate area around collection facilities. Couriers who travelled by foot carried a briefcase with enough room for ten 200-gram bottles or two litres of milk. Bicycle couriers usually had a bottle basket attached to their bikes. Bicycles and motorcycles or delivery vans were advantageous because they were not confined to specific routes, but a driver would be needed if a facility was going to use a motorcycle or van for collection, which added additional costs. If using the streetcar or public bus for collection purposes, it was appropriate, according to Kayser, for couriers to be allowed to ride free of charge or with a discount. She worked tirelessly to get reduced rates for the transport of

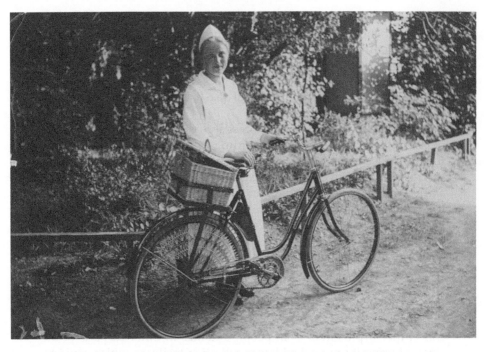

5.2 Milk pickup via bike courier. Stadtarchiv Erfurt Photo Archive.

breast milk. In light of the importance of breast milk collection facilities for population politics, Lufthansa offered the Erfurt facility a 50 per cent discount on the transport of breast milk and the Reich Train Management eventually created specific guidelines to address the reduced transport rates for breast milk.[38] The facility in Plauen, founded in 1938, worked out a 50 per cent discount with the public bus line to deliver milk daily to remote infant homes.[39] If funds increased, a collection facility could acquire its own car with an expanded back seat and metal sheet box with ice that could hold up to one hundred 200-gram bottles.[40] An individual facility often covered considerable distances depending on how big the city was. Travelling twenty, forty, or even one hundred kilometres in a day to retrieve milk was not a rarity. In Plauen, breast milk collectors covered 7,000 kilometres in one year.[41] Kayser suggested that nurses were the best people to do this collection work.

Doctors Friedrich Eckardt and Irma Feldweg, both heavily involved in advocating breast milk collection facilities and setting up their own facilities, wrote a history of the facilities and the process of collecting milk in 1954, entitled *Breast Milk Collection Facilities: The Meaning and Development of Breast Milk Collection Facilities*. They agreed that it had always been and always would be important for facilities to find assistants who had an interest in their activities. For them, this meant using people like midwives and nurses because of their professional backgrounds and "womanly approach." These women, they claimed, would likely know which mothers would produce a surplus of milk and would be best able to answer questions from donors about nutrition and the development of their children. When visiting homes on a daily basis, women leaders of the collection facilities – whether they were doctors, nurses, or midwives – developed friendly connections with donors and thus could educate and influence women within their own homes.[42] Eckardt and Feldweg also claimed that women in the medical profession were uniquely positioned to move their work from the breast milk collection facility into the home because of a strong convergence between their professional and personal lives. After all, the act of breastfeeding was a topic that many of them were familiar with either from their personal experiences as mothers or from conversations with their patients.

This rhetorical intrusion into the private sphere was analogous to women school doctors' conversations advocating for their own health parenting in people's homes during the Weimar period. The intrusion into private life happened as part of infant welfare measures even before the Weimar Republic and then accompanied the growth of the Weimar welfare state. As Mark Mazower demonstrates, "the idea that family health concerned society more generally" and that the "state should therefore intervene in private life to show people how to live" were characteristic of Weimar Germany and several other European states in the interwar period.[43] This became even more glaring under Nazism, as discourse sometimes turned to practice, for example, when women entered other women's homes to examine homes, pick up breast milk, and potentially advise mothers. For the most part, the blurring of public and private boundaries remained discursive under the Nazis and, as Elizabeth Whitaker shows, was characteristic of fascism in general, as medical ideas became connected to national, political, and demographic aspirations, therefore "justifying the intervention of experts in women's behavior in the home and opening the private sphere into the public domain."[44] Validating this idea, Joseph Goebbels, Hitler's propaganda minister, rallied women to put their personal comfort and private needs behind national duty in his famous 1943 speech on total war.[45]

Kayser also saw women and women's organizations as the most fitting advertising platform for breast milk collection. Midwives who worked in maternity hospitals monitored the great majority of births, and therefore could recruit women who were nursing to donate their surplus breast milk. Eventually, the Nazi Party's women's organizations, especially the Reich Mothers' Service, served as an excellent space to show instructional films and tables about the worth of breast milk collection. In at least one state, Thuringia, the Reich Mothers' Service showed an instructional film about breast milk collection during its mothers' training course.[46] The ideology of breast milk collection could be promoted in girls' schools, especially upper women's schools and in the League of German Girls, whose members could actually participate in the operation of facilities by bringing in the milk from donors who lived out of town. Kayser admitted that based on her own experience, "the advertising coming from the closest personally interested circles has considerably more success than calls aimed at the general public in the newspaper."[47] Kayser recognized the importance of human contact, especially between women, in promoting breast milk collection, and she even offered to rent out an instructional film and visual aids from the Erfurt facility to women's organizations to assist the cause.[48]

Once donors were identified, they underwent considerable screening before they were actually permitted to start donating to a breast milk collection facility. During their first visit to the facility, donors registered with a midwife, nurse, or doctor by filling out a form with personal information, including facts about the birth of their child and any past births or stillbirths. The donors had to produce a medical health certificate clearing them of any obstacles to donating breast milk. Because breast milk was to be used for a stranger's child, only donors who were medically cleared, according to Eckardt and Feldweg, should be allowed to donate milk. This meant that women should be free of infectious diseases of the skins, lungs, intestines, and blood.[49] While Kayser made no declarations about race in her book or publications, it would become clear that under the Nazis, only Aryans should be donating milk. If a woman was to become a donor, the leader of the facility would find a bed for her, give her a medical examination, discuss any questions about nursing, and show her the particulars of extracting excess breast milk. Facility leaders noted the domestic and social conditions of donors and knowledge of any diseases on index cards and stored them in the facility's donor files.[50] This included information about their husbands' professions and if they received unemployment support.

Aufnahme am *12. VIII 34.*

Name: *Lieselotte H.*   Wohnung: *Ottostr. 9.*

Tag der Entbindung: *2. VIII 34.*   Alter der Frau: *23 Jahr.*

Hebamme: *Schwester L.*

Zahl der Geburten: *1. Partus*   Zahl der lebenden Kinder: *1*

Fehlgeburten: *—*   Grund: *—*

Krankheiten: *Blinddarmoperation. Keine Hustenerkrankungen.*

Beruf des Mannes: *Kaufmann (Generalvertreter)*

Bemerkungen: *Mutter der Spend. 3 Kinder, viel Milch großmütter „ 8 „ alle gestillt.*

Zur Untersuchung bestellt: *15. VIII. 34.*

5.3 Admission card. Image from Kayser, *Frauenmilchsammelstellen*.

Class status was a consideration for the proper storage and donation of breast milk, perhaps because medical professionals had long assumed that working-class individuals did not always live in the most hygienic conditions. Within the course of the first week following registration, a nurse from the collection facility would visit the home of a potential donor and obtain information about the number of rooms in the house, the position of the rooms, especially the kitchen, and the location of milk storage. Such information was important so that facility leaders could give valuable pointers on the hygienic storage of milk. A living room that faced south, for example, frequently resulted in a higher risk of milk souring, and therefore women needed to take special measures to store milk properly.[51] This information and data from subsequent medical check-ups, which happened on a regular basis in order to ensure the health of the donor and the continued usage of her breast milk, were filed away with the registration forms.[52]

After donors went through this initial screening, they began the process of collecting their surplus breast milk. A donor would fully empty her breasts after each feeding by collecting excess milk in 200-gram bottles. The donor requested as many bottles as she wanted from the collector, who dropped off empty bottles and picked up full bottles on a daily basis. Each bottle was affixed with the registration number of the respective donor. Kayser found that, based on her experience, women learned to express their milk by hand quite easily. They would either collect extra milk in a water glass or funnel it directly into one of the bottles.[53] They would gather surplus milk from individual feedings in a single bottle. The complete emptying of the breast could not always be achieved by hand, and thus donors used small pumps for this purpose. Kayser, Eckardt, and Feldweg all recommended a few different brands. Clinics usually used an electronic pump, but at home, women used a couple of different small, glass hand pumps made to extract excess milk. They were easy to use and clean. Often, the breast milk collection facilities would loan out milk pumps for donors to use. In order to clean the milk pumps before use, donors had to rinse them and then boil them. Collection facilities always risked pumps shattering and had to account for this in terms of overall cost. Kayser also noticed that pumped milk was much more acidic than milk expressed by hand, and therefore, in the Erfurt facility, she allowed only milk obtained by hand.[54]

Once it was extracted, the donors were required to cool milk as quickly as possible. Therefore, they were instructed to store it in a cool and dark location until it was collected. Stone pots filled with cold water often proved the most useful for this purpose, according to Kayser.[55] Eckardt and Feldweg recommended sealing the breast milk in a cold pot with cold water and keeping it in the coldest room in the house, which in warm seasons meant storing it in the basement if one was available.[56] Cleanliness and storage had to be a top priority for donors in order to preserve breast milk from contamination and decomposition.

Once collectors retrieved the full bottles and replaced them with empty ones, they registered the amount of milk taken from each donor in the main collection book at the collection facility.[57] A page from the Erfurt collection book, for example, shows that in November 1936, fourteen different women donated an average of 15.2 litres of milk, with the majority of them (nine) donating milk daily.[58] Facilities also maintained index cards with the names of donors, the years they donated to the clinic, the amount of time they donated for, how many litres they donated, and how much they got paid. Women donated sometimes only a few days and at other times up to a year. For example, Frau Margarete donated 119.275 litres of milk between July 1932 and

5.4 Index card for Frau Margarete. Index cards from the donor index of the Erfurt collection facility, Stadtarchiv Erfurt.

April 1933, earning 289.19 Reichsmarks. Frau Ruth donated 77.650 litres between August 1932 and January 1933, earning 194.13 Reichsmarks.[59] Donors could also, naturally, keep their own record of the amount of milk donated. This made it easier to calculate the total number of litres donated at the end of each month. The daily amount of milk collected from one donor varied from 100 grams to 500 grams or even 1 or 2 litres; in exceptional cases, donors donated up to 3 litres a day. After the breast milk collection facility noted the amount of milk, the workers examined each bottle of milk for amount, acidity, bacterial content, and whether it contained any cow's milk or water additives. Kayser designed a procedure to determine if a bottle contained cow's milk, which entailed illuminating each bottle daily with a sunlamp in a dark chamber; breast milk would show up as a violet-blue colour versus cow's milk, which was yellow. Water additives could be tested by weighing the milk.[60] Once all bottles were individually tested, the milk from different donors was poured together and then refilled into fresh, sterilized bottles to be sent out for delivery.

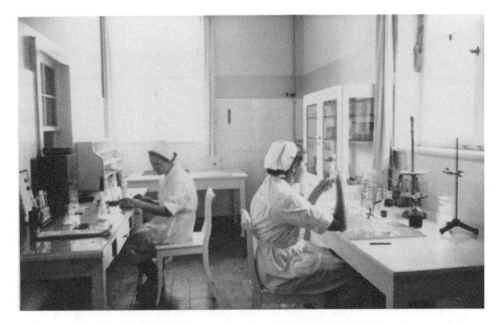

5.5   Examination room. Photograph material for the tenth anniversary of the Erfurt collection facility. Stadtarchiv Erfurt Photo Archive.

Breast milk was distributed in its natural form after being sterilized, but also in powder and frozen form. Prior to delivery, it was stored in a cool room or freezer at the facility. Facilities then delivered the milk to sick or vulnerable infants; this was, after all, the basis for the establishment of such institutions, according to Eckardt and Feldweg, and therefore, all precautions were taken to provide it only to mothers truly in need and to avoid giving milk to those who were simply lazy about nursing.[61] This was seemingly a rarity, given the high cost of cow's milk and the widespread promotion of nursing (over the use of formula) in popular medical and women's journals at the time. Although the class background of donors was unknown, Kayser remained committed to ensuring that women of all classes received the milk: "it was one of the basic conditions of the breast milk collection facility, on which it was built from the beginning, that the milk of the collection facility is available for children of all mothers, for the poor as well as for the rich."[62] Kayser's original altruistic idea of providing milk to women of all classes fit well with the Weimar welfare state, which favoured the

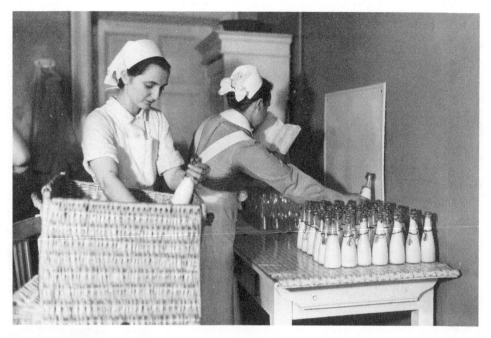

5.6 Nurses from the Erfurt collection facility packing sterilized milk for shipment. Stadtarchiv Erfurt Photo Archive.

community over the individual, and it was easily translatable to Nazi ideals of creating and serving a collective *Volk*.

Facilities issued milk to infants according to medical prescriptions, which were required in order to receive milk; if the prescription was not received, the milk delivery was cancelled. Facilities also supplied breast milk to the large children's clinics, infant homes, or women's hospitals with which they were often affiliated; recipients had to pay for the prescribed milk, but often the cost was fully covered by health insurance.[63] Private paying customers who lived in the cities of breast milk collection facilities had to pick up the milk themselves. Customers who lived outside the cities received milk in wooden crates either by car or often as express goods by train and, in rare cases, even by airplane. In the first six years of the Erfurt facility, milk was sent to ninety-nine different places, including the Rhine, the North Sea, and Upper Silesia.[64]

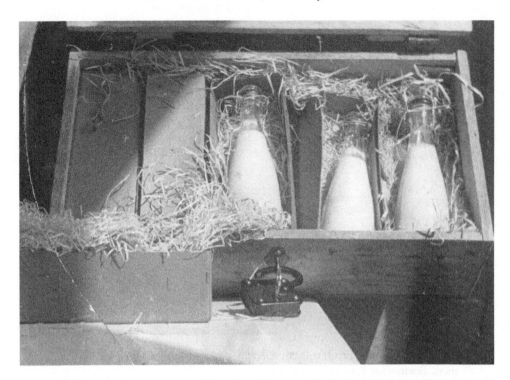

5.7 Erfurt transport crate with bottles of breast milk. Stadtarchiv Erfurt Photo Archive.

Eckardt and Feldweg noted that there were cases in which the Erfurt facility transported breast milk by airplane to the sick children of German families in Japan and South America.[65] In one case in which milk was sent with a German family to Tokyo, the family wrote from the Imperial Hotel there, stating that the milk, which was stored in a refrigerator, proved to be excellent, and confirmed that the child was "always cheerful and healthy."[66]

Proper packaging was essential and constituted a large portion of the daily work of a breast milk collection facility. Bottles were packaged with excelsior or corrugated cardboard and wood shavings in carefully prepared cartons so that they were unbreakable, and then placed in the wood crates. Each crate also contained return shipment instructions.[67]

Breast milk collection facilities compensated donors for the milk they donated. Eckardt and Feldweg thought this should be "obvious" even though they argued that no monetary sum was worth that of the donated milk.[68] When Kayser started the first breast milk collection facility after the First World War, she thought it was important to at least give mothers the equivalent nutrients to replace those lost when nursing. When the Magdeburg facility opened immediately after the war, she suggested that mothers be compensated in the form of food rations rather than money. For each litre of milk, at Kayser's request, the Food Administration offered donors half a pound of flour, corn flour, or sugar, and, regardless of quantity of milk donated, one pound of rice and an eighth of a pound of butter per week. Although "this seems little to us today ... at that time it was riches," Kayser wrote in *Hospital Social Service*, and it often spurred women to donate more milk, especially before Christmas and Easter because a loaf of bread made of flour, butter, and sugar was "an unattainable luxury."[69] It is unclear how long these contributions lasted, especially in light of the postwar food shortages, but it was clear that Kayser knew she needed to incentivize women to donate milk. Her hope was that women, regardless of class, would presumably donate more milk during times of crisis – for example, wartime – because basic foodstuffs and reliable salaries were scarce.

Over time, collection facilities compensated donors more frequently with money. By the end of the Second World War, the going rate for breast milk in all of Germany was consistently set at 2.50 Reichsmarks, which was about ten times the price of a litre of cow's milk. At the Erfurt facility, donors who were not local received 2.10 Reichsmarks per litre of breast milk because the collection facility paid the transportation expenses.[70] At the Pforzheim facility, established in 1935 and the seventh one founded in Germany, Dr Emmi Justi explained how they compensated donors 2.50 Reichsmarks per litre for milk that was brought in and 2 Reichsmarks if the milk had to be picked up.[71] Kayser specified that mothers earned an average of 30–40 Reichsmarks per month, and noted that, since an unemployed family with two children received about 70 Reichsmarks per month, "this revenue was a good contribution to livelihood."[72] Dr von Lölhöffel estimated that women could earn on average 60 to 80 Reichsmarks per month, occasionally upwards of 100 to 140 Reichsmarks if they had an abundance of milk.[73] Such appeals were likely aimed at lower-class women who may have found donating breast milk a consistent source of income.[74]

Kayser's manual on the establishment and operation of breast milk collection demonstrates just one example of her expertise on the subject. In addition, Eckardt, Feldweg, and many others praised Kayser's expertise and the Erfurt facility for setting an example for the establishment of other facilities within Germany and abroad. Once the Nazis came to power, Kayser and breast milk collection would become even more significant.

The Growth of Breast Milk Collection under Nazism

While Kayser's intentions for setting up breast milk collection facilities in 1919 in Magdeburg or even in 1926 in Erfurt were seemingly altruistic, after 1933 she was more resourceful. She recognized how the resources and authority of the Nazi regime could help broaden her efforts because nursing and breast milk collection fit seamlessly with Nazi ideology; similar to her colleagues working for the BDM and the RMD, she benefited from the increased attention on motherhood. As early as 1935, Kayser wrote to Dr Karl Astel, president of the Thuringia State Office for Racial Affairs, to schedule a meeting to discuss breast milk collection. Over the following year, she encouraged him on several occasions to visit the Erfurt facility in order to see the advantages of breast milk collection. The demand for milk all over Germany was now so great, she said, that she did not know how she would meet all requests, but she believed that if Astel showed interest in breast milk collection, they "would certainly gain the cooperation of a large portion of the population," and thus, could bring in significantly more milk and raise general awareness.[75] Kayser's appeals to this local Office for Racial Affairs indicate an early attempt to gain the support of regional leaders in order to expand her project. She was also pleading with Astel, one of the regime's leading racial hygienists, demonstrating that she at least tolerated the regime's racial ideology enough to want to work with him.

Her correspondence with state authorities in Thuringia then became more ambitious. The Erfurt facility received official approval from the Reich Ministry of the Interior in May 1937.[76] In September of that year, Kayser recognized the importance of her race in trying to solicit the attention of the *Reichsärzteführer* (Reich Physicians' Leader) Gerhard Wagner, as she highlighted her "pure Aryan descent" as well as her husband's in an inquiry to speak personally with him about breast milk collection. Such efforts clearly worked in her favour because Wagner appeared to grant her a meeting and asked for a summary of her thoughts and suggestions regarding breast milk collection. In her report, she highlighted the amount of milk disbursed over the past ten years as well as the number of donors, and she requested a follow-up meeting with Wagner to discuss how to increase the number of voluntary donors and the type of propaganda allowed from the medical point of view.[77] Kayser's appeals to the Reich Physicians' Leader demonstrate a change in her expectations of breast milk collection facilities; no longer did they merely exist to aid a community of women who could not produce enough milk for their sick, weak, or premature infants, but she now recognized how they might aid the entire *Volk*. More importantly, she grasped how the regime might help fuel her project. After all, she was trying to gain the ear of none other than the top medical leader – a strategy that would only help further breast milk collection efforts.

As Kayser's overtures toward the regime increased, so too did perceptions of her expertise and authority on breast milk collection. Kayser turned to writing reports for the Reichsgesundheitsamt (Reich Health Bureau) on the art of sterilization and the length of preservation.[78] At the beginning of 1936, on the suggestion of Dr Leonardo Conti, who was Prussian State Council and chairman of the Reichsarbeitsgemeinschaft für Mutter und Kind (Reich Working Group for Mother and Child; RAfMuK) at the time, a working committee formed to discuss the question of propagating breast milk collection facilities, to be affiliated with the RAfMuK. The Merseburg State Council, Dr Hans Tießler, and Conti sought Kayser's guidance in justifying the creation of new facilities. In her response, Kayser enthusiastically supported the affiliation with the RAfMuK in order to quickly help establish new facilities. "It will be a load off my mind if there are new collection facilities," she said, because the current facilities could no longer satisfy the demand for milk.[79]

By the fall 1936, breast milk collection had become a priority for the Nazis, who effectively took over its supervision and regulation. Although facilities could still be affiliated with private hospitals or institutions, the RAfMuK took over the supervision of all breast milk collection facilities, soliciting Kayser's expertise once again as they informed her of their intentions to draw up "Guidelines for the Establishment and Operation of Breast Milk Collection Facilities."[80] In 1937, the new leader of the RAfMuK, A. Schöbel, wrote to Kayser requesting a meeting to further orient himself with her work in breast milk collection and to discuss the guidelines. Whereas a couple of years earlier Kayser had had to plead with Astel to pay a visit to the Erfurt facility, this time Schöbel arranged to immediately travel to Erfurt.[81] After months of consulting with Kayser, in July 1939, the Reich Ministry of the Interior approved the guidelines, which aligned the work of all existing and new breast milk collection facilities throughout the Reich.[82] These guidelines included specifics about the goals, funding, support, and precise operation for such facilities, down to the exact number of bottles needed. After that, any new facility had to register with the RAfMuK, and all new leaders of breast milk collection facilities had to successfully complete training in Erfurt.[83] The medical profession credited Kayser for her "untiring work" to get these guidelines passed.[84] Kayser and Erfurt had been firmly established as the de facto centre of breast milk collection.

By July 1939, fourteen new breast milk collection facilities had been founded based on the Erfurt model. In addition, similar institutions abroad either sent someone to visit Erfurt or initiated written personal correspondence with Kayser and operated according to the same methods as the Erfurt facility. These included institutes in Switzerland, the Soviet Union, Hungary, Italy, Sweden, Argentina, Belgium, Holland, France, and the United States.[85] When Dr Irma Feldweg was setting up a breast milk collection facility in 1935 in Pforzheim at her husband's clinic, she wrote to Kayser with questions about how to build the facility based on the Erfurt model. A couple of months later, she reported back with news that the collection facility was up and running, "functioning completely after the Erfurt model."[86] Similarly, when Dr Friedrich Eckardt intended to create a new facility in Plauen in 1938, he asked Kayser if he could come to Erfurt to learn from her "infinite experience in this field."[87] A few months later, he reported to the RAfMuK that he "intend[ed] to build everything exactly as the [Erfurt] model."[88] Eckardt unabashedly praised the Erfurt facility and was critical of the RAfMuK's guidelines for not recognizing Erfurt as the nucleus of breast milk collection: "Through my experience, Erfurt was the practical correct and valuable teacher, through whose efforts we in Plauen had success ... I must say that in my eyes, Erfurt is and remains the spiritual centre for all FMS issues, and I mean for all FMS matters because it was there that I was shown the way to successfully develop an FMS."[89] Eckardt's endorsement of Erfurt and, by extension, of Kayser, resonated with Nazi higher-ups. The Reich Health Leader even asked if a Palestinian physician could visit Kayser's facility to learn about breast milk collection, showing how much credence it held.[90]

Further evidence of Kayser's perceived authority over all collection matters and her growing cooperation with the regime emerge in discussions about additional rations for breast milk donors. The Nazi government and even the postwar government(s) continuously informed Kayser how much additional rationing would be allotted to compensate donors, and Kayser consistently pushed for increasing this amount.[91] Kayser continued to emphasize that monetary compensation was not

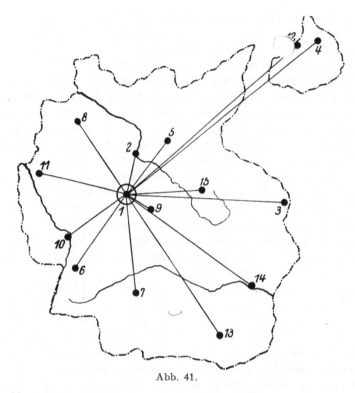

Abb. 41.

Nach Erfurter Muster wurden bis Juli 1939 Frauenmilch-sammelstellen gegründet in:

1. Erfurt 1927	6. Pforzheim 1935	11. Bochum 1939
2. Magdeburg 1929	7. München 1936	12. Königsberg . 1939
3. Gleiwitz....... 1934	8. Bremen 1937	13. Graz 1939
4. Insterburg..... 1934	9. Plauen 1938	14. Wien 1939
5. Berlin......... 1934	10. Mainz......... 1938	15. Reichenberg. 1939

5.8 Breast milk collection facilities in the German Reich, July 1939. Image from Kayser, *Frauenmilchsammelstelle.*

as important as replacing the nutrients that donors lost while nursing and donating their breast milk. During the Second World War, donors received 125 grams of fat and 350 grams of meat weekly in addition to financial compensation. Kayser and Eckardt both expressed surprise and disappointment by this amount and sought additional supplements for donors; Eckardt even wrote to the Reich Health Leader, Leonardo Conti, stating that the current allotments came to about only 1700 calories, which was not enough and could be seen as a "dangerous and irresponsible exploitation of milk donors."[92] Donors to the Erfurt facility also received smaller tokens of gratitude, such as a Christmas gift each year, purchased through voluntary donations from consumers and affixed with a card with the following saying: "A Christmas greeting to the helpful mothers from the thankful mothers!" This provided the breast milk collection facility a means to show donors thanks beyond the financial reward and highlighted the beneficial effects of their actions for a community of women – something that Kayser found to be "extraordinarily important."[93]

To a certain extent, Kayser's, Feldweg's, and even Eckardt's efforts to gain the approval of the regime and affiliating with the RAfMuK could be seen as resourceful. Not only were they working in a new, niche field, but Kayser and Feldweg, at least, were women still attempting to gain authority in the predominantly male domain of medicine. While Kayser, especially, worked to secure the endorsement of local, state, and national authorities, she slowly bought into the ideology, particularly the racial ideology of the regime. Questions regarding the racial purity of milk became a matter of concern after 1933, especially as doctors encountered non-Aryan donors in their facilities. Because Kayser was the de facto authority on all breast milk collection matters, others wrote to her to ask such questions. For example, after Feldweg's breast milk collection facility was up and running, she wrote to Kayser with her latest concern:

In recent weeks, we had a new unexpected concern for which we seek your advice. We have two non-Aryan deliverers and curious people have often questioned what happens to this milk. We have placed the milk separately and have given it only to a French woman up until now. Meanwhile the party has started to deal with the matter. Our local physician leader warns us of the "Stürmer."[94] What to do? The Nuremberg Laws leave us at this point in the lurch. Colonial Germans were often breastfed by blacks! Jewish milk is without a doubt easier to digest for nutritional disorders than cow's milk. For this reason, thus far I could not decide to refuse these deliveries.[95]

Feldweg was conflicted about whether or not to accept Jewish milk because in 1937, the regime, as she indicates in her letter, was still also formulating policies on the exclusion and inclusion of non-Aryans in Nazi society. She looked to guidance from the Nuremberg Laws, as this was the Nazi regime's most comprehensive legislation identifying Jews and forbidding them from citizenship. The Nazis often created other laws ad hoc and sometimes even undermined their own racial ideology, especially after the Second World War began.[96] Kayser, who would highlight her Aryan heritage to the Reich Physicians' Leader later that year, was clearly less conflicted about the issue of non-Aryan milk. She hastily responded to Feldweg a couple days later: "I would under no circumstances consciously use the milk of Jews for the collection facility. I know that this theoretical question has been discussed in Berlin, and although the view coincided with yours, it is necessarily better for the cause of the FMS itself, to demand the exclusion of Jews for the supply."[97] Even if decisions in Berlin were still under debate regarding the use of Jewish milk, Kayser condemns this and notes that it could be detrimental to the entire cause of collecting breast milk, which once had entailed providing it to women in all circles of the population.

Kayser, as the guru of breast milk collection, ostensibly subscribed to the racial hierarchy of the regime in terms of who should be included and excluded from the milk supply. Eckardt, too, condoned a racial hierarchy in breast milk collection, about which he also questioned Kayser:

> In the last week, a new problem has emerged, about which I would gladly like to compare notes with you. In Plauen, Volhynia-German families have been taken in.[98] Of these women, quite a number of them have a lot of milk; they rarely breastfeed their children over a year and could still donate a surplus, but the women were housed in camps, were sometimes heavily afflicted with vermin, and it is unclear which diseases they had previously, even when some of them leave a very clean impression after a thorough cleansing. At first, I do not have the impression that, under the particular conditions of their stay at the camp, if one applies the strict standard of our collection activities, that milk collection would be justifiable. Certainly, not a small amount of breast milk would be lost. But I am of the opinion: quality above everything, even if it is a pity to sometimes let breast milk go unused.[99]

Eckardt's hesitancy about using impure milk showcased his concerns about taking donations from mixed-race women, but also from diseased women. Both non-Aryans and unknown vermin could taint milk, and the Nazis were not unaccustomed to accusing them of being one and the same.[100] The question of whether or not to use foreign milk proved to be a balancing act for physicians between what they needed for their facilities to run, total war circumstances, and pressure to submit to racial hierarchies. Doctors like Feldweg remained more sceptical about buying whole-heartedly into Nazi anti-Semitism, even after the Nuremberg Laws had defined the racial, civic community; she recognized how important Jewish breast milk could be for her facility. Kayser, on the other hand, much more opportunistic as the leader of the breast milk collection project, seemed to recognize how submitting to the racial ideology of the regime might help her and her cause.

Preventing Infant Mortality

In addition to instances in which breast milk collection fit the mould of Nazi racial ideology, much of the rationale behind breast milk collection in Germany became linked to preventing infant mortality. Concerning rhetoric about infant mortality rates, especially among bottle-fed infants, became easy justification for the opening and expansion of breast milk collection facilities under Nazism. Fears of infant mortality dated back to well before the Nazis came to power. Around the turn of the century, fewer and fewer German mothers breastfed their newborns, but instead fed them unnaturally with formula. In Berlin, in 1885, out of every 100 newborns, only 55 were nursed by their mothers. In 1892, this number dropped to 44 and in 1900, it declined even further to 32 out of 100. Alarming infant mortality rates among these artificially fed infants followed, and thus, institutes began opening to reduce the damage caused by artificial feeding.[101] The first infant welfare centres opened in Berlin and Munich in 1905. By the outbreak of the First World War, there were 842 of these centres and their numbers grew very rapidly after that with the majority of centres opening between 1914 and 1920. By 1923, there were 4,529 centres throughout Germany. Before the war, these centres provided free medical examinations for the mother and child and also promoted breastfeeding by paying small premiums to needy mothers if they agreed to bring their infants in for regular examinations and to allow social workers to drop by unannounced to ensure they were nursing their children. In addition, they offered sterilized milk and advice on health and hygiene. The growth of these infant welfare centres in addition to the passage of the National Youth Welfare Law

(1922) helped reduce infant mortality overall, but infant mortality rates for bottle-fed children remained approximately five times higher than for breastfed children. Infant mortality was also considerably higher among the working class than the middle class because working-class women returned to work shortly after birth and had to supplement their milk, sometimes with "dubious surrogates" since cow's milk was so expensive. Thus, working-class women became the main targets of breastfeeding propaganda. The infant welfare movement worked diligently to convince working-class women of the importance of breastfeeding and now had the space to enlighten, persuade, and monitor many working-class individuals with the expansion of these centres.[102] The destruction of life during the war and the overall decline in fertility due to the shortage of German men after the war meant fears of infant mortality rates continued to grow, even if actual rates were declining. In the 1920s, about one in ten children died before their first birthday, but the public policy and rhetoric devoted to infant mortality were overwhelming.[103]

The fears of growing infant mortality rates among bottle-fed children created an opportunity for female physicians with the opening of breast milk collection facilities. The opening of these facilities during the Weimar Republic was part of a larger movement toward what David Crew has referred to as "an intrusive policing of mothers" couched in the language of protection. While pregnant and nursing women were collecting their maternity benefits, welfare authorities were creating "a medical surveillance network" and giving these mothers advice about pregnancy, the importance of breastfeeding, and "proper" childcare.[104] Elizabeth Whitaker has shown how "state and medical surveillance of maternal behavior was thought to account for the decline in infant mortality rates."[105] Pro-natalist movements that medicalized motherhood and were linked to infant mortality were not unusual throughout interwar Europe.[106] Patricia Stokes describes how "breastfeeding propaganda blamed women for selfishly dodging their maternal duties" and took on a moralistic and patriotic tone after the First World War.[107] Larry Frohman discusses how the infant welfare movement in Germany endorsed medical intervention into the once-natural practice of breastfeeding through the new infant welfare centres, where working-class mothers deferred to the knowledge of physicians and social workers rather than relying on old wives' tales or the experience of older, experienced mothers, in order to reduce infant mortality. Doctors and social workers admonished women's ignorance, negligence, and indifference about "modern scientific methods of child-raising," such as how to nurse properly or how to keep milk from spoiling. Their attempts to rationalize breastfeeding became part of larger efforts to teach good mothering in order to improve infant mortality rates.[108] The medical profession's campaign for breastfeeding coincided with an overall decline in infant mortality during the Imperial and Weimar periods.[109] The opening of breast milk collection facilities was also supposed to reduce the damage caused by artificial feeding. In fact, in a speech to the Hygiene Exhibition on 8 July 1934, Kayser claimed that "the greater death rate of artificially fed children was ultimately the reason for establishing a breast milk collection facility."[110]

The German doctors who advocated breast milk collection capitalized on the attention that the infant welfare movement was already allotting to breastfeeding and its promises of preventing infant mortality. Doctors Eckardt and Feldweg noted that a primary way to fight infant mortality was to prevent all dangers to the health of newborns and infants in their first year. They were quick to point out that one threat to infant health was unnatural feeding, and that infant mortality, in large part, was caused by incorrectly nursing infants with formula. They promoted a "breast is best" or natural nursing policy. They over-exaggerated statistics, claiming "it is a well-known fact that artificially fed infants die seven times more frequently from diseases in infancy or childhood than those who have been nursed naturally." Therefore, they thought it was essential to make every effort to breastfeed each infant for as long as possible.[111] Collecting surplus breast milk was one way to work towards naturally feeding every infant for as long as possible. Breast milk collection facilities, as Kayser envisioned them, provided milk for the infants of mothers who, despite their best efforts to nurse, could not do so or could not provide enough for their children. Such facilities also ensured that infants whose mothers died during birth or sick newborns who had to be separated from their mothers after birth still received breast milk, and therefore, obtained what Eckardt and Feldweg and others considered to be a preventative measure against infant mortality.[112] Without healthy children, the happiness of the family and the future of the people could not be guaranteed, according to Eckardt and Feldweg. They equated infant mortality with *Volkstod* (the people's death), adopting the rhetoric of the Nazis in which every individual act affected the whole and in which each individual was measured in terms of his or her health and value to the nation.[113] This language was akin to that which Detlev Peukert argues the Nazis used to distinguish between the healthy/unhealthy with reference to the *Volkskörper* (body of the nation).[114]

Borrowing ideologically infused rhetoric about infant mortality was a means for female physicians to raise consciousness about breast milk collection facilities, which were still relatively new, and perhaps helped draw the regime's attention to their collection efforts. These physicians were not only promoting the success of breast milk collection in preventing infant mortality, but they were also endorsing their own work in this new, cutting-edge field of medicine. Kayser, for example, claimed that over 100,000 infants died per year as a result of "unnatural nutrition" and that therein lay the important work of the breast milk collection facility. "Everywhere, day after day, in the places where no collection facilities exist, life-saving medicine is being wasted."[115] By indicating that their efforts saved lives, Kayser fashioned a rhetoric that elevated the work she and her colleagues performed in collection facilities. Similarly, Irma Feldweg highlighted the success of breast milk in preventing infant mortality in the Siloah women's clinic in Pforzheim. Between 1936 and 1938, the infant mortality rate there was about 4 per cent, which she advertised as being, on average, 2.4 per cent below the infant mortality rate throughout the Reich. Overall, the infant mortality rate had declined, a goal for which the Reich Health Leader was striving.[116] Feldweg and her colleagues could also market themselves to a regime that was increasingly preparing for war and a long future.

Infant mortality became a primary concern of the Nazi regime because of its overall concerns about the health and well-being of children. It aimed to build a thousand-year Reich and therefore needed a constant supply of fit and healthy individuals. Accordingly, the regime celebrated any decrease in infant mortality. The *NS-Volksdienst*, a party newspaper, claimed that the RAfMuK could be credited with reducing the infant mortality rate from 6.6 per every 100 living children to 4 by 1936. This was important to the Nazis because it corresponded to infant mortality rates in Holland, Norway, and Switzerland.[117] Clearly, it was essential for Germany to keep up with its European neighbours, especially with its plans for an upcoming war. Another party publication, *Völkisher Beobachter*, highlighted the decrease in infant mortality rates between 1932, when 7.9 per cent of children died in the first year of life, and 1936, when only 6.58 per cent of children died. That meant that, annually, 52,000 children of the Reich were being saved.[118] Between 1934 and 1936, this equated to 118,515 more children overall. The *Mitteldeutsche Nationalzeitung*, a regional newspaper, declared hope that "in a few years Germany will have the lowest infant mortality of all people."[119]

Maintaining low infant mortality rates remained a concern after the Second World War started. Before the war even began, Kayser wrote to the RAfMuK ensuring them that by expanding collection efforts, she could keep tens of thousands of infants alive annually. She faulted those who spoke against breast milk collection for indirectly and unintentionally contributing to the death of numerous infants.[120] "In 25 years – from 1919 to 1944 – 37,759 donors in Germany have given 577,173 litres of breast milk," according to Eckardt. With over half a million litres of breast milk, some 150,000 premature babies and sick infants could successfully be treated – a number that corresponded to the number of residents in Erfurt.[121] In thirty years of collecting breast milk, Eckardt and Feldweg estimated that around 70,000 donors had handed over approximately one million litres of breast milk, meaning that some 250,000 premature babies and sick infants could be successfully treated, healed, and kept alive. They made sure to emphasize that their work saved as many lives as the number of people living in Magdeburg, the founding city of breast milk collection. These findings showed that the prediction that Marie-Elise Kayser had made in 1919 – "I believe that the establishment of collection facilities for breast milk, especially in our time, would be able to contribute to the reduction of infant mortality" – had been realized.[122] Of course, infant mortality rates could have fallen due to a combination of factors – the promotion of breastfeeding, the crackdown on abortion, and better attention and funding for maternal and infant care. But these doctors were trying to garner public interest and support. By attempting to put an actual number on how many lives had been saved as a result of their efforts, advocates of breast milk collection provided further legitimacy to the general public and a ringing endorsement for their work.

The growth of breast milk collection facilities after 1939 also remained deeply connected to keeping infant mortality rates low, which remained on the National Socialist agenda after they started a war. In September 1939, there were fifteen breast milk collection facilities in Germany. Another two opened that fall and then five more in 1940, seven in 1941, eight in 1942, three in 1943, three in 1944, and one in 1945.[123] By the end of the war, there were a total of forty-four breast milk collection facilities throughout the Reich, with two-thirds of them opening after the start of the Second World War. This was no coincidence. For one, breast milk collection had been in existence for twenty years at that point, which was

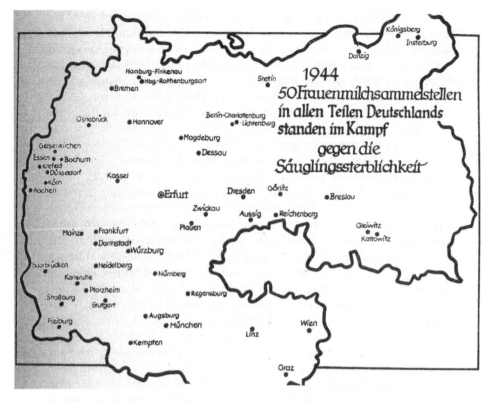

Königsberg
Insterburg
Danzig

Hamburg-Finkenau
Hbg-Rothenburgsort
Bremen

Stettin   1944

50 Frauenmilchsammelstellen
in allen Teilen Deutschlands
standen im Kampf
gegen die
Säuglingssterblichkeit

Osnabrück   Hannover
Berlin-Charlottenburg
Lichtenberg
Magdeburg
Dessau

Gelsenkirchen
Essen   Bochum
Krefeld
Düsseldorf   Kassel
Köln
Aachen

Erfurt   Dresden   Görlitz
Zwickau   Breslau
Aussig   Reichenberg

Mainz   Frankfurt   Plauen
Darmstadt
Würzburg   Gleiwitz
Kattowitz

Saarbrücken   Heidelberg
Karlsruhe   Nürnberg
Pforzheim
Straßburg   Regensburg
Stuttgart
Freiburg   Augsburg
München   Wien
Linz
Kempten

Graz

5.9 Breast milk collection facilities in the German Reich, 1944. Image from Eckardt and Feldweg, *Die Frauenmilchsammelstellen.*

a sufficient amount of time for it to gain popularity. Marie Elise-Kayser had published a significant number of articles, and her book would appear in 1940, thus spreading the word about breast milk collection in medical circles, women's circles, and among the general population.

Nutrition and Nursing Policies during the Second World War

The wartime mentality, which sought to preserve and use all of the Reich's resources, allowed breast milk collection to flourish during the Second World War, and it also influenced new nutritional and nursing policies. Joseph Goebbels outlined how important German resources were, especially once Germany turned toward total war after 1943: "The German people face the gravest demand of the war, namely of finding the determination to use all our resources to protect everything we have and everything we will need in the future."[124] Mark Cole has shown how the Nazis implemented heavily regulated nutritional campaigns throughout the country, including during the wartime period. Manipulating food consumption, he argues, was a means for the Nazis to achieve social, economic, and biopolitical goals. Part of their tripartite plan to achieve these goals involved "encouraging the frugal and proper use of foodstuffs."[125] Breast milk, already deemed a life-saving nutrient, presumably fell under this new Nazi nutritional policy.

Because of the heavy monitoring of food consumption, nutrition became a focal point for women physicians.[126] Dr Edith von Lölhöffel encouraged doctors to create the most sensible plan for nutrition and fully use the nutritional elements of the native soil. To her, this meant recognizing higher-quality food like whole-wheat bread, mushrooms, wild vegetables, wild salad, and wild fruits. This was partially a result of the practical realities of being unable to import many different types of food during wartime. Health concerns also played a role because, von Lölhöffel believed, many German-grown fruits and vegetables had medicinal purposes.[127] Restoring the productivity of seriously ill people as quickly as possible also proved to be "of great importance for the Volksgemeinschaft," according to Dr Ilse Szagunn. Szagunn presented a number of suggestions for how to nourish the Volk's sickest individuals in order to get them back to work as soon as possible.[128] The attention given to the nutrition and productivity of the German people was one side to what Cole has called "the paradox of Nazi consumption," which entailed boosting the German standard of living through its food policies while simultaneously causing the suffering and death of millions of people, often through starvation.[129]

To maximize labour efficiency in its factories during wartime, the Nazis focused their nutritional policies on increasing worker productivity, especially because of the hope that women would be returning to work.[130] As the war materialized, Cole suggests that "the Nazi regime became increasingly concerned with the rationalization of labour and the maximization of efficiency."[131] In addition to ensuring the proper nutrition of workers – a lesson not lost on them from the failures of the First World War – the regime also offered certain protections for pregnant women.[132]

This trend had begun in the late nineteenth century when movements all over Europe demanded protection for working women, particularly after childbirth. In the 1870s, coinciding with the second wave of industrialization, European powers passed laws prohibiting women from working laborious jobs for at least fifteen days after childbirth. Germany first introduced state-regulated health insurance maternity benefits for women workers in 1883. In 1887, the Reichstag passed a law that prohibited factory work for women for the first four weeks after childbirth; this was extended to six weeks in 1897 and eight weeks in 1908. In 1890, fourteen European nations met in Berlin to establish laws outlawing women's work in factories and workshops for the first month after childbirth. In 1903, an amendment to the health insurance law increased maternity benefits to seven weeks, and then the imperial insurance order of 1913 extended this to eight weeks. With the growth of women's employment during the First World War, European countries supported pro-natal policies to protect pregnant and nursing women, although sometimes resources were lacking. In Germany, maternity benefits were initially granted to soldiers' wives only and then extended to include unmarried women where a serviceman acknowledged paternity. Nursing mothers were entitled to twelve weeks of monetary allowance, which alongside the shortage of cow's milk, resulted in women's increased tendency to nurse their own children. In Hamburg, 75 per cent of mothers nursed their babies before the war, but this number increased to 96 per cent after the war. In 1917, Dr Marie-Elisabeth Lüders, a social worker and head of the Women's Section within the newly created War Office and then eventually head of the Central Office for Women's Work, introduced family and welfare measures, such as providing childcare for women in order to encourage them to work, but few came to fruition.[133] In 1916 in Italy, legislation established workplace nursing rooms, paid breaks to nurse either in the workplace or during longer breaks at home when nursing rooms were not available, and on-site childcare for children. Under the fascist regime, the number of childcare centres grew to over 7,000 in the late 1920s, but they were ill-equipped and poorly operated. Breast-feeding rooms in factories remained few and far between and many were unused.[134] Similarly, a 1917 law in France required employers to provide nursing rooms and to give women two half-hour breaks to nurse without suffering a loss of wages. French women, however, were reluctant to use the new facilities because they were thought to be hotbeds of contagious diseases, and most working

mothers preferred to leave their children with a neighbour or relative.[135] In 1927, Germany was the first major industrialized nation to
sign the Washington Convention on the employment of women before
and after childbirth, which permitted women who paid into the sickness insurance funds up to twelve weeks of maternity leave or eighteen weeks if they were not fully recovered. Nursing mothers also still
received a supplementary income for twelve weeks as part of the Family Maternity Benefit, given to female relatives of insured working
men, or Maternity Welfare, given to impoverished women and paid
for by the community.[136]

The Second World War exacerbated existing concerns about the
health and hygiene of Germany's women, especially in light of the fact
that so many women would be returning to work when the nation's
young soldiers went to war. Even prior to the outbreak of war, fears of
an imminent, unprecedented labour shortage loomed, and it became
clear to many in the Deutsche Arbeitsfront (German Labour Front) that
production in any field could not be managed without the participation
of women.[137] With this in mind, female physicians began to draw attention to how they could assist this new group of wage-earning women,
especially with regards to managing their health under the dual stress
of work and household activity.[138]

Szagunn, who reported on the state of working mothers who breastfed for the Ministry of Labour, highlighted the complications posed by
the increasing number of women in factories in the wartime economy,
particularly the lack of childcare and space for women to nurse in the
workplace. Such problems were becoming increasingly urgent in 1941,
according to Szagunn, and thus the first priority was to help mothers
understand that they could continue nursing upon returning to work.
She thought factories should be responsible for providing women a longer nursing break to go home or a place to nurse within the factory. If
women did not work too far from home, Szagunn argued they should
have the possibility of going home twice a day for nursing breaks,
which would be fifteen minutes longer than the two thirty-minute
breaks allotted by the German Labour Front. This extended nursing
break should be fully compensated to ensure that women were not
receiving reduced wages for "fulfilling their duty to nurse."[139] Rather
than allowing mothers to go home to nurse, factory owners had the possibility of allowing women to bring their children to work and providing a space for women to nurse either in a nursery or some sort of quiet
room. The advantage here was that nursing mothers could take shorter

breaks, therefore maximizing their time at work. This also helped out mothers by saving them the cost of childcare while they were at work.[140] Possibilities for company-sponsored nursing included either in-house nurseries within the factory, which was generally only possible in larger factories, or company nurseries in the same neighbourhood as the factory. In this latter case, the mother would drop her child off before work and pick him/her up after work. At the time of her writing, Szagunn claimed that there were not many of these in-house or neighbourhood nurseries, but they were increasing as women's work likewise grew.[141] Dr Margot Noack of the Obstetrics Department of the Kaiser-August-Victoria Home in Charlottenburg, Berlin, writing in 1943, stated that some factories had established nursing cribs or a calm room specifically for the purpose of pumping.[142]

Szagunn, in her 1941 article, also suggested possibilities for night nursing at more isolated factories. In this case, mothers who worked five days a week brought their children in Monday morning and took them home at noon on Saturday. Night nursing facilities were much more difficult for factories to establish under the current conditions due to the higher number of nursing personnel they required to staff the facilities. However, wherever night nursing existed, Szagunn suggested that such facilities had proven themselves in terms of the impeccable care they provided infants and mothers' desire and joy to work.[143]

Szagunn's demands to provide a space for women to breastfeed were part of a longer and larger European movement to gain rights for nursing mothers, but they also demonstrated her and other female physicians' dedication to the Nazi wartime economy. Dr Cläre Hellpap, who reported on her work in the Kassel breast milk collection facility in February 1941, was excited by the prospect that the facility could help wage-earning mothers who wanted to continue to breastfeed. She noted that the facility had gained the support of even the most reserved female farmers. This was "all the more important" because there were a number of women working in the countryside in the summer who frequently stopped nursing because they did not want to disrupt their work and leave their children at a relative's house.[144] Hellpap, like Szagunn, was pleased that women's work would not be interrupted during wartime. In two instances, the facility urged young workers to change jobs so that these mothers could continue to nurse. While the majority of donors were the wives of trained workers, Hellpap highlighted that donors came from all classes and included self-employed craft masters, academic professionals, and women in higher offices.[145] Hellpap, Szagunn, von Lölhöffel, Kayser, and others wanted to maximize what they could procure from Germany's natural resources, whether that meant feeding women and children German fruits and vegetables or pumping – literally – as much breast milk out of nursing mothers as they could and collecting it in facilities, ensuring that nothing would go to waste during wartime.

In addition to making the most of Germany's natural resources in a time of war, female physicians like Hellpap and Szagunn also contributed to the Nazi wartime economy by suggesting how to maximize female labour in Germany's factories. Hellpap saw value in collection facilities because they helped women balance nursing and wartime work, and she even advised two women to find new jobs that allowed them to better balance their maternal and professional lives. By advocating that factories provide nurseries for women workers, Szagunn sought to have nursing mothers return to work as soon as possible after childbirth and to minimize the time that women needed to nurse and be away from their work. She couched her demands for protections for nursing women workers in the urgency of wartime, in which Germany needed to capitalize on women's labour as soon as possible after they gave birth. While on one hand, Szagunn supported the Nazi regime's wartime agenda (including racial hygiene), on the other hand, she also demanded that factories provide their workers childcare and quiet spaces to nurse – rights for women that seemed radical for their time. After all, this previously private function was now receiving public discussion and attention.

Hellpap, too, suggested that women should have the ability to be both good mothers and good workers. Here, Szagunn and Hellpap reveal the complexities of female physicians' actions during the Nazi regime. Their practical work during the Second World War certainly supported the Nazi regime's wartime goals, but women doctors also used the context of war to expand their own professional roles in women's and children's health by fashioning these fields as even more central to the regime than the Nazis had already made them. At times, as the example of Szagunn clearly shows, they even demanded rights for women and children. This meant that it was often a group of middle- and upper-class doctors making claims that they knew what was best for women workers' bodies. While the war did not, in fact, bring about an overall change in the type of work that women doctors were doing – that is, in women's and children's medicine – the venues of their work changed, shifting from a focus on the home, marriage, the family, and schools to workplaces and the national agenda. The war and the confusion it created allowed them the freedom and flexibility to demand more for themselves and for their constituency than they might have been able to in a time of peace.

As the war raged on, the chaotic circumstances certainly affected the network of breast milk collection facilities. The Kassel collection centre, founded in the fall of 1939, catered to a number of families from the Saar-Palatinate who had been evacuated from the front in the first few weeks after the war began. Some of the first donors to the facility were mothers from the Saar region who had a large surplus of milk.[146] With Germany's borders constantly in flux for the next several years, breast milk collection facilities would face a flood of potential new donors and would often have to make difficult decisions about whose milk to accept, as the example from the Plauen facility described above indicates. When Eckardt questioned Kayser about accepting milk from Volhynia-German families, she referred him to the precedent set by mothers from the Saar region who were donating their milk to the Kassel facility.[147] The difference in the former case was that the mothers from Volhynia had been in resettlement camps – something that worried Eckardt. The Nazis also tended to view Poles as inferior, a designation that did not necessarily apply to women from the Saar, who were always considered German even when the British and French occupied the Saar following the First World War.[148]

Total war circumstances, moreover, exacerbated difficulties with milk delivery. In the pre-war years, breast milk collection facilities would often help each other out in the case of milk shortages.[149] When the situation became more dire, however, this was not always feasible. For example, Dr Herbert Bauer wrote to Kayser in January 1944 asking if the Erfurt facility could send breast milk to his extremely ill child at the city hospital in Bielefeld. Since December, his child had been receiving surplus breast milk, but that was now no longer available due to evacuation orders in the area. Kayser responded by stating that as much as they would like to send milk to his sick child, deliveries were no longer possible, and she instead advised him to turn to the Magdeburg or Plauen facilities for help.[150] In addition to desperately needing milk due to various wartime conditions such as evacuations or the bombing of certain facilities, one midwife even called for more facilities toward the very end of the war, stating that "the difficulties of wartime have, unfortunately, assumed a scale such that it is impossible for one to apply the peacetime standards. Breast milk collection facilities have now become more necessary than ever and each city should actually have their own collection facility, if only because the transport by rail has become so difficult."[151]

Near the end of the war, some breast milk collection facilities stopped operating altogether due to regular bombing raids. Midwife Fritzi Urschitz at the Vienna collection facility recounted the bombing that terrorized the city in October 1944 when they experienced air raid alarms two to three times each week.[152] She also described how they survived the wildest days of the war, the clinic luckily spared from bombing "by a miracle." They took in the sick – severely ill children and many other poor people; all the while they had "no water, no light, the wildest state of war."[153] The Plauen facility, which Dr Eckardt, one of the strongest advocates of breast milk collection, had built, was completely destroyed, and while he attempted to build a new facility, he was not always optimistic.[154] The Magdeburg facility was also significantly bombed, but there was good news coming out of the facilities in Essen, Bremen, Hamburg, and Berlin, which continued to operate.[155] The Erfurt facility – the centre of breast milk collection in Germany and worldwide – also met a positive fate by surviving the war unscathed.

Essentialist Rhetoric in Breast Milk Collection

It was during the chaos of the Second World War that female physicians strongly endorsed themselves as the leaders in the growing field of breast milk collection. The war exacerbated demands to preserve all of Germany's natural resources and to maximize the country's labour supply, but it also created a platform for female physicians to highlight the importance of breast milk collection as well as their essential role in the collection process. Although only a few women led breast milk collection facilities, others involved in the movement emphasized, in their writings, the essential qualities they embodied as women and mothers that made them particularly suitable to play a leading role in this relatively new field. Within the first few weeks of war, Dr Hellpap claimed that breast milk collection facilities had proven their indispensable worth for Germany, as it was increasingly important to protect the health and lives of the country's young infants.[156] Dr von Lölhöffel agreed that the establishment of breast milk collection facilities was more urgent than ever before, and she called on female physicians to make it their duty to boost mothers' abilities to breastfeed, both through their personal experience and through practical instruction.[157] She thought breast milk instruction was a task that female physicians were particularly suited for because they themselves had familiarity with breastfeeding. Indeed, Kayser *had* conceived of the idea while she herself was breastfeeding.

Female physicians highlighted their maternal abilities to encourage, coax, and empathize with mothers who were learning to breastfeed. Dr Margot Noack emphasized that female physicians served as psychological leaders to other women. Noack thought midwives and nurses could coach women in the technical aspects of nursing, but women doctors were essential to offer female patients psychological influence and leadership in the breastfeeding process. She claimed that in their clinic in Berlin, doctors had already achieved better results with regard to nursing. Noack pointed out that psyche and lactation were closely connected, and with wartime air raids and household difficulties, this became even more apparent. Women often opted out of breastfeeding more quickly because of these psychological burdens during the war. However, "the full personality of the doctor" could awaken and strengthen the self-confidence of mothers by helping them see their "full biological value." Noack said that mothers often had feelings that they could not breastfeed – an acquired complex that doctors would fight with all available means. In the obstetric ward at Noack's clinic, this meant that female doctors would address mothers personally and use persuasion therapy to teach them about the nursing process and convince them of its importance for the health of children. She claimed that "one can spare neither trouble nor time" in individually addressing mothers. "Thanks to her more empathetic psyche, the woman doctor can perhaps be more capable of influencing a young mother" because, after all, a woman is "especially receptive to the words of her doctor after childbirth, and therefore, this is the easiest time to influence a woman with regards to nursing." Noack had observed again and again how "the encouragement and coaxing from the side of physicians could fundamentally change the attitude of the mother" and how a "nursing talk" often led to an increase in milk. She called female physicians in particular to this task because they knew all the difficulties associated with nursing and were convinced they could be overcome.[158] The institutional training of female physicians proved just as essential as their personal experiences as mothers – something that they could offer to this new field that their male colleagues could not.

Another female physician from Marburg, Dr Cläre Sieberg, underlined the care and persuasive attitude that women doctors offered to nursing mothers. Calling on all health-care authorities to promote nursing and the collection of breast milk, she agreed that female physicians would be the best individuals to encourage women to nurse longer and to readily donate their surplus milk. This kind of guidance, she claimed, required a "very personal and a certain emotionally correct tone."[159] While midwives had successfully drawn donors to the breast milk collection facility in Kassel, for example, Sieberg insisted that the "doctor and particularly the female doctor should look after young mothers, to whom they have direct access, and not entrust health care to nursing assistants alone."[160] According to Sieberg, doctors, by nature of the profession they had chosen, were attracted to caring, but female physicians, she implied, showed empathy and care. These qualities were necessary when giving mothers – many of whom lacked insight about nursing – advice during this important time in their lives. She suggested that doctors could successfully promote nursing and even give mothers important medical advice since they would be advising them on a regular basis. Female physicians would have "countless opportunities to practically and scientifically intervene in this field. Physician encouragement can be more effective than the advising of nurses and other assistants."[161]

Conceivably, it was their combined professional and personal experiences that led Dr Kayser to assert that "breast milk collection was always intended to be one of the quintessential responsibilities of the female physician, particularly now."[162] She rallied female physicians to undertake this task, citing their expanded sphere of activity during wartime while male doctors were enlisting. Women doctors were already active in public clinics and welfare agencies, and therefore it was important for them to "pay great attention when they encounter[ed] wasted milk" in these places, according to Kayser. Wartime conditions demanded that female physicians take note when a nursing mother had a surplus of breast milk, awaken her interest in breast milk donation, and link her up with a particular collection facility. If no collection facility existed in their city of residence, donors could send their milk to the next closest collection facility in the form of express train parcels – something the breast milk collection facility would finance. Sterilizing milk before shipment also helped in the case of bad train connections – a likely occurrence during wartime. Overall, Kayser thought that women doctors played a crucial role in ensuring that during the war "nothing will perish and the general welfare will not be lost."[163] Certainly, she was emphasizing the Nazi regime's desire to preserve the well-being of its people and its natural resources during a time in which they were both under severe threat. She also allayed the anxieties of female physicians who might initially consider this work to be "trifling" by reassuring them that they were not going to be another cog in the breast milk collection operation; they would not, she ensured, become unskilled workers like their counterparts in paper or metal collection, but their qualifications and training would be necessary for the success of the facilities. Kayser was convinced that female physicians would be especially good for work in breast milk collection and that they would find much joy and satisfaction from their efforts in this field.[164]

Female physicians in addition to Kayser drew attention to their own experiences when they discussed breastfeeding and promoted collection efforts. Dr von Lölhöffel, for example, stated she had offered her own surplus milk to appropriate Berlin infant welfare centres during the Weimar years, and based on her own experience, she found that many healthy women had an abundance of milk but it went unused. In the vast majority of Berlin's women's clinics, instruction on nursing and increasing the amount of milk was unsatisfactory. She had determined through her own attempt at breastfeeding that it was possible to get milk flowing without even applying a child to her breast, but through expressing her milk. Four days after giving birth to twin premature babies, von Lölhöffel started expressing her milk, despite being discouraged from doing so at the clinic because she could not apply the babies to her breast. She was so successful that after being discharged, she could supply the daily amount needed for the one surviving child by expressing her milk three to four times a day. The baby was not applied to the breast until four months later, at which point it was released from the hospital, but it had been nourished naturally all along. Based on her experiences, the regular expression of breast milk was something that was easy to learn, and it actually provided relief for women who, after delivering premature babies, could not breastfeed but still had an abundance of breast milk.[165]

In her propaganda for breast milk collection facilities, which she claimed could provide this essential education about nursing for women, von Lölhöffel also highlighted her own experiences with breastfeeding as a means of connecting with a broader readership than was normal for *Die Ärztin*. Her attempts to encourage more women to breastfeed and donate their milk were much more effective when she shared her own personal success with both. "Even if every mother cannot provide milk for more than her own child," she wrote, "[breast milk collection facilities] still act as an example for mothers to donate a life-saving nutrient to other children and to directly stir healthy and simple feelings of motherhood, which no woman can fundamentally escape."[166] Here, von Lölhöffel relied not only on her own experiences as a mother, but assumed that all women had instinctive feelings of motherhood that were undeniable. Such strong presumptions again allowed von Lölhöffel to connect with mothers but also proved dangerous because she inferred that all women wanted to and could become mothers, which was most certainly not the case. She underscored her own experiential learning, as well as essential feminine qualities of empathy and care as a way to strengthen her own legitimacy as a leader of the movement and to embolden more mothers to contribute to the collection project.

The "Success" of Breast Milk Collection

Another means for women doctors to endorse themselves as the most suitable leaders for breast milk collection was to point to the success of the facilities. Investing their time and energy into encouraging "the joy of nursing" would surely generate positive results in facilities, according to Dr Cläre Sieberg.[167] In fact, statistics from Kassel indicate that it achieved its campaign goal to attract women to the facility there. Nursing or pumping breast milk took a considerable amount of time, leading Sieberg to assume that mothers with several children would rarely donate milk as readily as mothers with only one. However, an overview of monthly donors between January and September 1943 shows that the willingness to donate milk among mothers with one child was comparable to that of those with two or more.[168] Similarly, Friedrich Eckardt provided "striking proof of the joyful willingness of [Germany's] mothers to supply milk" to the collection facility in Plauen by collecting data from the site about the age distribution, social stratification, and performance of one thousand donors between 1939 and 1943. He noted that while it was obvious that the majority of donors had only one child, there were also mothers with four or more children, even with seven, eight, or nine, who were willing to donate their surplus milk – a demonstration of their willingness "to help other children" and of "the highest level of idealism of our German women with regards to population policy."[169]

Doctors working in breast milk collection often blamed any decrease in the number of litres collected on the war rather than their own recruitment efforts. The facility in Pforzheim collected 372 litres of breast milk the first year it opened, and 2,058 litres the following year – an increase of five and a half times. It reached its peak collection year in 1939, with 4,394 litres, before milk collection amounts began to drop off, unsurprisingly the same year the war started. Dr Emmi Justi insisted that this marked decrease in milk donations clearly demonstrated how the excitement and fright at the beginning of war could be detrimental to milk secretion. While the intake of milk did not rise again to this peak point in subsequent years, Justi accentuated an increase in the amount donated between 1940 (3,231 litres) and 1941 (3,336 litres). She was also careful to point out that although the amount of milk collected decreased, the number of donors increased from 39 women in 1935 to 325 women in 1943 – evidence, in her opinion, that even during wartime "our efforts have not failed."[170] Eckardt also noted that the low points of collection efforts at the Plauen facility were in the summer of 1940 and the winter of 1942–3. These numbers, he observed, corresponded to the war in France and the Battle of Stalingrad, respectively. According to Eckardt, "surely, the mental shocks of these events of the war did not *not* influence our mothers and their breastfeeding abilities and ability to donate milk."[171] Dr Noack, then, was correct in suggesting that women, psychologically affected by the war, had problems nursing.[172] Eckardt, like Justi and Noack, underscored that the war affected women's abilities to nurse and thereby the doctors' breast milk collection efforts; it had little, in other words, to do with their attempts or abilities to attract donors. In fact, Eckardt insisted that, contrary to expectations, the productivity of milk donors was even higher during the wartime years and had even increased.[173] Dr Sieberg agreed that "we can undoubtedly continue the work of the breast milk collection facility because it proved its legitimacy even under the difficult conditions."[174] Writing in 1944, she was presumably referring to the war.

Because the Nazi Party took over control of the publication of *Die Ärztin* in 1937, we must read these success stories with caution. Anything that did not favourably promote the Nazi war effort likely would have been omitted. That being said, it is perhaps telling that by advertising the impressive achievements of breast milk collection facilities, the Nazi

Party allowed female physicians to further validate their work within them. This is perhaps why they insisted that any failings on the part of breast milk collection – in terms of the number of either litres collected or donors – were no fault of their own, but of the extreme conditions under which they were operating.

In addition to highlighting slight increases in milk collection or reiterating the legitimacy of the facilities, doctors Sieberg and Hellpap emphasized that the donating mothers often long remembered the pride they felt at helping other children.[175] Dr Irma Feldweg described how "pleading letters, urgent telegrams come, weeping mothers and threatening fathers appear in person, sometimes from distant cities in order to secure vital breast milk for their sick infants. And later, touching thank-you letters with pictures of the chubby offspring prove, even after many years, that the breast milk collection facility has been able to resolve a serious concern."[176] Several photos of those chubby-cheeked, breastfed offspring exist in the photo archives in Erfurt.[177] Dr Kayser also received several such letters from mothers, fathers, and her colleagues throughout wartime Germany. Sometimes, these letters expressed thanks to Kayser for sending milk, and other times pleaded with her for milk. In one case, her colleague in Dresden requested milk for a family who had just had triplets. They already had another set of twins and eight children in total.[178] Personal letters reflect only positive feedback from mothers and customers, showing, on the one hand, how under the context of Nazism, such accounts may have been the only ones permitted. On the other hand, Kayser had received consistent positive affirmations since before the Nazi regime took over the breast milk collection industry, demonstrating that mothers and customers may have felt a sense of gratitude before they were pressured to express it.[179] These adulatory accounts from mothers may likely have been the only ones that Kayser and Feldweg kept and discussed in order to draw further attention to how vital breast milk collection facilities were to mothers, and therefore how essential their work was to the nation. Kayser claimed that the Christmas gift that milk consumers gave to milk donors in the Erfurt facility both before and during the war provided further evidence of how grateful customers were for the donations of other mothers.[180] Emphasizing the positive experiences that donors and customers took from the breast milk collection facilities legitimized breast milk collection and gave the doctors working in the facilities further rationale to continue this important work.

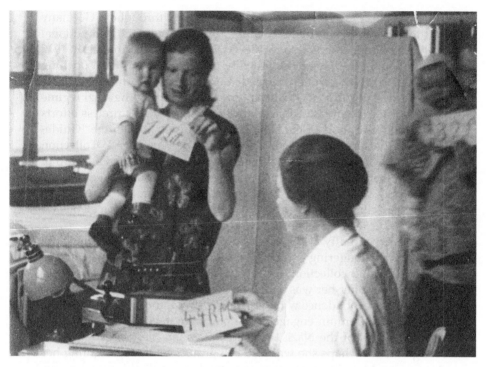

5.10 Donor with child, showing the amount of milk donated and the remuneration for donated milk. Stadtarchiv Erfurt Photo Archive.

Conclusions

By the end of the Second World War, breast milk collection had been underway in Germany for just over twenty-five years. By 1944, forty-four facilities were operating all over the Reich. In 1943, there were an estimated 11,401 donors, a large increase from the 45 in 1927, the first year the Erfurt facility was operational. Between 1919 and 1944, the facilities had collected 577,153 litres of breast milk. With this large supply, Dr Eckardt estimated that they had successfully treated 150,000 premature babies and sick infants.[181] Breast milk collection had proven its longevity, even with only twenty-nine facilities left standing at the end of war, and would continue into the postwar German states as well.

Erfurt and, by extension, Dr Marie-Elise Kayser were at the centre of these collection efforts. Kayser's persistence and productivity paid off.

She was determined to help mothers in all classes throughout Germany and to eventually gain the recognition of local, regional, and national authorities, both of which she achieved. Her humanitarian aims in 1919 when opening the Magdeburg facility or even in 1926 when opening the Erfurt facility certainly turned more ideological throughout the 1930s, especially after she realized how the support of the Nazi regime could bolster the breast milk collection cause. Kayser's tireless efforts to secure the support of the Nazi government resulted in the "Guidelines for the Establishment and Operation of Breast Milk Collection Facilities," RAfMuK support and administration, and even a stamp of approval from the Reich Ministry of the Interior. Simultaneously, the regime may have used her breast milk collection project to realize its own goal to continue to decrease infant mortality and exploit all of Germany's natural resources during wartime.

Kayser eventually showed signs of allying with an ideologically tainted, war-mongering regime, certainly not her intent when she initiated breast milk collection. Her attitude toward the Nazi regime and what it could offer her was ambiguous and complicated. Based on her personal correspondence with Dr Irma Feldweg and Dr Friedrich Eckardt, she at minimum engaged with and may have subscribed to the racial ideology of the Nazis, as she condemned the use of Jewish or foreign milk. Perhaps she was also being cautious by highlighting her Aryan race. More likely, she was expedient. After all, this was a means of obtaining the recognition and support she thought breast milk collection merited. She, and other women doctors working alongside her, couched much of their rhetoric in the context of Germany's war, with the understanding that breast milk was a sacred natural resource that needed to be preserved and maximized. The same could be said of Germany's nursing mothers, whose bodies and labour were vital to the war effort and who needed to return to work as soon as possible after giving birth.

Some members of the second generation of female doctors, who started their careers as the Nazis came to power yet still experienced discrimination, especially prior to the war, gained professional opportunities for themselves by claiming they knew what was best for other women and their bodies. Moreover, these doctors were advocating that other women's bodies (and their resources) should be used for the war effort. While this makes them complicit with Nazi war aims, or at least culprits for adopting the regime's rhetoric, they pushed the boundaries of their own professional space and demanded unprecedented rights, such as nursing rooms and extended breaks for working mothers who were still nursing. Kayser, for one, widened her work as a pediatrician by creating a new field, not to mention the first facility of this kind in Germany. Certainly, she can also be viewed as a role model for others in breast milk collection both at home and abroad; after all, she trained 80 per cent of all the leaders at facilities throughout Germany, and the other 20 per cent were regarded as the so-called "grandchildren of the mother institute in Erfurt."[182] In other words, she produced two new generations of leaders, demonstrating a long-lasting legacy beyond pediatrics.

Women physicians working in breast milk collection fashioned a rhetoric that emphasized the feminine qualities of empathy and care in order to justify the leading role that they thought they should take in breast milk collection. On the one hand, they essentialized all women, reducing them to characteristics that the male medical profession often used to push female doctors out of mainstream positions during the Nazi regime. On the other hand, members of the League of German Female Physicians were claiming a new space for themselves in breast milk collection by embracing these maternal and feminine characteristics – something they did precisely *because* they were exiled to fields of medicine in which they were primarily treating women and children. Making such maternalist arguments allowed female physicians to participate in and become leaders in a burgeoning medical field during the war. It also gave them the freedom to influence their patients by intervening in critical decisions that had implications for the fate of Germany's children and, therefore, for Germany's future.

Conclusion

Women doctors worked to create a space for themselves in the Weimar and Nazi medical profession. How they came to accomplish this has been the focus of this book. Their struggle to be admitted to medical study was a long one, as they faced the hostility of men who feared that the caring and healing aspects of medicine made women more naturally suited for this profession. Men already encountered competition from lay healers and midwives for authority over the profession in the late nineteenth century and therefore initially encouraged women onto medical tracks where they would serve only women and children. German feminists Helene Lange and Mathilde Weber called attention to the need for women doctors, citing women's modesty as an important factor in allowing women to study medicine. Female physicians, they argued, were necessary to treat women patients and women's diseases, and medicine was well suited to the qualities and talents they acquired in motherhood.[1] Women finally achieved entrance to German universities, and thereby medical study, in the first decade of the twentieth century – relatively late compared to women in other Western European countries and the United States. The number of female physicians continued to grow, and after the First World War the Weimar Constitution promised them full professional equality. Male discrimination in the medical profession, however, did not cease in the interwar period. Men now faced the new threat of an overcrowded profession with many individuals returning from war and many newly licensed women doctors. As a result, men continued their efforts to steer women into marginal fields by discriminating against them in the most elite areas of employment like the health insurance practices. In the final year of the republic, the profession's bias against women became state-sanctioned with the passage of a *Doppelverdiener* law against married women civil servants who were second wage earners. Just two years later, the Nazi regime passed another law that forbade married women whose husbands had adequate income from working for the choice health insurance practices. The Nazi Party also initially made it clear that it wanted to limit women's access to medical study and to employment in general.[2]

Women doctors were by no means passive observers of their own careers. Female physicians also made choices about the employment paths they took. While working in marriage counselling centres, schools, in the anti-alcohol and anti-VD campaigns, breast milk collection facilities, or the BDM or RMD meant they made less money or worked part-time or even voluntarily, they certainly did not see this work as inferior. Rather, these medical spaces offered them the opportunity to showcase their expertise in women's and children's health based on their biological training and their personal experiences as women and mothers. This latter fact was also what they claimed made them more qualified for these positions than their male colleagues. In addition, because of their part-time or irregular hours, these jobs offered female doctors the flexibility to pursue professional careers, especially in fields that were of a personal interest to many of them, as well as motherhood. The nature of the work they performed in these spaces was akin to their domestic responsibilities, meaning they could use this fact to prove their professional worth and could straddle their obligations as mothers and workers under a similar rubric of activities. They solved their own work-family dilemma by pursuing this sensible, less resistant path. They certainly were not getting any resistance from men in the profession, many of whom agreed they should be serving in these fields.

Female doctors became autonomous and authoritative in what became their own secluded medical spaces. Places like marriage counselling centres, girls' vocational schools, breast milk collection facilities, the BDM, and the RMD often gave female physicians more control and allowed them to be more active than they might have been in spaces where they were under the watch of outsiders. They demonstrated their command of such fields by broadening their duties from being mere medical advisers, teachers, or collaborators to becoming political, educational, and social leaders for their patients and students. As a result, they arrogated professional authority within the medical profession under two different regimes.

During the Weimar Republic, female physicians redefined and expanded the practice of medicine. Within various medical spaces – counselling centres, schools, VD clinics – they worked to acquire political, educational, and social rights for their underprivileged and often overlooked lower-class female and youth patients. Especially in light of the failed professional promises for women during the Weimar Republic, acquiring access to birth control for women in marriage counselling centres, equalizing girls' physical education curriculum in schools, and achieving equivalent treatment for women in VD counselling centres gave them meaningful work.

They also fostered an atmosphere of trust between patient and doctor, resulting in a nurturing and maternal relationship. Women, they maintained, were more likely to trust doctors with their intimate marital problems and visit marriage clinics if they employed a female counsellor, especially one who was married. Similarly, female doctors argued that venereal disease clinics would attract more women if they knew that they could trust a woman physician to protect their modesty and shame. Female vocational school students, they asserted, were more likely to discuss embarrassing issues like menstruation if they could turn to a female school doctor. The trusting relationship that developed between doctors and their patients and students emerged from their experiential commonalities as women. These relationships are what female physicians claimed gave them more legitimacy and clout among their patients, and thereby made them highly qualified to assist the Weimar regime achieve its goals in the areas of marriage counselling or in the anti-alcohol or anti-VD campaigns. Although the Weimar state may not have officially acknowledged their abilities to do so, women doctors asserted that they could be more effective promoters of premarital health certificates or could more easily draw women into the anti-alcohol or anti-VD campaigns.

After 1933, female doctors became even more explicit about how their innate abilities, first-hand experiences, and the trusting relationships they built with patients could help the Nazi state accomplish its health goals. The members of the BDÄ who did not fall victim to Hitler's anti-Semitic policies unashamedly advertised themselves as *Volksärztinnen* (people's doctors) who could lure apolitical women to support National Socialism and could indoctrinate them to its ideology. During the BDM-sponsored mother evenings, BDM physicians, who were ideally also married mothers themselves, bonded with mothers, informing them about the activities their daughters were involved in and providing advice about how to answer their daughters' health and sexual questions. In addition to gaining the trust of these mothers, BDM physicians earned the trust of BDM leaders by offering them emotional guidance and support. Gaining the confidence of mothers and leaders allowed BDM physicians to exert influence over them, subsequently allowing them to help doctors indoctrinate young girls to Nazi ideology. A deeper trust developed between BDM physicians and *Mädels* when they all wore the same uniform and participated in the same activities, thereby giving BDM physicians direct influence over the members when it came to state and political matters. Dr Marie Elise-Kayser and others in breast milk collection facilities highlighted how female physicians' personal experiences in nursing made them more capable of drawing women into the breast milk collection movement, which fit the Nazi regime's agenda of preserving natural resources and preventing infant mortality. In contrast to the Weimar state, the Nazis recognized the value women doctors provided to the regime and openly employed them for these larger medical objectives in national organizations such as the BDM and the RMD. The Reich Ministry of the Interior gave Kayser's breast milk collection initiative a stamp of approval, and facilities became state sponsored by 1939. Although women doctors continued to direct women's and children's medicine using the same maternalistic language under Nazism, the face of the medicine they practised changed to incorporate the ideological goals of the state – something the Weimar version had lacked.

Through the work they did during the Nazi period, women doctors helped to create a micro *Volksgemeinschaft* (people's community) in the BDM or in breast milk collection facilities, and they also became more inclusive, equal members of the larger *Volksgemeinschaft* through the opportunities presented to them in women's and children's medicine. This study demonstrates, then, that the *Volksgemeinschaft* was inclusive, created more equality, and opened up opportunity for a group of German female physicians.[3] Women physicians could freely interpret and appropriate the notoriously vague rhetoric of the *Volksgemeinschaft* and apply it to the girls in the BDM or to the community of breast milk donors. Because there was no clear-cut definition of what the concept meant, it could be applied to almost anything, and thus, "there was … hardly a field of social action or cultural production during the National Socialist dictatorship in which *Volksgemeinschaft* did not play a part."[4] Consequently, these doctors became complicit in spreading Nazi ideology, which entailed excluding others – that is, the racially "unfit" – from joining the BDM or donating their breast milk. They also became *Volks-genossin* (comrades) or full-fledged members of the *Volksgemeinschaft* through this work. Their belonging in a larger *Volksgemeinschaft* of doctors, women, and Nazis fulfilled them, empowered them, legitimized them, and charged them "to make a personal and active contribution to the realization of the utopia."[5] In other words, once they had a sense of belonging in the national *Volksgemeinschaft*, they could help perpetuate and create local or regional communities among specific groups of women, girls, and mothers.

Women doctors continued to find ways to carve novel professional spaces even as circumstances and contexts changed. They made a claim – one that was accepted by the higher-ups, especially under Nazism – that because they were women, and especially if they were mothers, they had a special role to play in aiding and advising girls and women. This unique perspective and their natural-given abilities, they asserted, meant they could improve medicine in a number of different areas, namely those centred on the well-being of women and children. Girls and women trusted women physicians and believed they knew from experience what they were talking about. This is an important point of continuity from the Weimar to Nazi periods, but even more generally this was women's claim to access to the profession from the very beginning.

There was continuity between the types of work women doctors claimed they could best perform for both regimes and also in their mobilization methods. The women in this nascent profession carved and cultivated their niche by recognizing and reflecting so-called "social problems" and new social structural opportunities presented by each regime. In the Weimar Republic, doctors became involved in curtailing divorce rates and promoting healthy marriages, reducing alcoholism, preventing the spread of VD, and providing adequate health education to girls in schools. In the Nazi era, they worked to prevent infant mortality in breast milk collection facilities, taught about the preservation of the Reich's resources in mothers' training courses, and actually maximized natural resources with the collection and redistribution of breast milk. These two states certainly differed significantly, especially with regards to their motivations for intervening into women's and children's health. In the Weimar Republic, a social welfare agenda linked to curbing perceived national crises was the primary motivation for its social programs related to women and children. Under Nazism, the strengthening of the nation, the fulfillment of ideological goals, and the creation of an exclusionary, racial *Volksgemeinschaft* were the reasons for the regime's focus on women and children. While their motivations may have varied, both regimes provided the space (even if only discursively) for female physicians to create and expand their work as physicians.

In allying with these various health projects, women physicians often stated that they were doing much more than the tasks required of them. In municipal, religious, and private marriage counselling centres, they saw themselves as providing much more than the premarital health exams mandated by certain states like Prussia, and instead primarily distributed birth control and marital advice to women, based on their cited reasons for visiting clinics in the first place. In some cases, they performed abortions or sterilization, or even offered legal or economic advice. More often than not, they served as a source of comfort to women who came to them with intimate problems, such as domestic violence or sexual dysfunction. In schools, too, female doctors claimed to go above the call of duty to administer annual fitness exams for students. They advised girls about healthy clothing choices and supported them as they confronted menstruation. In addition, they moved their discourse from the schoolhouses into the home, writing instructional pamphlets and holding workshops for mothers about proper childcare. They also extended their work to the larger public sphere by convening conferences, such as the 1925 Conference on the Physical Education of Women. In the anti-VD campaign, women doctors became political activists for women, as they fought the double standard embedded in state-regulated prostitution. Under Nazism, they incorporated Nazi ideologies like *Blut und Boden* (blood and soil) and comradeship into the activities of the BDM, and trained mothers in the RMD to be aware of their larger obligations to the German *Volk* and German state through *Mütterschulung* courses. And Kayser, a pediatrician, changed course by initiating Germany's breast milk collection efforts, redirecting it to infants in need and devoting countless hours to vying for the regime's attention. These women physicians were certainly mobilized, demonstrating how a professional group, notwithstanding systematic discrimination or perhaps even *because* of it, found ways to showcase their talents and often claimed to perform their jobs more eagerly and more comprehensively than required.

While their maternalistic strategy allowed them to grow professionally, they advanced at the expense of lower-class individuals. Their rhetoric was often denigrating toward their primarily lower-class patients and students. They criticized parental negligence in matters of health and, at times, attempted to impose their own middle-class values of health onto their patients and students. However, middle- and upper-class female physicians also worked in medical spaces where they helped break down class barriers. In marriage counselling centres, vocational schools, and VD clinics, they established intimate contact and developed relationships with women of the lower class. In the BDM, RMD, and breast milk collection facilities, they worked with girls and mothers of all classes. One of the stated aims of Nazism, as David Schoenbaum showed over fifty years ago, was to eliminate the class divide, but Nazi promises never met reality.[6] The medical spaces discussed in this study, however, suggest areas where the National Socialists, in fact, achieved some degree of success in eradicating the class divide. And female physicians played a role in erasing this gap. In the BDM – a space that is well known for class divisions, especially between BDM leaders, who were primarily middle-class, and the girls – doctors participated in all activities wholeheartedly, even wearing the same matching uniforms.[7] In breast milk collection facilities, Kayser insisted that donors and recipients come from all classes. Historically, more lower-class and socially disadvantaged people were suppliers of body products like breast milk, and more rich people were recipients.[8] However, in addition to Kayser's commitment to ensuring that women of all classes received milk, Drs Hellpap and Eckardt reported that while the majority of donors to the Kassel and Plauen facilities were from worker families, donors came from all classes.[9] This book's focus on class or, better yet, the interrelationship between class and gender, shows how a group of women both reinforced the class divide to advance professionally (because of the gendered discrimination they faced) and helped to eradicate it by creating trusting relationships among women of different classes in female medical spaces.[10]

Much of the work that women physicians became involved in (or at least proposed becoming involved in) had to do with restoring national health in the Weimar and Nazi years. They used the rhetoric of the nation and its health to legitimize their work and draw attention to their causes. After the First World War, the Weimar state started to intervene in marriage to create healthier marriages and to prevent divorce at a time when divorce rates were rising. When ideas of voluntary marriage health certificates were being debated in the Reichstag and the first private and municipal clinics opened, female doctors stated that they would be the best suited to serve the majority female clientele who visited the clinics. As the republic became overly concerned with youth and their welfare, female physicians suggested crafting a girls' physical education program focused on restoring and strengthening female bodies. Also, growing problems in the post–First World War era, prostitution, VD, and alcoholism were perceived as threats and the campaigns against them focused on strengthening the German national body. The Nazi regime was not shy about bolstering the *Volksgesundheit* (people's health) and especially the health of Germany's mothers, who would produce the next generation for the thousand-year Reich. The BDM and RMD, where female physicians claimed a presence, were just two of several welfare bureaucracies aimed at improving the health of the regime's mothers and youth. And lastly, with fears about infant mortality rates affecting the already vulnerable German nation, breast milk collection became one means to help prevent this.

Both the Weimar and Nazi states provided attention and health care to women and children for divergent reasons, and female physicians' efforts in garnering additional attention to these fields is particularly noteworthy and useful in light of current debates about women's access to health care and the role of the state in providing it. As the women at the centre of this book have shown, they were quite successful at drawing the state's attention to women's issues. They demonstrate how women, deemed the guardians of future generations, often have more influence over promoting women's and children's issues as national concerns, particularly if they are medical authorities.

To take the recent political issue of breastfeeding as just one example, it is often women and women physicians who have organized the cause and have drawn regional, state, and national authorities into debates about the collection of milk, nursing in public, or "breast is best" policies. As Kara Swanson has shown, in breast milk banks, doctors have become the main actors. Doctors, she claims, have an incredible amount of discretion as to when body products like breast milk should be used to treat a patient.[11] They also have authority over who should receive this life-saving nutrient. As Dr Kayser has shown us, this kind of authority, which could be vital or detrimental to one's life, has existed for some time and often became augmented in times of crisis – in wartime, for example. In 1944, when she received a request at the Erfurt facility to send breast milk to an extremely sick child who had previously been receiving it but no longer had access to it because of evacuations in the area, Kayser turned him down.[12] She certainly held a position of authority over this life-saving nutrient and people's access to it, evidenced by the letters she received from people pleading for milk.[13] The once private, intimate act of breastfeeding has become not only politicized today, but also scientized, collectivized, and scrutinized by medical authorities and average women alike. The discourse from the Weimar and Nazi eras about becoming involved in people's private lives and intervening in the private act of mothering still endures and fuels current debates about nursing. Similar to the Weimar and Nazi eras, much of the rhetoric today is only rhetoric and not active or physical intervention. Instead, it plays out primarily on motherhood blogs and social media in the same way that it once played out in a medical journal. Interestingly, the debate about whether public authorities should facilitate mothering in private has been reversed, and it is now a question of whether women should be partaking in this once private act in public.

There is also a usable past to these physicians' breast milk collection efforts, even if they flourished under Nazism. Bernhard Rieger has argued that "recent research has demonstrated that recasting the gender order and embracing innovative technology played crucial roles in Nazi plans to shape a radically new, powerful 'modern' Germany."[14] Doctors like Kayser, Feldweg, Eckardt, and others, in their creation of and participation in breast milk collection, were also helping shape what was deemed to be modern in Nazi Germany, much of which came in the form of technological and scientific innovation.[15] Along with studies linking smoking to lung cancer and positive strides in environmentalism, breast milk collection was one of the many scientific achievements of the Nazi regime.[16] Both Germany and other Western countries, including the US, still use a method of collecting and redistributing breast milk. Now, more than ever, breast milk is deemed to be liquid gold.

So the question remains whether female doctors advanced their own professional ambitions or the medical rights of their patients. In other words, did their maternalistic strategy work? Yes, these women were certainly pioneers in the German medical profession, especially during the Weimar period. For one, they made women's and children's health, which was already a national topic of concern, even more prominent. While a few men were also engaged in women's and children's health (most notably, Dr Friedrich Eckardt), it is unlikely that many women's concerns would have received the attention they did in medical discourse without the tireless work of many women in the profession. They centred women's issues like menstruation, access to birth control, healthy nursing, proper clothing, and motherhood in medical discourse. They advocated for a separate physical education program for girls in schools and accomplished their goal of getting certain states to provide female physicians for female patients in VD clinics. They also collected over 577,000 litres of breast milk and, by some estimates, helped approximately 150,000 premature babies and sick infants.[17] It is also safe to assume that their patients, who now had someone to turn to with their intimate, embarrassing problems, felt at ease knowing there was a woman doctor on hand to assist them. Lower-class women who previously lacked a voice or a place to turn for medical help, found solidarity with other women in the atmosphere of the waiting room as well as empathy and comfort from women doctors.[18] Women physicians made political, educational, and social demands on behalf of their patients and students, thereby making gains for these individuals and for women's and children's health more broadly.

They also did a service for their own professional objectives. They became experts in women's and children's health, and thereby valuable to the Weimar and later to the Nazi state. They reconciled their own career ambitions with their motherhood roles by finding a niche that allowed them the flexibility to do both. They found or created spaces in which they could be autonomous and could develop meaningful relationships with their colleagues and patients, resulting in their activism and their expanded, influential medical roles. Female physicians, then, through their use of the rhetoric of motherhood, opened up new discursive spaces to achieve political and social results for their patients and for themselves. After 1933, the BDÄ remained advocates for women's and children's health, and for their own position in medicine, but the maternalist impulses that served the cause of social reform in the Weimar years became the handmaidens to the purposes of the Nazi regime.

Notes

Introduction

1 Dr Marie-Elise Kayser, "Frauenmilchsammelstellen," *Die Ärztin* 4, no. 2 (1928): 28–9.
2 Marie-Elise Kayser, "Frauenmilchsammelstellen!," *Die Ärztin* 11, no. 2 (1935): 23.
3 Koven and Michel, *Mothers of a New World*, 4.
4 Ibid.; Mazower, *Dark Continent*, 83–4. Ann Taylor Allen shows how the middle-class women's movement used maternalist rhetoric before the war in *Feminism and Motherhood in Germany*.
5 Benjamin Ziemann highlights gender and class as important, relational analytical categories of Germany in the 1920s. See "Weimar Was Weimar." The following are the most important medical histories of Weimar and Nazi Germany: Kater, "The Burden of the Past"; Kater, *Doctors under Hitler*; Kater, "Professionalization and Socialization of Physicians"; Michalczyk, *Medicine, Ethics, and the Third Reich*; Proctor, *Racial Hygiene*; and Weindling, *Health, Race and German Politics*. There has also been recent interest in examining Weimar and Nazi health policies from a gendered perspective: Allen, "German Radical Feminism and Eugenics"; Bock, "Racism and Sexism in Nazi Germany"; Eckelmann, *Ärztinnen in der Weimarer Zeit*; Grossmann, "Berliner Ärztinnen und Volksgesundheit"; Grossmann, *Reforming Sex*; Mouton, *From Nurturing the Nation*; Schleiermacher, "Ärztinnen zwischen Sozialhygiene und Eugenik"; Schleiermacher, "Rassenhygienische Mission"; Timm, *The Politics of Fertility*; Usborne, *Cultures of Abortion*; Usborne, *The Politics of the Body*; and Usborne, "Women Doctors and Gender Identity in Weimar Germany."

6 Sonya Michel argues that maternalist practices were "most frequently deployed by middle-class women to justify their own political participation as well as the establishment of institutions, policies, or legislation directed at poor or working-class women and children." See "Maternalism Reconsidered," 4.

7 Weindling, "Bourgeois Values, Doctors and the State," 213.

8 Ibid., 198–9.

9 Grossmann, *Reforming Sex*, 136.

10 Grossmann, "German Women Doctors from Berlin to New York," 66.

11 Mouton, *From Nurturing the Nation*, 15, 35.

12 Dickinson, "Biopolitics, Fascism, Democracy," 15–16.

13 Marhoefer, *Sex and the Weimar Republic*, 176; and Roos, *Weimar through the Lens of Gender*, 213.

14 Usborne, *Cultures of Abortion*; Usborne, *The Politics of the Body*, 204.

15 Timm, *The Politics of Fertility*, 31–2, 319.

16 Koven and Michel, "Womanly Duties," 1079.

17 Seth Koven and Sonya Michel initially used "maternalism" in their discussion of large-scale social welfare programs and policies that emerged in France, Germany, Great Britain, and the United States in the late nineteenth and early twentieth centuries. See Koven and Michel, *Mothers of a New World*, and "Womanly Duties." They were responding to definitions of "familial feminism" and "relational feminism" posed by Karen Offen in her discussion of welfare states in France and by Theda Skocpol in her discussion of the US as a unique maternalist welfare state. See Offen, "Depopulation, Nationalism, and Feminism," and "Defining Feminism"; and Skocpol, *Protecting Soldiers and Mothers*.

18 Weindling, *Health, Race, and German Politics*, 2, 577.

19 Helmut Walser Smith explores the deep continuities of German history through the lens of vanishing points in *The Continuities of German History*, especially 13–38.

20 Kater shows that a male doctor had almost twice the chance to establish himself in health insurance practice, especially in the early years of the Weimar Republic and the Third Reich. Things improved slightly for female doctors working in health insurance practices in the latter half of the Weimar Republic. Kater, *Doctors under Hitler*, 90, 248.

21 See Remy, *The Heidelberg Myth* for a discussion of professors at the University of Heidelberg, and Walker, *Nazi Science*, for an investigation of physicists working on the atomic bomb. Female professionals such as

secretaries and prostitutes also faced few changes from the Weimar to Nazi transition. See Lower, *Hitler's Furies*, and Harris, *Selling Sex in the Reich*, for a discussion of secretaries and prostitutes, respectively.

22 Article 119 read: "Marriage, as the foundation of the family and the preservation and expansion of the nation, enjoys the special protection of the constitution. It is based on the equality of both genders. It is the task of both the state and the communities to strengthen and socially promote the family. Large families may claim social welfare. Motherhood is placed under state protection and welfare."

23 Koonz, "Mothers in the Fatherland," 447–8.

24 Timm, *The Politics of Fertility*, 9.

25 See the standard definitions in Kevles, *In the Name of Eugenics*. See also Timm, *The Politics of Fertility*, 86.

26 Usborne, *The Politics of the Body*, 5–6.

27 Weindling, *Health, Race, and German Politics*, especially 123–54.

28 Kevles, "Eugenics Then and Genetics Now," 190; Kevles, *In the Name of Eugenics*.

29 Timm, *The Politics of Fertility*, 9.

30 Grossmann, "Berliner Ärztinnen und Volksgesundheit"; Grossmann, "German Women Doctors from Berlin to New York"; Schleiermacher, "Ärztinnen zwischen Sozialhygiene und Eugenik"; Schleiermacher, "Rassenhygienische Mission"; and Usborne, "Women Doctors and Gender Identity in Weimar Germany."

31 Stokes, "Contested Conceptions," 146.

32 Mouton, *From Nurturing the Nation*, 12.

33 Kater, "Professionalization and Socialization of Physicians," 686–7.

34 Mazón, *Gender and the Modern Research University*, 95, 104, 107. See also Eckelmann, *Ärztinnen in der Weimarer Zeit*, 16. Both Eckelmann and Mazón note that in its demands for women to be permitted to study medicine, the women's movement highlighted the "feminine" nature of practising medicine, which made it especially fitting for women's helping, healing, and nurturing qualities.

35 Huerkamp, "The Making of the Modern Medical Profession," 66–7.

36 Koblitz, "Science, Women, and the Russian Intelligentsia," 207.

37 Judith-Maria Rüger, "Der weibliche Nachwuchs der deutschen Aerzteschaft," *Monatsschrift deutscher Ärztinnen* 6, no. 3 (1930): 45. See also Eckelmann, *Ärztinnen in der Weimarer Zeit*, 16; Kater, "Professionalization and Socialization of Physicians," 686–7; and Mazón, *Gender and the Modern Research University*, 59, 112.

38 Dr Ursula Romann, "Vor 40 Jahren. Erinnerungen an den Berufsweg der ersten in Deutschland approbierten Ärztin, Frau Dr med. Ida Democh-Mauermeier," *Die Ärztin* 17, no. 4 (1941): 154–5.

39 "Berufszählung: Die berufliche und soziale Gliederung des deutschen Volkes. Textliche Darstellung der Ergebnisse," in *Statistik des Deutschen Reichs* 408 (Berlin: Reimar Hobbing, 1931), 301–4; "Berufszählung: Die berufliche und soziale Gliederung der Bevölkerung des Deutschen Reichs. Die Erwerbstätigkeit der Reichsbevölkerung," in *Statistik des Deutschen Reichs* 453, no. 2 (Berlin: Verlag für Sozialpolitik, Wirtschaft und Statistik, Paul Smidt, 1936), 192; "Die Berufstätigkeit der Bevölkerung des Deutsche Reichs. Die Reichsbevölkerung nach Haupt- und Nebenberuf," in *Statistik des Deutschen Reichs* 556, no. 1 (Berlin: Verlag für Sozialpolitik, Wirtschaft und Statistik, Paul Smidt, 1942), 162.

40 van Kann, "Die Zahl der Ärzte 1942 und ein Rückblick bis 1937," 300–3. Dr Ilse Szagunn, "Die Zahl der Ärztinnen in der Gegenwart," *Die Ärztin* 19, no. 1 (1943): 24. Szagunn admits that most of her statistics come from van Kann's article. This number accounted for the new regions of the Reich, which included the so-called German Ostmark (Austria), the Sudetenland, and the Kattowitzer region, which brought in about 1,200 new female doctors. See also Kater, *Doctors under Hitler*, 89. Kater's statistics are from van Kann's article in *Deutsches Ärtzeblatt* and from another article: van Kann, "Zahl und Gliedergung der Fachärzte Deutschlands im Jahre 1940," 285. Van Kann's numbers show a more gradual increase of women physicians than the *Statistik des Deutschen Reichs* – 6.5 per cent in 1932, 7.9 per cent in 1937, 9.8 per cent in 1939, 12.4 per cent in 1942 – but still demonstrate that within a short amount of time, women doubled their numbers in medicine.

41 Dr med. Marie Unna-Boehm, "Bericht über die Gründungsversammlung des Bundes Deutscher Ärztinnen am 26. und 27. Oktober 1924," *Vierteljahrsschrift deutscher Ärztinnen* 1, no. 3 (1924), 74; Anne Marie Durand-Wever and Laura Turnau, "Die deutsche Aerztin. Statistische Notizen," *Vierteljahrsschrift deutscher Ärztinnen* 2, no. 3 (1926): 92; Usborne, "Women Doctors and Gender Identity in Weimar Germany," 112.

42 Dr Helene Börner, "Rundfrage an die Aerztinnen über ihre Stellungnahme zur Schwangerschaftsunterbrechung," *Die Ärztin* 8, no. 1 (1932): 4.

43 For more on the political and religious affiliations, medical backgrounds, and professional fields of the first generation of female physicians, see Bleker and Schleiermacher, *Ärztinnen aus dem Kaiserreich*, and the

accompanying database: Buchin, "Dokumentation: Ärztinnen aus dem Kaisserreich." Their figures indicate that close to fifty female doctors were active as full-time or part-time school doctors, eighteen were active in counselling centres, and six worked for local police authorities. In welfare institutions, health offices, or in their capacity as auxiliary municipal doctors, there were sixty active female physicians. A few administered several functions. Out of the 792 doctors who, to their knowledge, had been licensed by 1918, Bleker and Schleiermacher found that only 28 had achieved civil servant status in public health care. For more about the goals of Bleker's and Schleiermacher's project, see Sach, "Gedenke, daß du eine deutsche Frau bist!," 8.

44 Grossmann, "German Women Doctors from Berlin to New York," 74.
45 Benz, *Das Tagebuch der Hertha Nathorff*, 29, 36–7.
46 Eckelmann, *Ärztinnen in der Weimarer Zeit*, 24.
47 The DDP, DVP, and DNVP lost most of their supporters to the Nazis. Evans, *The Feminist Movement in Germany*, 244, 253.
48 This is an argument also made by Eckelmann, *Ärztinnen in der Weimarer Zeit*, 47, 63.
49 Evans, *The Feminist Movement in Germany*, 254, 256–7. The BDF, unlike the BDÄ, dissolved itself in 1933.
50 On the complex relationship between liberals, including the DDP (the party of liberal democracy) and the BDF (the liberal feminist movement), see Kurlander, *Living with Hitler*, especially 195.
51 Sach, "Gedenke, daß du eine deutsche Frau bist!," 50.
52 For histories on the *Gleichschaltung* (coordination) of the BDÄ, or those women doctors who left Germany, either by choice or coercion, or those forced out of the profession, see Bleker, "Anerkennung durch Unterordnung?"; Bleker and Eckelmann, "Der Erfolg der Gleichschaltungsaktion"; Eckelmann, *Ärztinnen in der Weimarer Zeit*; Grossmann, "Berliner Ärztinnen und Volksgesundheit"; Grossmann, "German Women Doctors from Berlin to New York"; Schleiermacher, "Rassenhygienische Mission."
53 Stephenson, "Women and the Professions in Germany," 275–6. For a similar argument that female legal equality and suffrage did not yield substantial changes for women professionally, see Bridenthal, "Beyond Kinder, Küche, Kirche," and Bridenthal and Koonz, "Beyond Kinder, Küche, Kirche." For the larger history of how the Weimar Republic failed to live up to the welfare commitments outlined in its constitution, see Hong, *Welfare, Modernity, and the Weimar State*.
54 Usborne, "Women Doctors and Gender Identity in Weimar Germany," 109.

55 In March 1917, women outnumbered men at work for the first time. See Bridenthal, "Beyond Kinder, Küche, Kirche," 155.

56 "Warnung vor dem ärztlichem Studium," *Deutsche Tageszeitung*, 9 April 1925, in BArch, NS/VI.7089.

57 Bleker, "Anerkennung durch Unterordnung?," 126–7.

58 Stephenson, "Girls' Higher Education in Germany in the 1930s," 49.

59 Kater, *Doctors under Hitler*, 93; Pauwels, *Women, Nazis, and Universities*, 24; Stephenson, *Women in Nazi Society*, 166.

60 Richard Grün, "Frauenerziehung, die Schicksalfrage des deutschen Volkes," *Deutsches Bildungswesen* 2 (1934): 151–3, as quoted in Pauwels, *Women, Nazis, and Universities*, 16. See also Adelsberger, "Die Frau als Ärztin," 198–9. As a female doctor herself, Adelsberger claimed that these arguments could be rebutted by the fact that women had the physical capability to bear and raise children on their own.

61 See, for example, Dr med. Max Grünewald, "Die Frau als Ärztin," *Frau und Gegenwart*, 4 September 1928, in BArch, NS/VI.7089.

62 Usborne, "Body Biological to Body Politic," 144.

63 Richards, "Huxley and Woman's Place in Science."

64 Adelsberger, "Die Frau als Ärztin," 200.

65 "Zahl und Familienstand der Ärztinnen," *Die Ärztin* 11, no. 9 (1935): 147, 150.

66 Bleker and Schleiermacher, *Ärztinnen aus dem Kaiserreich*, 110.

67 Usborne, "Women Doctors and Gender Identity in Weimar Germany," 112–13.

68 Grossmann, "German Women Doctors from Berlin to New York," 79.

69 Recent work that discusses the question of women's role as perpetrators, agents, actors, or opportunists during the Third Reich and the Second World War includes: Harvey, *Women and the Nazi East*; Kramer, *Volksgenossinnen an der Heimatfront*; Lower, *Hitler's Furies*; Steinbacher, *"Volksgenossinnen"*; and von Saldern, "Innovative Trends in Women's and Gender Studies."

70 Evidence that doctors viewed motherhood as an instinctive and natural role for women: Nathorff, "Zum Problem der Geburtenregelung," 863; Heusler-Edenhuizen, "Eheberatungsstellen," 187. For more on the socially constructed belief that womanhood equals motherhood, see Campbell, *Childfree and Sterilized*.

71 Zegenhagen demonstrates how female pilots emphasized their femininity in "The Holy Desire to Serve the Poor and Tortured Fatherland," 584–5. Further examples of women scientists emphasizing their femininity to make their mark in certain scientific, medical, and

engineering professions can be found in: Cowan, *More Work for Mother*; Cowan, "Parlors, Primers, and Public Schooling"; Kohlstedt, "Nature, Not Books"; Morantz-Sanchez, *Sympathy and Science*, especially chapter 3, "Bringing Science into the Home"; Oldenziel, "Man the Maker, Woman the Consumer"; Pycior, "Marie Curie's 'Anti-Natural Path'"; Schiebinger, *Has Feminism Changed Science?*; Schiebinger, "Maria Winkelmann at the Berlin Academy"; Shteir, "Botany in the Breakfast Room"; Terrall, "Salon, Academy and Boudoir." This topic was a primary theme of the conference "Women of Science, Women in Science: Figures and Representations, 18th Century to Present," 4–6 June 2009, in Grenoble, France, and in the subsequent publication, Andréolle and Molinari, *Women and Science*.

72 Keller, *A Feeling for the Organism*. See also: Barinaga, "Is There a Female Style of Doing Science?"; Oreskes, "Objectivity or Heroism?"; and Rosser, *Female-Friendly Science*.

73 Rossiter designates fields of science as "marginal" when between 5 and 15 per cent of the participants are women. This means that this group is generally the second or third generation of women to enter that field, as access to the field is unproblematic (although still restricted in areas). This group is also generally professionalized with a club or organization. See "Which Women? Which Science?," 171–2.

74 Foucault, *The History of Sexuality*; Foucault, *The Archaeology of Knowledge*; Foucault, *The Birth of Biopolitics*.

75 Walther, *Sex and Control*, 2–3.

76 Frevert, *Women in German History*, 203.

77 Herf, *Reactionary Modernism*.

78 On the theory of equality *and* difference, see Scott, "Deconstructing Equality-versus-Difference," 44, and Scott, *Only Paradoxes to Offer*.

1. Promoting Marriage, Motherhood, Eugenics, and Health Care

1 "In der Geburtenberatungsstelle der IAH," *Der Weg Der Frau*, August 1931, in ADE, CA/GfSt 247, 43.

2 Ibid.

3 On the longer history of population policy, see Timm, *The Politics of Fertility*, 5–8.

4 Dr Lotte Fink, "Schwangerschaftsunterbrechung und Erfahrungen aus Ehe- und Sexualberatung," *Die Ärztin* 7, no. 3 (1931): 71.

5 Timm, *The Politics of Fertility*, 5–12.

6 In the late 1800s, there were 40 live births per 1,000 Germans and 29.8 in 1910. By 1920, this number had dropped to 25.9, to 19.6 by 1926, and to 14.7 by 1933, at which point it started to increase again. Pauwels, *Women, Nazis, and Universities*, 15. Pauwels's statistics (outlined in table 1 on page 144) come from the *Statistisches Jahrbuch* from 1917, 1921/22, 1930, 1935, and 1941/42. See also Knodel, *The Decline of Fertility in Germany*, 5.

7 Hoffmann and Timm, "Utopian Biopolitics," 88. On concerns about depopulation in post–First World War France, see Roberts, *Civilization without Sexes*, especially chapter 4.

8 See, for example, Dr Helene Lange, "Axmann: 'Der Schiksalweg studierter Frauen,'" *Vierteljahrsschrift deutscher Ärztinnen* 2, no. 3 (1926): 58; Dr Hertha Riese, "Soll der Staat Heiratsvermittler werden? Ueber die Notwendigkeit der Einrichtung staatlicher Ehevermittlungsstellen," *Berliner Tageblatt*, 8 January 1928, in BArch, R 86/5620.

9 See, for example, "Ehescheidungsgründe," *Heirat und Ehe* 2, no. 7 (1927), in ADE, CA/G 397, 6/7, and "Eheschließungen und Ehescheidungen in Essen," *Heirat und Ehe* 2, no. 11 (1927), in ADE, CA/G 397, 7/9.

10 Timm, *The Politics of Fertility*, 81.

11 Ibid., 82.

12 The following are the major studies of German eugenics: Proctor, *Racial Hygiene*; Weindling, *Health, Race and German Politics*; Weiss, *Race Hygiene and National Efficiency*; Weiss, "The Race Hygiene Movement in Germany"; Weingart, Kroll, and Bayertz, *Rasse, Blut und Gene*.

13 This was emphasized, among other places, in the RGA's *Merkblatt für Eheschließende* from 1920. See several copies of the final version, in BArch, R 86/5618 or BArch, R 86/2372, Bl. 472 or the various draft versions, in BArch, R 86/5623.

14 As Dr med. Georg Hartwich, the acting district medical officer in Einbeck, emphasized in a brochure, "a state's interest always exists both in terms of the quality and the number of offspring." See Hartwich, "Deutschlands größte Gefahr (Der Geburtenrückgang)," September 1923, in BArch, R 86/5636.

15 Timm, *The Politics of Fertility*, 81.

16 Petition from the Berlin Society for Racial Hygiene to RMI, 5 September 1917, in BArch, R 86/2372, Bl. 30–1. See also letter from Bumm to RMI, 11 December 1917, in BArch, R 1501/9379, Bl. 5.

17 Letter from Bumm to RMI, 11 December 1917, in BArch, R 1501/9379, Bl. 6–7.

18 Allen, "Feminism, Venereal Disease, and the State in Germany," 39, and Dickinson, "Biopolitics, Fascism, Democracy," 10.

19 Letter from Bumm to RMI, 11 December 1917, in BArch, R 1501/9379, Bl. 8–12. See also Timm, *The Politics of Fertility*, 97–8.

20 Letter from Reichkanzler (Reichsamt des Innern) to RMI, 1 February 1918, in BArch, 1501/9379, Bl. 70.

21 See Schubart letters to RMI, Reich Ministry of Justice, and Prussian Ministry of the Interior and their responses, in BArch, R 1501/9379, especially Bl. 320–2.

22 See Weindling, *Health, Race and German Politics*, 361.

23 See, for example, a letter from the BDF to all its district and local associations from 28 December 1920, in which it asked local leaders to ensure the distribution of leaflets in their registry offices, in BArch R 1501/9379, Bl. 247. See also Timm, *The Politics of Fertility*, 98–9.

24 Timm, *The Politics of Fertility*, 100–1.

25 Runderlaß des Ministers für Volkswohlfahrt, betr. Einrichtung ärztlich geleiteter Eheberatungsstellen in Gemeinden und Kreisen, 19 February 1926, in BArch, R 86/5618, Bl. 7–10. See also Leitsätze des Reichsgesundheitsrates, 26 February 1920, in BArch, R 86/5618, Bl. 243.

26 Press coverage in the months following the ordinance recognized that doctors were simply making a recommendation to marriage candidates as to whether or not they were healthy enough to enter marriage, based on genetic or other health reasons. See especially "Die Errichtung von ärztlich geleiteten Eheberatungsstellen," *Berliner Tageblatt*, 24 March 1926, and P. Merz, "Aerztlich geleitete Eheberatungsstellen," *Köln Volkstg.*, 3 April 1926, in BArch, R 86/5624. See also Runderlaß des Ministers für Volkswohlfahrt, in BArch, R 86/5618, Bl. 7–8.

27 Timm, *The Politics of Fertility*, 103. The second quote appeared in a letter from Hans Harmsen to the Minister für Volkswohlfahrt, December 1927, in ADE, CA/GfSt 247, 2–4, and ADE, CA/G 397, 18/1–18/3.

28 Timm, *The Politics of Fertility*, 82.

29 See Reinert, *Frauen und Sexualreform*, 193.

30 von Soden, *Sexualberatungsstellen der Weimarer Republik*, 68–70.

31 Proctor, *Racial Hygiene*, 138.

32 The professionalization of eugenics in Germany happened primarily via Alfred Ploetz, one of the co-founders of the German eugenics movement, who coined the term "racial hygiene" (*Rassenhygiene*) in his 1895 book *The Fitness of Our Race and the Protection of the Weak*, which became a German synonym for eugenics. In 1904, he established the first journal in the world dedicated to eugenics, the *Archiv für Rassen- und Gesellschaftsbiologie (Journal of Racial and Social Biology)*, and in 1905, he established the world's first eugenics organization, the Society for Racial

Hygiene. See Weiss, "German Eugenics, 1890–1933," 4, and Proctor, *Racial Hygiene*, 15–17.

33 *Wohin des Weges? Merkblatt für erwachsene Mädchen*, in BArch, R 86/5618, Bl. 284.

34 Dr F.K. Scheumann, the leader of the municipal marriage counselling centre in Prenzlauer Berg in Berlin, insisted that doctors' psychological and social knowledge as well as their social mentality made them ideal candidates for marriage counselling work. See "Gesundheitspflege: Wer darf heiraten?," *Stadt-Anzeiger*, Köln, 15 January 1928, in BArch, R 86/5625.

35 See Runderlaß des Ministers für Volkswohlfahrt, in BArch, R 86/5618, Bl. 7–8, or "Die Errichtung von ärztlich geleiteten Eheberatungsstellen," in BArch, R 86/5624.

36 Grossmann, "Berliner Ärztinnen und Volksgesundheit in der Weimarer Republik," 189, 200.

37 These centres concentrated on social, psychological, and legal marriage counselling. People could inquire about marriage contracts, get information about divorce questions, and receive psychological help for marriage conflicts and economic problems. They did not intend to give out information about birth control, but in practice, this did not hold. The first clinic of this type opened in 1927 in Berlin. Reinert, *Frauen und Sexualreform*, 194.

38 Dr E. Heffe, "Eheberatungsstellen," *Handwörterbuch der Wohlfahrtspflege* (Berlin: Carl Heymanns Verlag, 1928), in BArch, R 86/5622.

39 These included organizations like Helene Stöcker's Bund für Mutterschutz und Sexualreform (League for the Protection of Mothers and Sexual Reform; founded in 1905), the Reichsverband für Geburtenregelung und Sexualhygiene (National Association for Birth Control and Sexual Health; founded in 1921), the Internationale Arbeiterhilfe (International Worker's Aid; founded in 1921), the Bund für Geburtenregelung und Volksgesundheit (League for Birth Control and Volksgesundheit; founded in 1924), and the Liga für Mutterschutz und soziale Familienhygiene (League for the Protection of Motherhood and Social Family Health; founded in 1928).

40 This came from an announcement about Hirschfeld's new marriage counselling centre in *Deutsche Medizinische Wochenschrift* 4 (June 1924), in BArch, R 1501/9380, Bl. 54.

41 Timm, *The Politics of Fertility*, 88–9. On Stöcker's enthusiasm for eugenics, see Allen, *Feminism and Motherhood in Germany*; Allen, "German Radical Feminism and Eugenics"; and Hackett, "Helene Stöcker: Left-Wing Intellectual and Sex Reformer."

42   von Soden, *Sexualberatungsstellen der Weimarer Republik*, 9.
43   Timm, *The Politics of Fertility*, 85–93; von Soden, *Sexualberatungsstellen der Weimarer Republik*, 31.
44   Max Hirsch, "Das Chaos der Eheberatung," *Deutsche Medizinische Wochenschrift* 18, no. 57 (1931): 766.
45   Dr Pfeiffer sent a copy of the report from Dr Rabe to the medical officer of the Danzig Health Office, 25 October 1924, in BArch, R1501/9380, Bl. 100–1.
46   Letter from Bumm to RMI, 20 April 1925, in BArch, R 1501/9380, Bl. 98–9.
47   Dickinson, "Biopolitics, Fascism, Democracy," 14.
48   Letter from Hirtsiefer to Regierungspräsidenten, 19 February 1926, in BArch, R 1501/9380, Bl. 155–6.
49   Timm, *The Politics of Fertility*, 113–14.
50   The Kommunistische Partei Deutschlands (KPD) had demanded the abolition of Paragraph 218 (the law that forbade abortion in Germany) since its founding in 1919, viewing the law as an example of "class injustice and bourgeois hypocrisy" because "sanitoria doors stood open to women who could pay for therapeutic abortion justified as 'medically necessary' while working-class women were condemned to quacks and hazardous, potentially deadly, 'self-help.'" The KPD believed safe abortions should be available to *all* women, not just bourgeois women, and they thought coercive abortion aimed at the working class was just another example of political injustice. See Grossmann, *Reforming Sex*, 21, 35–6, 92–5.
51   "Sexual- und Eheberatungsstellen. Was die Kommunisten dazu fordern," *Die Rote Fahne*, 5 March 1928, in BArch, R 86/5622.
52   Timm, *The Politics of Fertility*, 104.
53   Letter from Harmsen to Hirtsiefer, December 1927, in ADE, CA/G 397, 18/1–18/3.
54   Timm, *The Politics of Fertility*, 104.
55   Ibid., 104–6.
56   Ibid., 105.
57   See the 1932 and 1933 annual reports for the Protestant Marriage Counselling Centre in Berlin-Friedenau, in ADE, CA/GfSt 247, 3a-8, 10 and 14–23; the 1934 annual report in ADE, CA/G 399, 9–18; and the 1935 annual report, in ADE, CA/G 401, 8–14.
58   Timm, *The Politics of Fertility*, 105.
59   For more on Harmsen and his work, see Grossmann, *Reforming Sex*, 145, 190; Schleiermacher, "Racial Hygiene and Deliberate Parenthood: Two

Sides of Demographer Hans Harmsen's Population Policy," 201–10; and Schleiermacher, *Sozialethik im Spannungsfeld von Sozial- und Rassenhygiene*.

60 Letter from Harmsen to Pastor Dr Beckmann, 14 May 1932, in ADE, CA/G 398, 26.

61 See various letters between Harmsen and doctors working in evangelical marriage counselling centres from 1932, in ADE, CA/G 400.

62 Timm, *The Politics of Fertility*, 105.

63 Ibid., 107.

64 See meeting minutes of the Association of Public Marriage Counselling Centres, 9 September 1928, in BArch, R 1501/26239, Bl. 22–4.

65 Dr Hertha Nathorff, "Zum Problem der Geburtenregelung," *Die Medizinische Welt* 4, no. 24 (1930): 862.

66 One gynecologist thought the growing number of birth control clinics throughout Germany would lead to the dissolution of the family, the state, and ultimately, to the decline of the West, a familiar rhetoric used by eugenicists concerned about the *Geburtenrückgang*. See Grossmann, *Reforming Sex*, 60.

67 Heuseler-Edenhuizen, "Eheberatungsstellen," 187.

68 Höber, "Zweck, Erfahrungen und Ziele der Eheberatung," 143.

69 Fink, "Schwangerschaftsunterbrechung und Erfahrungen aus Ehe- und Sexualberatung," 71.

70 Grossmann, *Reforming Sex*, 66, 70.

71 See, for example, Fink, "Schwangerschaftsunterbrechung und Erfahrungen aus Ehe- und Sexualberatung," 72.

72 Usborne, "Women Doctors and Gender Identity in Weimar Germany," 116–17. The VsÄ, which had about 1,500 members by the beginning of the 1930s, undertook a campaign to legalize abortion on health, socio-economic, and eugenic grounds. Doctors within the VsÄ were not all united about a total repeal of the law, but they all believed in legalized abortion for medical and socio-economic reasons. See Usborne, "Abortion in Weimar Germany," 190–1.

73 Usborne, *The Politics of the Body in Weimar Germany*, 196–7.

74 Grete Albrecht, "Zur Lage der Aerztinnen in Deutschland," *Die Ärztin* 9, no. 12 (1933): 260–1.

75 Schleiermacher, "Rassenhygienische Mission," 90.

76 For more on Szagunn's numerous activities, see Buchin, "Dokumentation: Ärztinnen aus dem Kaiserreich," or Sach, "Gedenke, daß du eine deutsche Frau bist!"

77 Dr M. Wiederhold, "Zur Geschichte der Eheberatungsstellen," in ADE, CA/G 397, 24/6.

78 Grossmann, *Reforming Sex*, especially 136–65; Grossmann, "German Women Doctors from Berlin to New York," 83. In this article, Grossmann discusses where many of the doctors who staffed these clinics fled to and what they did after emigrating. See also Timm, *The Politics of Fertility*, 125.

79 Weindling, *Health, Race, and German Politics*, 430.

80 Timm, *The Politics of Fertility*, 149–52.

81 See the 1932 and 1933 annual reports for the Protestant Marriage Counselling Centre in Berlin-Friedenau, in ADE, CA/GfSt 247, 3a-8, 10 and 14–23. See the 1934 annual report, in ADE, CA/G 399, 9–18. See the 1935 annual report, in ADE, CA/G 401, 8–14.

82 The Protestant marriage counselling centre in Stuttgart, founded in 1929, reported that since 1 October 1930, they had 46 advice seekers, 34 women and 12 men. See the report from a 1931 survey on Protestant marriage counselling centres in Germany, in ADE, C/G 398, 6–9. The Protestant marriage counselling centre in Charlottenburg reported that out of 128 visitors in 1933, 97 were women and 31 were men. See ADE, CA/GfSt 247, 27/1–27/2.

83 See several copies of the *Merkblatt für Eheschliessende*, in BArch, R 86/5618 and several early drafts, in BArch, R 86/2372.

84 Dr Margarete Riderer-Kleemann, "Ehefragen bei inneren Krankheiten der Frau," *Vierteljahrsschrift deutscher Ärztinnen* 3, no. 2 (1927): 38.

85 Dr Helene Fritz-Hölder, "Ehefragen," *Vierteljahrsschrift deutscher Ärztinnen* 3, no. 1 (1927): 8–10.

86 See Dr Eva Wendorff, "Frauen-Beratungsstellen," *Saarbrücker Zeitung*, 3 February 1929, in BArch, R 86/5622.

87 Hermine Heusler-Edenhuizen, "Ehefragen. Zum Programm der Eheberatungsstellen," *Vierteljahrsschrift deutscher Ärztinnen* 3, no. 1 (1927): 8.

88 Dr Anne-Marie Durand-Wever, "Ehe und Erziehungsberatung," 574, 577.

89 Heusler-Edenhuizen, "Ehefragen. Zum Programm der Eheberatungsstellen," 8.

90 Dr med. Josephine Höber, "Zehn Monate städtische Eheberatungsstelle für weibliche Ratsuchende," *Vierteljahrsschrift deutscher Ärztinnen* 3, no. 2 (1927): 41.

91 Usborne, "Women Doctors and Gender Identity in Weimar Germany," 111.

92 Grossmann, "German Woman Doctors from Berlin to New York," 77, 79.

93 Ibid., 70–1.

94 Ilse Szagunn, "Aus dem praktischen Arbeit einer evangelischen Eheberatungsstelle," in ADE, C/G 399, 32. The annual reports from the Friedenau marriage counselling centre also confirm this.

95 Durand-Wever, "Ehe und Erziehungsberatung," 574–5.

96 Höber, "Zehn Monate städtische Eheberatungsstelle für weibliche Ratsuchende," 41–3.

97 Fink, "Schwangerschaftsunterbrechung und Erfahrungen aus Ehe- und Sexualberatung," 71. These numbers were based on a survey of advice seekers.

98 Durand-Wever, "Ehe und Erziehungsberatung," 574–5; Szagunn, "Aus der praktischen Arbeit einer evangelischen Eheberatungsstelle," in ADE, C/G 399, 32.

99 Ilse Szagunn, "Bericht über meine Tätigkeit als Ärztin an der Eheberatungsstelle Berlin-Friedenau im Jahre 1933," in ADE, CA/GfSt 247, 7a.

100 Ilse Szagunn, "Bericht über meine Tätigkeit als Ärztin an der Eheberatungsstelle Berlin-Friedenau im Jahre 1932," in ADE, CA/GfSt 247, 20.

101 Höber, "Zehn Monate städtische Eheberatungsstelle für weibliche Ratsuchende," 43.

102 Grossmann, "German Women Doctors from Berlin to New York," 70.

103 For examples on how these clinics offered contraceptive options see: Drs Frankenthal and Flake, meeting minutes, Association of Public Marriage Counseling Centres, 9 September 1928, in BArch, R 1501/26239, Bl. 22–4; Heusler-Edenhuizen, "Eheberatungsstellen," 187; and Nathorff, "Zum Problem der Geburtenregelung," 862. Nathorff thought the most effective measure to prevent unwanted pregnancy was to eliminate all laws against abortion. Her views, she claimed, stemmed from her experience in an infant and maternity home and a municipal family and marriage counselling centre, where she saw women from the poorest and most abject economic circles, who, met with the toughness of Paragraph 218, were forced to have quack abortions, which then made them unable to have children and sometimes cost them their lives. See Nathorff, "Zum Problem der Geburtenregelung," 862–3. Fink, speaking from her experience in a private clinic, also agreed that any woman could simply pay 50–100 Marks to find a doctor to give her an abortion, but then she ran the risk of death or sickness. Fink also noted the large number of women who came to her counselling centre asking for abortions; of those who received operations, she did not observe a single death. See Fink, "Schwangerschaftsunterbrechung und Erfahrungen aus Ehe- und Sexualberatung," 70–1.

104 Durand-Wever, "Ehe und Erziehungsberatung," 576.

105 Riderer-Kleemann, "Ehefragen bei inneren Krankehiten der Frau," 40.

106 Grossmann, "German Women Doctors from Berlin to New York," 72–3.
107 Fritz-Hölder, "Ehefragen," 11.
108 Dr Karl Kautsky, "Fünf Jahre öffentliche Eheberatung," *Monatsschrift deutscher Ärztinnen* 4, no. 2 (1928): 24.
109 Dr Heinrich Lottig, "Die rassenhygienischen Aufgaben der Eheberatungsstellen," *Vierteljahrsschrift deutscher Ärztinnen* 3, no. 2 (1927): 33–4.
110 Durand-Wever, "Ehe und Erziehungsberatung," 573–4.
111 Höber, "Zehn Monate städtische Eheberatungsstelle für weibliche Ratsuchende," 41–4.
112 Heusler-Edenhuizen, "Ehefragen. Zum Programm der Eheberatungsstellen," 5–7.
113 Ibid., 8.
114 Grossmann, "Berliner Ärztinnen und Volksgesundheit in der Weimarer Republik," 205, and Schleiermacher, "Ärztinnen zwischen Sozialhygiene und Eugenik in der Weimarer Republik," 1.
115 Szagunn, "Bericht über meine Tätigkeit als Ärztin an der Eheberatungsstelle Berlin-Friedenau im Jahre 1932," in ADE, CA/GfSt 247, 17–18.
116 Both Sach and Schleiermacher address Szagunn's eugenic leanings. Sach, "Gedenke, daß du eine deutsche Frau bist!," 35; Schleiermacher, "Ärztinnen zwischen Sozialhygiene und Eugenik in der Weimarer Republik"; Schleiermachar, "Rassenhygienische Mission und berufliche Diskriminierung."
117 Grossmann, "German Women Doctors from Berlin to New York," 72.
118 Szagunn, "Bericht über meine Tätigkeit als Ärztin an der Eheberatungsstelle Berlin-Friedenau im Jahre 1932," in ADE, CA/GfSt 247, 18.
119 Timm, "The Politics of Fertility," 236.
120 Grossmann, "German Women Doctors from Berlin to New York," 75.
121 Prinz, "Ehe- und Sexualreform," 159–62. See also Grossmann, "Berliner Ärztinnen und Volksgesundheit in der Weimarer Republik," 206.
122 Fink, "Schwangerschaftsunterbrechung und Erfahrungen aus Ehe- und Sexualberatung," 71. As far as I can tell, the patients consented to these sterilizations after Fink and Riese suggested them.
123 Ibid., 72.
124 Fink admitted to both these motivations. She subscribed to both social and medical reasons for abortion and birth control. Ibid., 74.
125 Ibid., 72.
126 Timm, "The Politics of Fertility," 236.

127 Fritz-Hölder, "Ehefragen," 8–9.
128 Although she does not specify these circumstances, her eugenic language (*Minderwertigkeit, Verkümmerung*) and her continuous discussion of a responsibility to future generations in the remainder of the article, suggest that she means inferior or unqualified people here.
129 Ilse Penning, "Warum brauchen wir weibliche Aerzte?," *Die Ärztin* 10, no. 6 (1934): 105.
130 Isle Szagunn, "Vita von Ise Szagunn. Ein Lebensbild in der Zeit," *Berliner Medizin* 12, no. 11 (1961): 261. See also Sach, "Gedenke, daß du eine deutsche Frau bist!," 19.
131 Timm, *The Politics of Fertility*, 83.
132 Nathorff, "Zum Problem der Geburtenregelung," 862–3.

2. Preparing Girls for Motherhood

1 For more on the gendering of the global health movement, see Petchesky, *Global Prescriptions*.
2 Heusler-Edenhuizen, "Die sexuelle Not unserer Jugend."
3 Jensen, *Body by Weimar*, 6.
4 Harvey, *Youth and the Welfare State*, 35.
5 Ibid., 30. Harvey has identified the boundaries of what constituted youth in interwar Germany. The upper age limits of the phase designated as youth were difficult to define, but fourteen- to eighteen-year-olds were the relevant group as far as juvenile justice and vocational schooling were concerned (ibid., 15).
6 Most accounts dealing with youth placed the onset of puberty at twelve for girls and fourteen for boys. Some even claimed that puberty started as early as eleven for girls. See, for example, Hermine Heusler-Edenhuizen, "Die körperliche Erziehung der Frau vom ärztlichen Standpunkt," Vortrag für die erste Magdeburger Fauenwoche, 4 March 1926, 9, in LArch-Berlin E Rep.300-52, Bd. 2, uncatalogued, copy, original collection in Niedersächsisches Landesarchiv (NLA)-Staatsarchiv Aurich, Rep. 220/30.
7 Harvey, *Youth and the Welfare State*, 30.
8 Harvey differentiates between *Jugendpflege*, which sought to keep delinquent children out of trouble, and the more coercive *Jugendfürsorge*, which targeted children with definable social, educational, and physical deficiencies. Ibid., 41–4.
9 *Soziale Praxis* 20, no. 19 (1911), in BArch, R 86/5671.

10 Donson, *Youth in the Fatherless Land*, 3.
11 "Abteilung V. Pflege der weiblichen Jugend," Zentralstelle für Volkswohlfahrt, in BArch, R 86/5671.
12 Weindling, *Health, Race and German Politics*, 213.
13 Dr Agnes Bluhm, "Weibliche Jugendpflege und Volksgesundheit" (Zentralstelle für Volkswohlfahrt, Abteilung IV, 1913), in BArch, R 86/5671.
14 Ibid.
15 Ibid.
16 Buchin, "Dokumentation: Ärztinnen aus dem Kaisserreich."
17 Bluhm, "Weibliche Jugendpflege und Volksgesundheit," in BArch, R 86/5671.
18 For a good discussion of the *Lebensreform* movement, see Hau, *The Cult of Health and Beauty in Germany*, and Williams, *Turning to Nature in Germany*, 11.
19 Profé, "Zur Hygiene der Frauen- und Mädchenkleidung," 2.
20 Ibid., 1–3.
21 Fischer-Dückelmann, *Die Frau als Hausärztin*, 132.
22 Profé, "Zur Hygiene der Frauen- und Mädchenkleidung," 2–3.
23 Hau, *The Cult of Health and Beauty in Germany*, 72.
24 For more on the Weimar New Woman see: Bridenthal, Grossmann, and Kaplan, *When Biology Became Destiny*; Frevert, *Women in German History*; Grossmann, "*Girlkultur* or Thoroughly Rationalized Female"; Grossmann, "The New Woman and the Rationalization of Sexuality in Weimar Germany"; Peukert, *The Weimar Republic*; Usborne, "The New Woman and Generational Conflicts"; Weitz, *Weimar Germany*.
25 Profé, "Zur Hygiene der Frauen- und Mädchenkleidung," 1.
26 Ibid., 3–4.
27 Profé, "Mädchen – Kinder zweiter Klasse?," 105–6.
28 Ibid., 105, 108.
29 Ibid., 106–7.
30 Ibid., 105, 109.
31 Fischer-Dückelmann, *Die Frau als Hausärztin*, 6–10.
32 Profé, "Unsinn im Mädchenturnen," 84–7. See also Profé, "Unser Mädchenturnen," 404–9, and Profé, "Die körperliche Erziehung unsere Mädchen," 135–9.
33 Profé, "Unsinn im Mädchenturnen," 85–6.
34 Profé, "Unser Mädchenturnen," 405.
35 Profé, "Unsinn in Mädchenturnen," 87.
36 Profé, "Unser Mädchenturnen," 405.

37 Profé, "Unsinn in Mädchenturnen," 87.

38 On physical education discourse throughout Europe and the US see: Grant, *Physical Culture and Sport in Soviet Society*; Mangan and Park, *From 'Fair Sex' to Feminism*; McIntosh, *Physical Education in England since 1800*; Meinander, *Towards a Bourgeois Manhood*. On the sexual education of youth throughout Europe, see Sauerteig and Davidson, *Shaping Sexual Knowledge*.

39 Jensen, *Body by Weimar*, 4.

40 Peukert, *The Weimar Republic*, 89–90.

41 Bessel, *Germany after the First World War*, 252.

42 Harvey, *Youth and the Welfare State*, 165. The full description of Articles 120 and 122 of the Weimar Constitution can be found in "Die Verfassung des Deutschen Reichs," 11 August 1919, *Reichsgesetzblatt* (1919), ii, 1383–1418, 1406.

43 Harvey, *Youth and the Welfare State*, 167–8.

44 Ibid., 171–2.

45 Ibid., 173.

46 Lamberti, *The Politics of Education*, 1. Peukert agrees that the Weimar years were a time of great educational reform. See Peukert, *The Weimar Republic*, 142–3.

47 Lamberti, *The Politics of Education*, 7.

48 von Lölhöffel, "Die Frau im Sport," 450.

49 Invitation, in LArch-Berlin B Rep.235-01, MF 3136–3143.

50 Dr Erna Corte, "Erste öffentliche Tagung für die körperliche Erziehung der Frau," *Nachrichtenblatt* 5, no. 4 (1925), in LArch-Berlin B Rep.235-01, MF 3136–3143.

51 Ibid. See also correspondence between the individuals and parties from 1924 to 1925, in LArch-Berlin B Rep.235-01, MF 3136–3143.

52 Ibid.

53 Invitation, in LArch-Berlin B Rep.235-01, MF 3136–3143.

54 See correspondence, conference minutes, and subsequent publication, in LArch-Berlin B Rep.235-01, MF 3136–3143.

55 Corte, "Erste öffentliche Tagung für die körperliche Erziehung der Frau," in LArch-Berlin B Rep.235-01, MF 3136–3143.

56 Bertha Sachs, "Die körperliche Erziehung der Frau vom ärztlichen Standpunkt," in *Die körperliche Ertüchtigung der Frau. Neun Vorträge gehalten auf der Ersten öffentlichen Tagung für die körperliche Ertüchtigung der Frau* (Berlin: F.A. Herbig Verlagsbuchhandlung, 1925), 15, in LArch-Berlin B Rep.235-01, MF 3136–3143.

57 Ibid., 16–17, 23–4.

58 Donson argues that it was the First World War that initially undermined adult authority over youth. See *Youth in the Fatherless Land*, 154–75, 227.

59 Weindling, "Eugenics and the Welfare State during the Weimar Republic," 135.

60 Sachs, "Die körperliche Erziehung der Frau vom ärztlichen Standpunkt," 16–17 and 23–4, in LArch-Berlin B Rep.235-01, MF 3136–3143.

61 Dr Hermine Heusler-Edenhuizen, "Erfahrungen und Wünsche einer Frauenärztin," in *Die körperliche Ertüchtigung der Frau. Neun Vorträge gehalten auf der Ersten öffentlichen Tagung für die körperliche Ertüchtigung der Frau* (Berlin: F.A. Herbig Verlagsbuchhandlung, 1925), 28, in LArch-Berlin B Rep.235-01, MF 3136–3143.

62 Sachs, "Die körperliche Erziehung der Frau vom ärztlichen Standpunkt," 19, in LArch-Berlin B Rep.235-01, MF 3136–3143.

63 Ibid.

64 Heusler-Edenhuizen, "Erfahrungen und Wünsche einer Frauenärztin," 26, in LArch-Berlin B Rep.235-01, MF 3136–3143.

65 Heusler-Edenhuizen, "Eheberatungsstellen," 187.

66 The Medical Association in Berlin, for example, enthusiastically recommended a mandatory year of home economics training for all fourteen-year-old girls before they left school. See "Das hauswirtschaftliche Pflichtjahr im Urteil der Aerzte," *Rheinisch-Westfälische Zeitung*, 10 June 1926, in BArch, R 86/2395.

67 Heusler-Edenhuizen, "Erfahrungen und Wünsche einer Frauenärztin," 26–8, in LArch-Berlin B Rep.235-01, MF 3136–3143.

68 Ibid.

69 Ibid., 26.

70 Sachs, "Die körperliche Erziehung der Frau vom ärztlichen Standpunkt," 21–2, in LArch-Berlin B Rep.235-01, MF 3136–3143.

71 Jarausch, "The Crisis of German Professions," 387.

72 Koven and Michel, "Womanly Duties," 1079.

73 See, for example, *Soziale Praxis* 20, no. 19 (1911), and Dr Agnes Bluhm, "Weibliche Jugendpflege und Volksgesundheit" (Zentralstelle für Volkswohlfahrt, Abteilung IV, 1913), in BArch, R 86/5671.

74 McIntosh, *Physical Education in England since 1800*, 216, and Manthorpe, "Science or Domestic Science?," 196.

75 Sauerteig, "Sex Education in Germany," 12–15, 24–5. Grossmann also discusses the increased medicalization and politicization of the sex reform movement, which included sex education, in *Reforming Sex*, chapter 2.

76 The Munich Physician's Organization, for example, wanted to expand the medical supervision of youth to all higher schools. See

Dr Dornberger, "Hebung der Volkskraft durch Kräftigung unserer Jugend," *Münchener medizinische Wochenschrift* 64, no. 1 (1917): 10–11, in BArch, R 86/5675.

77 Ibid.

78 Harvey, *Youth and the Welfare State*, 62–4, 78–80. On educational debates about girls' vocational education in interwar France, see Roberts, *Civilization without Sexes*, especially chapter 7.

79 Ibid., 82–3.

80 Ibid., 81.

81 Heusler-Edenhuizen, "Die körperliche Erziehung der Frau vom ärztlichen Standpunkt," 9, in LArch-Berlin E Rep.300-52, Bd. 2.

82 Dr Paula Heyman, "Schularzt oder Schulärztin in den höheren Schulen?," *Monatsschrift deutscher Ärztinnen* 4, no. 5 (1928): 84.

83 Dr phil. Agnes Molthan, "Zur Frage der Schulärztin," *Monatsschrift deutscher Ärztinnen* 5, no. 5 (1929): 85–6.

84 Heusler-Edenhuizen, "Die körperliche Erziehung der Frau vom ärztlichen Standpunkt," 8–9, 14, in LArch-Berlin E Rep.300-52, Bd. 2.

85 Dr med. Josephine Höber, "Warum Unterricht in Gesundheitslehre von Ärzten und Ärztinnen gegeben werden soll," *Monatsschrift deutscher Ärztinnen* 5, no. 8 (1929): 157. She was responding to Hertel, "Wer soll den Unterricht in Gesundheitslehre erteilen?," *Monatsschrift deutscher Ärztinnen* 5, no. 5 (1929): 86–7, and Molthan, "Zur Frage der Schulärztin," 86.

86 Dr Susanne Altstaedt, "Hygienische Volksaufklärung. Ueber sexuelle Aufklärung in der Berufsschule," *Vierteljahrsschrift deutscher Ärztinnen* 2, no. 3 (1926): 71.

87 Hermine Heusler-Edenhuizen, "Die sexuelle Not unserer Jugend," *Die Frau* 35, no. 10 (1928): 606.

88 Dr Edith von Lölhöffel, "Körpererziehung in der Familie," *Monatsschrift deutscher Ärztinnen* 5, no. 8 (1929): 157–8. Other lectures by von Lölhöffel included "Housewife Diseases and Their Prevention," "Importance and Technique of Air and Sun Baths," and "First Aid in the Nursery."

89 "Ein Schulmerkblatt," *Vierteljahrsschrift deutscher Ärztinnen* 1, no. 5 (1925): 141–3.

90 Grossmann, "The New Woman and the Rationalization of Sexuality in Weimar Germany," 165.

91 Dr Ilse Szagunn, "Probleme der schulärztlichen Versorgung der Berufsschulen," *Monatsschrift deutscher Ärztinnen* 5, no. 5 (1929): 90–1.

92 Ibid.

93 Dr med. Josephine Höber, "Aufgaben der Schulärztin einst, jetzt, und in Zukunft," *Monatsschrift deutscher Ärztinnen* 5, no. 4 (1929): 64.

94 Dr Käte Gaebel, "Schulärzte für die Berufsschulen," *Monatsschrift deutscher Ärztinnen* 4, no. 7 (1928): 122. Szagunn provides further evidence that female students preferred a female doctor. See Szagunn, "Untersuchung und Behandlung von Studentinnen durch Ärztinnen," *Monatsschrift deutscher Ärztinnen* 6, no. 3 (1930): 53–6.

95 Höber, "Aufgaben der Schulärztin einst, jetzt, und in Zukunft," 64.

96 Grossmann, *Reforming* Sex; Mouton, *From Nurturing the Nation*; Usborne, *Cultures of Abortion*; Usborne, *The Politics of the Body*; von Soden, *Sexualberatungsstellen der Weimarer Republik.*

97 Höber, "Aufgaben der Schulärztin einst, jetzt, und in Zukunft," 63–5.

98 Grossmann, *Reforming Sex*; Mouton, *From Nurturing the Nation*; Usborne, *Cultures of Abortion*; Usborne, *The Politics of the Body*; and Weindling, *Health, Race and German Politics.*

99 For more on how physical activity became linked to German national identity in the nineteenth and twentieth centuries, see Goltermann, *Körper der Nation.*

100 "Ein Schulmerkblatt," 141–3.

101 See von Lölhöffel, "Körpererziehung," 157–8.

102 Profé, "Mädchen – Kinder zweiter Klasse?," 105–9; Dr E. Michaelsen, "Leibesübungen in den Berufsschulen," *Monatsschrift deutscher Ärztinnen* 5, no. 5 (1929): 92.

103 Between 45 and 50 per cent of female students in Görlitz vocational schools expressed their desire for physical education. See Michaelsen, "Leibesübungen in den Berufsschulen," 92.

104 Gaebel, "Schulärzte für die Berfusschulen," 119–20. In Frankfurt, 10 per cent of the children leaving school were in remedial classes or a *Hilfsschule.*

105 Dr Lotte Landé, "Die schulärztliche Betreuung psychisch und intellektuell anormaler Kinder," *Monatsschrift deutscher Ärztinnen* 5, no. 5 (1929): 88.

106 Ibid.

107 Ibid., 88–9.

108 Grossmann makes this argument in "Berliner Ärztinnen und Volksgesundheit," 189, 205, and "German Women Doctors from Berlin to New York," 67.

109 Laura Turnau, "Frauensport und Sportärztin," *Vierteljahrsschrift deutscher Ärztinnen* 1, no. 5 (1925): 146.

110 Dr Gertrud Heckler, "Körperkultur der berufstätigen Frau," *Vierteljahrsschrift deutscher Ärztinnen* 2, no. 4 (1926): 106–8. Male physicians generally felt that "any education beyond the pablum of

the typical higher girls' school curriculum would irrevocably damage girls' health and reproductive development." See Mazón, *Gender and the Modern Research University*, 80.

111 See Verbrugge, *Active Bodies*.

112 Dr med. Clara Bender, "Aerztliches über weibliche Gymnastik und Körperkultur," *Vierteljahrsschrift deutscher Ärztinnen* 2, no. 4 (1926): 100.

113 Hau, *The Cult of Health and Beauty in Germany*, 73.

114 See Mazón, *Gender and the Modern Research University*.

115 Heusler-Edenhuizen, "Die körperliche Erziehung der Frau vom ärztlichen Standpunkt," 1, in LArch-Berlin E Rep.300-52, Bd. 2.

116 Bender, "Aerztliches über weibliche Gymnastik und Körperkultur," 100.

117 Dr Elisabeth Hoffa, "Mädchenschulturnen und Schulärztin," *Monatsschrift deutscher Ärztinnen* 5, no. 4 (1929): 68.

118 Heusler-Edenhuizen, "Die körperliche Erziehung der Frau vom ärztlichen Standpunkt," 10–11, in LArch-Berlin E Rep.300-52, Bd. 2; Sachs, "Die körperliche Erziehung der Frau vom ärztlichen Standpunkt," 18, in LArch-Berlin B Rep.235-01, MF 3136–3143.

119 Bender, "Aerztliches über weibliche Gymnastik und Körperkultur," 101; Heusler-Edenhuizen, "Die körperliche Erziehung der Frau," 10–11, in LArch-Berlin E Rep.300-52, Bd. 2.

120 Heusler-Edenhuizen, "Die körperliche Erziehung der Frau vom ärztlichen Standpunkt," 17, in LArch-Berlin E Rep.300-52, Bd. 2; Bender, "Aerztliches über weibliche Gymnastik und Körperkultur," 104.

121 Heusler-Edenhuizen, "Erfahrungen und Wünsche einer Frauenärztin," 26, in LArch-Berlin B Rep.235-01, MF 3136–3143; Heusler-Edenhuizen, "Die körperliche Erziehung der Frau vom ärztlichen Standpunkt," 18, in LArch-Berlin E Rep.300-52, Bd. 2.

122 For more on the discipline of female bodies prior to the Second World War, see Zweiniger-Bargielowska, *Managing the Body*.

123 On the history of menstruation, see McClive, *Menstruation and Procreation in Early Modern France*, and Read, *Menstruation and the Female Body in Early-Modern England*.

124 Heusler-Edenhuizen, "Die körperliche Erziehung der Frau vom ärztlichen Standpunkt," 13–14, in LArch-Berlin E Rep.300-52, Bd. 2.

125 Bender, "Aerztliches über weibliche Gymnastik und Körperkultur," 101.

126 Profé, "Frauensport aus Ärztliche Sicht," 115.

127 Heusler-Edenhuizen, "Die körperliche Erziehung der Frau vom ärztlichen Standpunkt," 14, in LArch-Berlin E Rep.300-52, Bd. 2.

128 Ibid., 15. Profé also addressed the issue of cleanliness during menstruation in "Frauensport aus Ärztliche Sicht," 115.

129 Heusler-Edenhuizen, "Die körperliche Erziehung der Frau vom ärztlichen Standpunkt," 15, in LArch-Berlin E Rep.300-52, Bd. 2.

130 Sauerteig, "Sex Education in in Germany," 24, and Sauerteig and Davidson, *Shaping Sexual Knowledge*, 9.

131 Hoffa, "Mädchenschulturnen und Schulärztin," 69.

132 Sauerteig, "Sex Education in Germany," 20.

133 Dr Helene Börner, "Ueber sexuelle Aufklärung im Rahmen der Schule," *Monatsschrift deutscher Ärztinnen* 5, no. 4 (1929): 66.

134 Ibid., 66–7.

135 Altstaedt, "Hygienische Volksaufklärung," 72.

136 Dr Erna Janzen, "Hygienische Volksaufkärung. Ueber sexuelle Aufklärung in den Berufsschulen," *Vierteljahrsschrift deutscher Ärztinnen* 3, no. 2 (1927): 53.

137 Altstaedt, "Hygienische Volksaufklärung," 72.

138 Heusler-Edenhuizen, "Erfahrungen und Wünsche einer Frauenärztin," 26, in LArch-Berlin B Rep.235-01, MF 3136–3143.

139 Szagunn, "Vita," 261–2. The Law Governing the Legal Status of Female Civil Servants and Public Officials, passed in 1932, stated that women who were second wage earners could be dismissed from public service. See Peukert, *The Weimar Republic*, 97.

140 Szagunn, "Vita," 262.

141 Ibid., 263.

142 Ibid., 261.

143 von Lölhöffel, "Körpererziehung in der Familie," 157–8.

144 Sauerteig, "Sex Education in Germany," 12, 18, 26.

145 See Ziemann, "Weimar Was Weimar."

146 The only notable exceptions in *Die Ärztin* were articles about the general problems of physical education and medical care in the schools. However, males wrote these articles, which focused on male and female physical education. See Dr Theobald Fürst, "Probleme der schulärztlichen Versorgung der Berufsschulen," *Monatsschrift deutscher Ärztinnen* 5, no. 8 (1929): 154–6, and Prof. Dr Eugen Matthias, "Aufgaben und Probleme der Körpererziehung in der Schule," *Monatsschrift deutscher Ärztinnen* 5, no. 9 (1929): 170–6.

3. Fighting the Vices That Threatened Women

1 Bleker and Schleiermacher, *Ärztinnen aus dem Kaiserreich*.

2 For an excellent discussion of feminist and abolitionist criticisms, see Roos, *Weimar through the Lens of Gender*, 97–136.

3 Weindling, *Health, Race and German Politics*, 11–13.

4 For example, in Berlin, over a one-year period, 7,872 marriages ended in divorce (one-fourth of all of Prussia's divorces), and 50 per cent of the divorces in Prussia were due to adultery. "Ehescheidungsgründe," *Heirat und Ehe* 2, no. 7 (1927), in ADE, CA/G 397, 6/7.

5 In various brochures, the German Society for Combating Venereal Disease emphasized the link between alcohol abuse and freer extramarital sexual encounters, especially with prostitutes infected with VD. See *Beratungsstelle für Geschlechtskranke Merkblatt* and *Kleines Merkblatt*, in BArch, R 1501/11874, Bl. 115 and 118.

6 According to Anita de Lemos, a police doctor in Hamburg, middle-class families and youth saw the monetary profits of prostitution in light of postwar economic and housing needs. See de Lemos, "Das gegenwärtige Prostitutionswesen in Hamburg in seinen Beziehungen zur Abschaffung der Bordelle," *Vierteljahrsschrift deutscher Ärztinnen* 2, no. 1 (1926): 16–17.

7 Widdig, *Culture and Inflation in Weimar Germany*, 214.

8 Letter from RMI to the Reich Chancellor, 25 January 1919, and letter from RMI to the governments of the German free states outside of Prussia, 17 February 1919, in BArch, R 1501/11874, Bl. 13–15 and Bl. 19.

9 Letter from the DGBG to the State Secretary of the Interior, 14 February 1918, in BArch, R 1501/11874, Bl. 21.

10 Timm, *The Politics of Fertility*, 35.

11 Walther, *Sex and Control*, 14.

12 Letter from Kriegsministerium to Reichskanzler (Reichsamt des Innern), 2 February 1918, in BArch, R 86/1064.

13 Timm, *The Politics of Fertility*, 36.

14 Ibid., 40–3.

15 Roos, *Weimar through the Lens of Gender*, 43.

16 Sauerteig, "'The Fatherland Is in Danger,'" 77.

17 Letter from the Association for the National Hygiene Museum and the DGBG to RMI regarding an exhibit for education about VD, 25 September 1919, in BArch, R 1501/11875, Bl. 134–5.

18 "Zunahme der Geschlechtskrankheiten. Beispiel Pfalz. Statistik der in den Krankenhäusern behandelten Fälle (Nur Neuzugänge)," in LArch-Berlin B Rep.235-01, MF 3380–3389.

19 "Bericht Nr. 1: Die bisherigen Ergebnisse der Reichsstatistik der Geschlechtskranken vom Nov./Dez. 1919 und ihre Bedeutung," 15 January 1921, in BArch, R 1501/11885, Bl. 108–16 and "Bericht Nr. 2: Die bisherigen Ergebnisse der Reichsstatistik der Geschlechtskranken vom November/Dezember 1919 und ihre Bedeutung," 1 April 1921, in BArch,

R 1501/11885, Bl. 137–9. Sauerteig states that the survey estimated that about half a million Germans caught VD each year. See "'The Fatherland Is in Danger,'" 76.

20 In a 1 October 1920 article of *Vorwärts*, Dreuw claimed to have an informant regarding these statistics. See Letter from Bumm to RMI, 30 November 1920, in BArch, R 1501/11885, Bl. 99–100. By 1922, Dreuw asserted that some 10 million Germans had a venereal disease. See Dr med. Dreuw, "Gesetzliche Bekämpfung der Geschlechtskrankheiten," *Zeitschrift für Medizinalbeamte* 35, no. 10 (1922): 249.

21 See Letter from Bumm to RMI, 30 November 1920, in BArch, R 1501/11885, Bl. 99–100. For Bumm's estimate, see Letter from Bumm to RMI, 8 December 1921, in BArch, R 1501/11877, Bl. 198.

22 See, for example, the complaint of the RGA that the numbers reported in the press were "fantastic," in "Bericht Nr. 1," in BArch, R 1501/11885, Bl. 110.

23 Timm, *The Politics of Fertility*, 45. See similar arguments in Bessel, *Germany after the First World War*, and Usborne, *The Politics of the Body*.

24 Timm has an excellent overview of the provisions of the 1927 law in *The Politics of Fertility*, 58–60.

25 "Der Reichsgesetz zur Bekämpfung der Geschlechtskrankheiten," *Korrespondenz Frauenpresse*, 24 July 1923, in LArch-Berlin B Rep.235-01, MF 3380–3389.

26 de Lemos, "Das gegenwärtige Prostitutionswesen in Hamburg," 16.

27 On the class background of prostitutes: Abrams, "Prostitutes in Imperial Germany," 189–209; Evans, "Prostitution, State and Society in Imperial Germany," 115; Harris, *Selling Sex in the Reich*, 40–6; and Roos, *Weimar through the Lens of Gender*, 72–5.

28 See Evans, "Prostitution, State and Society in Imperial Germany" for more on the debate about state-regulated prostitution in Imperial Germany.

29 On the regulation of prostitution in other European states: Corbin, *Women for Hire*; Gibson, *Prostitution and the State in Italy*; Harris, *Selling Sex in the Reich*, 10–11; and Walkowitz, *Prostitution and Victorian Society*.

30 Roos, *Weimar through the Lens of Gender*, 16–17.

31 de Lemos, "Das gegenwärtige Prostitutionswesen in Hamburg," 18.

32 Evans, "Prostitution, State and Society in Imperial Germany," 113.

33 Roos, *Weimar through the Lens of Gender*, 17, and Evans, "Prostitution, State and Society in Imperial Germany," 108.

34 In Hamburg, 3,117 unregistered prostitutes were arrested in 1913. In 1921, however, this number had increased to 8,700, a 179 per cent

increase. In 1922, 8,064 unregistered prostitutes were arrested there. Similarly, in Frankfurt, 990 unregistered prostitutes were arrested in 1913, but in 1921 and 1922, this number increased to 1,669 and 1,698 respectively. See Roos, *Weimar through the Lens of Gender*, 61–2.

35 In places like Munich and Leipzig, arrests for unregistered prostitutes either stabilized or slightly decreased in the early Weimar years. In Leipzig, for example, arrests decreased between 1918 (2,380) and 1925 (1,731). See Roos, *Weimar through the Lens of Gender*, and Evans, "Prostitution, State and Society in Imperial Germany," 108.

36 Buchin, "Dokumentation: Ärztinnen aus dem Kaiserreich."

37 Roos, *Weimar through the Lens of Gender*, 16–18.

38 The most comprehensive history of prostitution that does not solely focus on discourse is Harris, *Selling Sex in the Reich*. For histories that focus more on the discourse of prostitution: Freund-Widder, *Frauen unter Kontrolle*; Jenders and Müller, *Nur die Dummen sind eingeschrieben*; Marhoefer, *Sex and the Weimar Republic*; Roos, "Backlash against Prostitutes' Rights"; Roos, *Weimar through the Lens of Gender*; Smith, *Berlin Coquette*; Timm, *The Politics of Fertility*; Timm, "Sex with a Purpose."

39 de Lemos, "Das gegenwärtige Prostitutionswesen in Hamburg," 18.

40 Ibid., 19.

41 Dr Hildegard Canon, "Kritische Betrachtungen über die verschiedenen Systeme der Ueberwachung der Prostitution und der Bekämpfung der Geschlechtskrankheiten," *Die Ärztin* 10, no. 3 (1934): 52.

42 For a good discussion of how the women's movement was involved in prostitution reform, see Roos, *Weimar through the Lens of Gender*, 97–136.

43 Ibid., 107–8. See also Allen, "Feminism, Venereal Diseases, and the State in Germany."

44 Anna Pappritz, "Das Gesetz zur Bekämpfung der Geschlechtskrankheiten," *Vierteljahrsschrift deutscher Ärztinnen* 1, no. 6 (1925): 157–9.

45 "Aufruf!," *Vierteljahrsschrift deutscher Ärztinnen* 1, no. 1 (1924): 2. In this article, the BDÄ stated that in its affiliation with the International Medical Women's Association, there would be no political questions addressed at their annual congresses.

46 Dr med. Meta Oelze-Rheinboldt, "Zum neuen Gesetzenwurf zur Bekämpfung der Geschlechtskrankheiten," *Vierteljahrsschrift deutscher Ärztinnen* 1, no. 6 (1925): 161.

47 Dr med. Marie Kaufmann-Wolf, "Zur Bekämpfung der Geschlechtskrankheiten," *Die Frau* 27, no. 8 (1920): 233–4.

48 Ibid., 233–5.

49 Meeting minutes, "Bekämpfung der Geschlechtskrankheiten, der Gewerbsunzucht und der Kriminalität durch soziale Massnahmen," in BArch, R 1501/11876, Bl. 106.

50 Einladung, Konferenz zur Frage der beforstehenden Gesetzgebung zur Bekämpfung der Geschlechtskrankheiten, 15 September 1920, in LArch-Berlin B Rep.235-01, MF 3153–3161.

51 Marie Stritt, "Die Bundeskonferenz zur Frage der Bekämpfung der Geschlechtskrankheiten," *Die Frauenfrage. Zentralblatt des Bundes Deutscher Frauenvereine* 22, no. 3 (1920), in LArch-Berlin B Rep.235-01, MF 3153–3161. See also the minutes from the conference from 2 October 1920, in LArch-Berlin B Rep.235-01, MF 3153–3161.

52 Roos, *Weimar through the Lens of Gender*, 90–2.

53 On some of the nuanced approaches to coercive and emancipatory aspects of the law, see Marhoefer, *Sex and the Weimar Republic*, 82–3; Roos, *Weimar through the Lens of Gender*, 8, 91–2, 133; and Timm, *The Politics of Fertility*, 2. On the coercive aspects of the law, see Freund-Widder, *Frauen unter Kontrolle*, 104–5, and Harris, *Selling Sex in the Reich*, 162–5.

54 Anna Pappritz, "Die Wirkungen des neuen Gesetzes zur Bekämpfung der Geschleskrankheiten," *Monatsschrift deutscher Ärztinnen* 5, no. 2 (1929): 22–4.

55 Dr Eva Hensel, "Die bisherige Durchführung des Reichgesetzes zur Bekämpfung der Geschlechtskrankheiten," *Die Ärztin* 7, no. 10 (1931): 238–43; and Dr Eva Hensel, "Die bisherige Durchführung des Reichsgesetzes zur Bekämpfung der Geschlechtskrankheiten," *Die Ärztin* 7, no. 11 (1931): 261–5.

56 Marhoefer, *Sex and the Weimar Republic*, 88–9.

57 Harris, *Selling Sex in the Reich*, 32–4.

58 For more on the establishment and tasks of welfare offices, see Roos, *Weimar through the Lens of Gender*, 114–21.

59 For this work, de Lemos earned 3.80 Marks per hour. See Bleker and Schleiermacher, *Ärztinnen aus dem Kaiserreich*, 110.

60 Ibid., 110–11. They collected this information from the personal files of Hildegard Menzi in the Staatsarchiv Hamburg.

61 Ibid., 109–10.

62 Schleiermacher, "Rassenhygienische Mission und berufliche Diskriminierung," 95–6.

63 Timm, *The Politics of Fertility*, especially chapter 1; Sauerteig, "'The Fatherland Is in Danger,'" 86.

64 Timm, *The Politics of Fertility*, 54.

65 Allen, "Feminism, Venereal Diseases, and the State in Germany," 45.

66 Meeting minutes, "Bekämpfung der Geschlechtskrankheiten, der Gewerbsunzucht und der Kriminalität durch soziale Massnahmen," in BArch, R 1501/11876, Bl. 102–3.
67 Timm, *The Politics of Fertility*, 54.
68 This is indicated by the 223 people who visited the clinics in the first five months of their opening (until the end of 1916).
69 The 223 advice seekers in 1916 increased to 797 in 1917, 2,216 in 1918, and 10,194 in 1919.
70 During the first three years in which the counselling centres were in existence, there were almost 13,500 people with VD reported in Westphalia (9,047 men and 4,384 women). See Meeting minutes, "Bekämpfung der Geschlechtskrankheiten, der Gewerbsunzucht und der Kriminalität durch soziale Massnahmen," in BArch, R 1501/11876, Bl. 103–4.
71 Prof. Dr Pinkus, leader of the Beratungsstelle für Geschlechtskranke der Landesversicherungsanstalt Berlin, "Bericht über das Jahr 1920," in BArch, R 1501/11877, Bl. 67.
72 Meeting minutes, "Bekämpfung der Geschlechtskrankheiten, der Gewerbsunzucht und der Kriminalität durch soziale Massnahmen," in BArch, R 1501/11876, Bl. 104.
73 Sauerteig, "'The Fatherland Is in Danger,'" 85.
74 Letter from Katharina Scheven to RMI, 7 June 1919, in BArch, R 1501/11874, Bl. 142.
75 Sauertig, "'The Fatherland Is in Danger,'" 78.
76 Dr Hildegard Canon, "Zur Frage der Tätigkeit weiblicher Aerzte an Beratungsstellen für Geschlechtskrankheiten," *Die Ärztin* 10, no. 2 (1934): 31.
77 Hermine Heusler-Edenhuizen, president of the BDÄ, to RMI, 22 September 1926, in BArch, R 1501/11880, Bl. 32.
78 This is a hypothetical family but was quite close to some of the patients that Ilse Szagunn saw in her role as a doctor in the marriage counselling centre in Berlin-Friedenau, described in chapter 1.
79 Letter from the BDF to RMI, 31 December 1927, in BArch, R 1501/11880, Bl. 278–9.
80 Kaufmann-Wolf, "Die Reglementierung der Prostitution," 100.
81 Allen shows that dating back to the Imperial period, feminist campaigns argued for equal treatment for men and women. See "Feminism, Venereal Diseases, and the State in Germany."
82 Letter from Bumm to RMI, 19 July 1919, in BArch, R 1501/11875, Bl. 81.

83 Canon, "Zur Frage der Tätigkeit weiblicher Aerzte an Beratungsstellen für Geschlechtskrankheiten," 31.

84 Timm, *The Politics of Fertility*, 63.

85 Canon, "Zur Frage der Tätigkeit weiblicher Aerzte an Beratungsstellen für Geschlechtskrankheiten," 30–1. One of her colleagues who fell in line with the views of the new regime condemned her "liberal-individualistic thoughts." See Dr Helfriede Schmidt-Meyer, "Zurückweisung der Canon'schem 'Kritischen Bemerkungen über die verschiedenen Systeme der Ueberwachung der Prostitution und der Bekämpfung der Geschlechtskrankheiten,'" *Die Ärztin* 10, no. 4 (1934): 65–6.

86 It was not uncommon for female physicians to serve on the corresponding committees in the BDÄ and BDF. For example, letters between BDÄ and BDF members demonstrate that Anne-Marie Durand-Wever served on the Committee for the Physical Education of Women for both organizations, and in fact, the BDÄ chose her for this committee because of her analogous work in the BDF. See letters from March 1926 regarding this matter, in LArch-Berlin B Rep.235-01, MF 2158–2168. "Der Wortlaut des Gesetzes," was part of a special issue of *Nachrichtenblatt*, the journal of the BDF, called "Bekämpfung der Geschlechtskrankheiten. Das neue Gesetz. Welche Aufgaben erwachsen den Bundesverbänden und deren Vereinen?," 5 September 1927, in LArch-Berlin B Rep.235-01, MF 2158–2168.

87 Marhoefer, *Sex and the Weimar Republic*, 88–9, 102. She also states that, at least in Berlin, many clients came to the clinics voluntarily.

88 Walther, *Sex and Control*, 13–14.

89 Proctor, *The Nazi War on Cancer*, 141.

90 Weindling, *Health, Race and German Politics*, 71–2.

91 Ibid., 90.

92 Ibid., 72–3, 185–6.

93 Ibid., 170, 246.

94 Ibid., 176, 185.

95 Kevles, "Eugenics Then and Genetics Now," 191. See also Kevles, *In the Name of Eugenics*.

96 Weindling, *Health, Race and German Politics*, 265.

97 Ausschuß für Alkoholverbot in Deutschland, "Tatsachen," in LArch-Berlin B Rep.235-01, MF 2158–2168.

98 See, for example, Dr Reinhard Straecker, "Was ist gegen den deutschen Alkoholismus gegenwärtig möglich und nötig?," *Vierteljahrsschrift deutscher Ärztinnen* 1, no. 5 (1925): 136–9, and Dr Röder, "Zur

Alkoholfrage," *Aerztliches Vereinsblatt für Deutschland* 38, no. 730 (1909), in BArch, R 86/5196. Röder reported on the anti-alcohol movements in England, Sweden, Switzerland, Australia, and the United States.

99 Weindling, *Health, Race and German Politics*, 353–5.

100 Taking only 20 cases in 1917 and 76 cases in 1918, the welfare office saw over 100 cases in 1919, over 200 cases in 1920, 442 cases in 1921, and 365 cases in only the first quarter of 1922, of which approximately 353 were reported due to the drinkers' various criminal acts. "Die Zunahme des Alkoholismus," *Soziale Praxis* 31 (1922), in BArch, R 86/5189.

101 The hospital in Bremen admitted 98 people as alcoholics in 1921, an increase of almost two-thirds compared with the previous year and an eleven-fold increase from 1918. The asylum there documented 5 cases of alcohol-caused mental illness in 1919, 12 in 1920, and 26 in 1921. In a Munich asylum, 43 people were admitted due to mental disorders from alcohol abuse in 1919, and this number rose to 72 people in 1920 and 128 people in 1921 – almost a 200 per cent increase. In the asylums and hospitals of the present Prussian states (with the exception of some institutions in Düsseldorf), the number of admittances of alcoholic mental disorders was 1,034 in 1918 and reached 1,366 in 1919 and 1,979 in 1920. See "Die Zunahme des Alkoholismus," *Soziale Praxis* 31 (1922), in BArch, R 86/5189.

102 Ausschuß für Alkoholverbot in Deutschland, "Tatsachen," 1922, in LArch-Berlin B Rep.235-01, MF 2158–2168.

103 A few examples from medical journals and anti-alcohol organizations: Röder, "Zur Alkoholfrage," in BArch, R 86/5196; Dr Max Fischer, "Ärzteschaft und organisierte Arbeit gegen den Alkoholismus," *Deutsches Ärzteblatt* 60, no. 12 (1931): 158; Deutscher Frauenbund für alkoholfreie Kultur, "Frauen hört!," in BArch, R 1501/26382, Bl. 42; Ausschuß für Alkoholverbot in Deutschland, "Tatsachen," in LArch-Berlin B Rep.235-01, MF 2158–2168. See also Weindling, *Health, Race and German Politics*, 71.

104 Proctor, *The Nazi War on Cancer*, 127, 141. Proctor highlights that while the Nazi anti-alcohol campaign was strong, it failed to stem the tide of drinking, perhaps because the economy recovered throughout the 1930s and people could once again afford alcohol and because people turned to alcohol as a refuge from Nazi terror. See *The Nazi War on Cancer*, 148–9.

105 The Women's Working Group for the Fight against Alcohol Adversity demanded a seat and voice in the Reich Central Office against Alcoholism in November 1928, but was denied. See Dr Margarete Riderer-Kleemann, "Bericht über die Gründung der

Frauenarbeitsgemeinschaft zur Bekämpfung der Alkoholnot," *Die Ärztin* 4, no. 1 (1928): 15–16.

106 Deutscher Frauenbund für alkoholfreie Kultur, "<u>Warum</u> ist die Alkoholfrage Frauensache?," in BArch, R 1501/26382, Bl. 33.

107 Letter from the Deutscher Frauenbund für alkoholfreie Kultur to RMI, 24 January 1928, in BArch, R 1501/26382, Bl. 12–14. See several other letters from the League petitioning the RMI for money, in BArch, R 1501/26382.

108 "Frauen hört!," in BArch, R 1501/26382, Bl. 42.

109 "<u>Warum</u> ist die Alkoholfrage Frauensache?," in BArch, R 1501/26382, Bl. 33.

110 "Frauen hört!," in BArch, R 1501/26382, Bl. 42. This ad noted that the welfare office booked 50 per cent of poor relief on the account of alcohol. Some 1,900,000 people were lacking homes, another 9,000,000 did not have beds, and "400,000 drinking families with more than one million innocent suffering children burden[ed] the community."

111 For an example of this type of thinking, see Wilhelmine Lohmann, "Die Frau ist zur Mitarbeit an der Trinkerfürsorgestelle berufen," in BArch, R 86/5196.

112 For example: Elisabeth Boehm, "Was können wir Frauen tun, um den Alkoholmißbrauch einzuschränken? Bekämpfung des Alkoholmißbrauches durch die Frauen," in LArch-Berlin B Rep.235-01, MF 2158–2168.

113 Lohmann, "Die Frau ist zur Mitarbeit an der Trinkerfürsorgestelle berufen," in BArch, R 86/5196.

114 Dr Alfred Korach, "Die Trinkerfürsorge," *Vorwärts*, 5 August 1927, in BArch, R 86/5196.

115 Ironically, the anti-alcohol campaign also became closely connected to the life reform movement, which criticized the mainstream medical profession and experimented with new methods of combating illness. For more on life reform, see Hau, *The Cult of Health and Beauty*, and Williams, *Turning to Nature in Germany*.

116 Dr med. Röder, "Der Arzt ist zur Mitarbeit an der Trinkerfürsorgestelle berufen," 1909, in BArch, R 86/5196.

117 Fischer, "Ärzteschaft und organisierte Arbeit gegen den Alkoholismus," 157.

118 Letter from Verein Freiburger Ärzte to the Reich Ministry, the Reichstag, medical associations, daily newspapers, and the medical press, 27 January 1923, in BArch, R 86/5200.

119 Röder, "Zur Alkoholfrage," in BArch, R 86/5196. In his article, he cites Dr Graf Haeseler, "Zur Alkoholfrage," *Aerztliches Vereinsblatt für Deutschland* 38, no. 726 (1909): 705–8.

120 Weindling, *Health, Race and German Politics*, 23–4.
121 Fischer, "Ärzteschaft und organisierte Arbeit gegen den Alkoholismus,"
     157–8.
122 Letter from Verein Freiburger Ärzte, in BArch, R86/5200.
123 One article in *Die Ärztin* cited that only twelve to fifteen female
     colleagues were involved in the struggle against alcoholism. See Emil
     Abderhalden, "Die Ärztin und die Alkoholfrage," *Vierteljahrsschrift
     deutscher Ärztinnen* 1, no. 4 (1925): 81. In unpublished data for their book
     Ärztinnen aus dem Kaisserreich, Bleker and Schleiermacher identified
     nine female physicians licensed before 1918 who were involved in
     the abstinence movement: Clara Bender, Agnes Bluhm, Anna Fischer-
     Dückelmann, Agnes Hacker, Ottilie Hoffmann, Lotte Landé, Else
     Liefmann, Margarethe Riderer-Kleemann, and Marie Charlotte Anna
     Snell. Five of them (Bender, Landé, Leifmann, Riderer-Kleemann, and
     Snell) were members of the BDÄ's Committee to Combat Alcohol. Sabine
     Schleiermacher gave me this unpublished data from her personal files on
     24 February 2009.
124 Abderhalden, "Die Ärztin und die Alkoholfrage," 81.
125 Grossmann, "Berliner Ärztinnen und Volksgesundheit in der Weimarer
     Republik," 205.
126 See Grossmann, *Reforming Sex*.
127 The author claimed that in his time (presumably within the first two
     decades of the twentieth century), all female medical students had
     abstained from alcohol and were involved in the movement. See
     Abderhalden, "Die Ärztin und die Alkoholfrage," 81.
128 Ibid., 81–2.
129 Members of the committee in 1928, when Liefmann was chair, included
     Dr Clara Bender (Breslau: now Wrocław, Poland), Dr Elisabeth
     Soecknick (Elbing: now Elbląg, Poland), Dr Riderer-Kleemann
     (Berlin-Charlottenburg) Dr Maria Snell (Dresden), Dr Lotte Landé
     (Frankfurt am Main), Dr v. Schütz (Erfurt), and Dr Hedwig Rohling
     (Cologne). See Riderer-Kleemann, "Bericht über die Gründung der
     Frauenarbeitsgemeinschaft zur Bekämpfung der Alkoholnot," 15.
130 Dr Else Liefmann, "Die Frau und der Alkohol," *Vierteljahrsschrift
     deutscher Ärztinnen* 3, no. 4 (1927): 117–18.
131 The Association of Abstaining Physicians, which *Die Ärztin* encouraged
     female doctors to become involved in, made alcohol-free youth education
     one of its main goals. The Women's League for an Alcohol-Free Culture
     also promoted this as one of its goals.

132 Theo Gläß, "Die deutsche Jugend und die Alkoholfrage," *Die Ärztin* 8, no. 2 (1932): 33.
133 Leitsätze der Vorträge. Zweiter deutscher Kongreß für alkoholfreie Jugenderziehung, 21–5 May 1922, in BArch, R 86/5187.
134 Gläß, "Die deutsche Jugend und die Alkoholfrage," 36. Bluhm's study can be found in *Zum Problem "Alkohol und Nachkommenschaft"* and "Sind Alkoholschäden vererbbar?"
135 *Die Ärztin* stated that one could recognize the frightening increase of alcohol-caused disease, misfortune, and violence that was spreading among the masses. See Straecker, "Was ist gegen den deutschen Alkoholismus gegenwärtig möglich und nötig?," 136.
136 Gläß, "Die deutsche Jugend und die Alkoholfrage," 36.
137 Liefmann, "Die Frau und der Alkohol," 118.
138 Gläß, "Die deutsche Jugend und die Alkoholfrage," 36. See also Stelzner, *Weibliche Fürsorgezöglinge.*
139 See, for example, Többen, "Gefährdung, Verwahrlosung und Kriminalität der Jugend in ihren Beziehungen zum Alkoholismus"; Gläß, "Die deutsche Jugend und die Alkoholfrage," 36.
140 Gläß, "Die deutsche Jugend und die Alkoholfrage," 36. See also Riese, *Die sexuelle Not unserer Zeit.*
141 Kaufmann-Wolf, "Zur Bekämpfung der Geschlechtskrankheiten," 233–5.
142 Dickinson, "Biopolitics, Fascism, Democracy," 6. See also Foucault, *The History of Sexuality.*
143 Sauertig, "'The Fatherland Is in Danger,'" 87.
144 Oelze-Rheinboldt, "Zum neuen Gesetzenwurf zur Bekämpfung der Geschlechtskrankheiten," 161–2.
145 de Lemos, "Das gegenwärtige Prostitutionswesen in Hamburg," 18.

4. Building the *Volksgemeinschaft*

1 Dr med. Emmi Drexel, "Über schulärztliche Arbeit," *Die Ärztin* 13, no. 7 (1937): 206–11.
2 On the formation of the *Volksgemeinschaft*, see Kühne, *Belonging and Genocide*; Wildt, *Hitler's Volksgemeinschaft and the Dynamics of Racial Exclusion*; Wildt, *Volksgemeinschaft als Selbstmächtigung* (German version). For a recent debate on the usefulness of *Volksgemeinschaft* as an analytical term, see Steber and Gotto, *Visions of Community in Nazi Germany.*

3 The following are the most important works that handle the question of professionals, especially doctors and other civil servants, being increasingly attracted to and overrepresented in the Nazi Party: Childers, *The Formation of the Nazi Constituency*; Childers, *The Nazi Voter*; Hamilton, *Who Voted for Hitler?*; Jarausch, "The Crisis of German Professions"; Kater, *The Nazi Party*. For female professionals: Bock, *Zwangssterilisation im Nationalsozialismus*; Harvey, *Women in the Nazi East*; Lower, *Hitler's Furies*. Michael Kater has written extensively about the proclivity of doctors to welcome and support Hitler: Kater, *Doctors under Hitler*; "Hitler's Early Doctors"; "The Nazi Physicians' League of 1929"; "Physicians in Crisis at the End of the Weimar Republic"; and "Professionalization and Socialization of Physicians in Wilhelmine and Weimar Germany."

4 Kater, *Doctors under Hitler*, 106–7. Most of these women became affiliated through their work in the BDM or their membership in Nazi women's organizations, rather than party membership per se. While 49.9 per cent of male physicians joined the party, only 19.7 per cent of female physicians did. See table in Kater, *Doctors under Hitler*, 252.

5 Dr G. Becker-Schäfer, "Die Aerztin im neuen Staat. Ein Aufruf," *Die Äztin* 9, no. 8 (1933): 169–70, and Agnes Bluhm, "Aerztin und Rassenhygiene," *Die Ärztin* 9, no. 10 (1933): 209.

6 See Bleker, "Anerkennung durch Unterordnung?"; Bleker and Eckelmann, "Der Erfolg der Gleichschaltungsaktion"; Eckelmann, *Ärztinnen in der Weimarer Zeit*; Grossmann, "Berliner Ärztinnen und Volksgesundheit"; Grossmann, "German Women Doctors from Berlin to New York"; Schleiermacher, "Rassenhygienische Mission."

7 See, for example, Bluhm, "Aerztin und Rassenhygiene," 209, and Dr Lea Thimm, "Agnes Bluhm: Die rassenhygienischen Aufgaben des weiblichen Arztes," *Die Ärztin* 12, no. 7 (1936): 135–9.

8 Becker-Schäfer, "Die Aerztin im neuen Staat," 168–70, and Monheim, "Offener Brief an die Mitglieder des Bundes Deutscher Aerztinnen," *Die Ärztin* 9, no. 6 (1933): 122–4. See also Bleker and Eckelmann, "Der Erfolg der Gleichschaltungsaktion," 91.

9 Bleker and Eckelmann, "Der Erfolg der Gleichschaltungsaktion," 95.

10 The total number of physicians in Germany is based on my findings in the *Statistik des Deutschen Reichs*. The number of BDÄ members comes from Grossmann, "German Women Doctors from Berlin to New York," 67–8, and corresponds to numbers in Bleker and Eckelmann, "Der Erfolg der Gleichschaltungsaktion," 88, and Eckelmann, *Ärztinnen in der Weimarer Zeit*, 4.

11 Bleker and Eckelmann, "Der Erfolg der Gleichschaltungsaktion," 88.

12 Bleker claims that every fifth woman doctor was Jewish, which she concludes from the fact that about 300 doctors of the 1,500 panel practice female physicians were barred in 1933. See "Anerkennung durch Unterordnung?," 127, 135. Grossmann, based on numbers from *Die Ärztin* and *Statistik des Deutschen Reichs*, claims that 722 of the 6,785 physicians in Berlin were women, and of these, 270 were Jewish (approximately 38 per cent of women doctors). See Grossmann, "German Women Doctors from Berlin to New York," 67–8. See also Stephenson, *Women in Nazi Germany*, 63, and Kaplan, *Between Dignity and Despair*, 26.

13 "Mitteilungen des Vorstandes," *Die Ärztin* 9, no. 5 (1933): 102.

14 Bleker and Eckelmann, "Der Erfolg der Gleichschaltungsaktion," 88.

15 Benz, *Das Tagebuch der Hertha Nathorff*, 35, 40.

16 "Die Ereignisse," *Die Ärztin* 9, no. 6 (1933): 117.

17 Ibid.

18 In the news section from the first issue of *Die Ärztin*, the BDÄ reaffirmed its apolitical stance, even on popular issues such as the abolishment of Paragraph 218. The editors stated they would be taking no position on the question of the abolishment of Paragraph 218 and would consider both pro and con arguments. See "Bundesnachrichten," *Vierteljahrsschrift deutscher Ärztinnen* 1, no. 1 (1924): 13.

19 "Aufruf!," 2.

20 Ibid.

21 Schleiermacher, "Rassenhygienische Mission," 100–1. See also Bleker and Eckelmann, "Der Erfolg der Gleichschaltungsaktion," 90.

22 Bleker and Eckelmann, "Der Erfolg der Gleichschaltungsaktion," 90.

23 "Die Ereignisse," 117.

24 Ibid., 118.

25 See Monheim's report in ibid.

26 Ibid.

27 Ibid.

28 Monheim, "Offener Brief," 123–4.

29 Schleiermacher, "Rassenhygienische Mission," 97.

30 Szagunn, "Vita," 26, and Sach, "Gedenke, daß du eine deutsche Frau bist!," 35.

31 Szagunn, "Vita," 261–2.

32 Schleiermacher, "Ärztinnen zwischen Sozialhygiene und Eugenik," 3; Szagunn, "Probleme der schulärztlichen Versorgung der Berufsschulen," 90–2; and Szagunn, "Vita," 262.

33 The annual reports I found in the ADE, which run through 1935, confirm this. See Sach, "Gedenke, daß du eine deutsche Frau bist!," 21.

34 Timm, *The Politics of Fertility*, 151–2.

35 Schleiermacher, "Ärztinnen zwischen Sozialhygiene und Eugenik," 4.

36 Sach, "Gedenke, daß du eine deutsche Frau bist!," 41.

37 Kaplan, *The Making of the Jewish Middle Class*, 150.

38 Szagunn, "Vita," 263.

39 Sach, "Gedenke, daß du eine deutsche Frau bist!," 22.

40 Buchin, "Dokumentation: Ärztinnen aus dem Kaisserreich."

41 Sach, "Gedenke, daß du eine deutsche Frau bist!," 50.

42 Szagunn, "Vita," 264.

43 On the coordination of German schoolteachers, see Lansing, *From Nazism to Communism*. On the coordination of German professors, see Remy, *The Heidelberg Myth*.

44 Lena Ohnesorge, "Kurzgeschichte des 'Deutschen Ärztinnenbundes,'" *Mitteilungsblatt des deutschen Ärztinnenbundes e.V.* 17, no. 12 (1970): 10, as quoted in Eckelmann, *Ärztinnen in der Weimarer Zeit*, 46.

45 "Bericht über die 5. Ordentliche Mitgliederversammlung des Bundes Deutscher Ärztinnen am 28. Januar 1934," *Die Ärztin* 10, no. 2 (1934): 25.

46 Turnau remained available to her successor to pass on knowledge and experience. See "Die Ereignisse," 118.

47 "Mitteilungen des Vorstandes," 102. In the Berlin chapter, the *Gleichschaltung* affected six of the board members. See Eckelmann, *Ärztinnen in der Weimarer Zeit*, 47.

48 Grossmann, "German Women Doctors from Berlin to New York," 81–2.

49 Kater, *Doctors under Hitler*, 105.

50 Nathorff reported this experience in her diary on 5 August 1938. See Benz, *Das Tagebuch der Hertha Nathorff*, 112.

51 Bleker, "Anerkennung durch Unterordnung?," 127. The number of doctors eliminated from the BDÄ is unknown because member lists are unavailable. See Eckelmann, *Ärztinnen in der Weimarer Zeit*, 47.

52 Kater, *Doctors under Hitler*, 105–6.

53 The RÄK also had to approve the choice of all leaders, according to the new by-laws. See Eckelmann, *Ärztinnen in der Weimarer Zeit*, 46.

54 Koonz, "Mothers in the Fatherland," 447–8.

55 Kater, *Doctors under Hitler*, 106.

56 "Bundesnachrichten," *Die Ärztin* 13, no. 1 (1937): 22.

57 Ursula Kuhlo, "Das Referat Ärztinnnen," *Die Ärztin* 16, no. 5 (1940): 114.

58 Kater, *Doctors under Hitler*, 106.

59 Kühne, *Belonging and Genocide*, 143.

60 Historians have debated to what extent the *Volksgemeinschaft* was specific to Nazism. Michael Wildt argues that the concept was not originally a National Socialist one and existed well before 1933. Ulrich Herbert claims that the ideal of the *Volksgemeinschaft* was not a specifically German phenomenon. What was seemingly unique were the ways in which the Nazis radicalized the *Volksgemeinschaft* concept and other pre-existing ideas, such as the myth of comradeship. See Kühne, *Belonging and Genocide*, 166, and Steber and Gotto, *Visions of Community in Nazi Germany*, especially the essays by Ian Kershaw, Wildt, and Herbert.

61 Becker-Schäfer, "Die Aerztin im neuen Staat," 168–70. See also Bleker and Eckelmann, "Der Erfolg der Gleichschaltungsaktion," 91.

62 Becker-Schäfer, "Die Aerztin im neuen Staat," 169–70.

63 Monheim, "Offener Brief," 123.

64 Outside of the distinctions between the three age groups that follow in this paragraph, I use BDM throughout the chapter to refer to all three age groups.

65 The most recent comprehensive English account of the BDM is Reese, *Growing Up Female in Nazi Germany*. See Pine's work on the BDM in *Hitler's "National Community"* and "Creating Conformity." Other important works on the BDM include: Jürgens, *Zur Geschichte des BDM*; Kinz, *Der Bund Deutscher Mädel*; Klaus, *Mädchen im Dritten Reich*; Klaus, *Mädchen in der Hitlerjugend*; Miller-Kipp, *"Auch du gehörst dem Führer"*; Reese, "Bund Deutscher Mädel"; Reese, *"Straff, aber nicht stramm – herb, aber nicht derb."* On "Glaube und Schönheit," see Hering and Schilde, *Das BDM-Werk*.

66 Mahlendorf, *The Shame of Survival*, 96.

67 Mouton, "Sports, Song, and Socialization," 67.

68 Pine, "Creating Conformity," 371–4.

69 Dr med. Lore Heidepriem-Friedel, "Bericht über die Arbeitstagung der Obergauärztinnen des BDM," *Die Ärztin* 10, no. 11 (1934): 196–7.

70 Kater, *Doctors under Hitler*, 108–9. See Dr med. Ulla Kuhlo, "Gesundheitsdienst im Bund deutscher Mädel," *Die Ärztin* 17, no. 5 (1941): 199.

71 Dr Auguste Hoffmann, "Die Aufgaben der Aerztin im Bund Deutscher Mädel," *Die Ärztin* 10, no. 2 (1934): 31–3.

72 Dr Anneliese Panhuizen, "Wie mache ich die Schularzttätigkeit fruchtbar für die ärztliche Tätigkeit im Bund Deutscher Mädchen," *Die Ärztin* 13, no. 1 (1937): 7–8.

73 Hoffmann, "Die Aufgaben der Aerztin im Bund Deutscher Mädel," 31–2.

74 Steber and Gotto claim because there was a lack of clear-cut definition of what the *Volksgemeinschaft* concept meant, it could be applied to almost anything. See *Visions of Community in Nazi Germany*, 20.

75 Heidepriem-Friedel, "Bericht über die Arbeitstagung der Obergauärztinnen des BDM," 197.

76 Ibid., 198.

77 Grossmann, "German Women Doctors from Berlin to New York," 81.

78 Reese, *Growing Up Female in Nazi Germany*, 25–6.

79 Hoffmann, "Die Aufgaben der Aerztin im Bund Deutscher Mädel," 31–2.

80 Heidepriem-Friedel, "Bericht über die Arbeitstagung der Obergauärztinnen des BDM," 198.

81 Dr Auguste Hoffmann, "Die erzieherische Aufgabe der Aerztin im BDM," *Die Ärztin* 10, no. 12 (1934): 205.

82 Dr med. Josephine Bilz, "BDM.-Ärztin und BDM.-Führerin," *Die Ärztin* 17, no. 5 (1941): 212–14.

83 Ibid., 213–14.

84 Hoffmann, "Die erzieherische Aufgabe der Aerztin im BDM," 205.

85 Kuhlo, "Gesundheitsdienst im Bund deutscher Mädel," 197.

86 Both Hoffmann, "Die Aufgaben der Aerztin im Bund Deutscher Mädel," 32, and Dr med. Erika Geisler, "Ziel und Wege in der Gesundheitserziehung des Mädels," *Die Ärztin* 17, no. 5 (1941): 201, made this argument.

87 Kater, *Doctors under Hitler*, 109.

88 Geisler, "Ziel und Wege in der Gesundheitserziehung des Mädels," 201.

89 Kuhlo, "Gesundheitsdienst im Bund deutscher Mädel," 195.

90 Ibid., 197–8.

91 Ibid., 198. It is unclear how many mothers were reached during these mother evenings.

92 Dr med. Grete Deicke-Busch, "BDM.-Ärztin und Elternhaus," *Die Ärztin* 17, no. 5 (1941): 217.

93 Ibid.

94 Stephenson, *The Nazi Organization of Women*, 188.

95 Deicke-Busch, "BDM.-Ärztin und Elternhaus," 217.

96 Ibid., 218.

97 Mahlendorf, *The Shame of Survival*, 91.

98 Kuhlo, "Gesundheitsdienst im Bund deutscher Mädel," 196.

99 Mahlendorf, *The Shame of Survival*, 121.

100 Geisler, "Ziel und Wege in der Gesundheitserziehung des Mädels," 201–2.

101 According to a decree introduced on 15 February 1938 by Hermann Göring, it was compulsory for all single women under the age of twenty-five to prove they had done a year of service working in agriculture or domestic service in order to be employed in private or state factories or offices as blue-collar or white-collar workers. See Reese, *Growing Up Female in Nazi Germany* 24.

102 Geisler, "Ziel und Wege in der Gesundheitserziehung des Mädels," 204–5.

103 Dr Grete Deicke-Busch, "Aerztliche Arbeit im B.d.M," *Die Ärztin* 10, no. 1 (1934): 8.

104 Geisler, "Ziel und Wege in der Gesundheitserziehung des Mädels," 201–2.

105 Mahlendorf, *The Shame of Survival*, 69, 85, 119–42.

106 Maschmann, *Account Rendered*, 23.

107 Deicke-Busch, "Aerztliche Arbeit im B.d.M," 7. See also Kuhlo, "Gesundheitsdienst im Bund deutscher Mädel," 194.

108 On the building of comradeship in Nazi Germany, see Kühne, *Belonging and Genocide*, and *Kameradschaft*.

109 Deicke-Busch, "Aerztliche Arbeit im B.d.M," 7.

110 Kuhlo, "Gesundheitsdienst im Bund deutscher Mädel," 195.

111 See, for example, Mahlendorf, *The Shame of Survival*, 92; Maschmann, *Account Rendered*, 12; Mouton, "Sports, Song, and Socialization," 68–71.

112 Kuhlo, "Gesundheitsdienst im Bund deutscher Mädel," 199.

113 Bilz, "BDM.-Ärztin und BDM.-Führerin," 212.

114 Hoffmann, "Die erzieherische Aufgabe der Aerztin im BDM," 205.

115 Kuhlo, "Gesundheitsdienst im Bund deutscher Mädel," 199.

116 Hoffmann, "Die erzieherische Aufgabe der Aerztin im BDM," 205.

117 Kühne, *Belonging and Genocide*, 144.

118 Kuhlo, "Gesundheitsdienst im Bund deutscher Mädel," 199–200.

119 Deicke-Busch, "Aerztliche Arbeit im B.d.M," 7–8.

120 Kuhlo, "Gesundheitsdienst im Bund deutscher Mädel," 197.

121 Hoffmann, "Die Aufgaben der Aerztin im Bund Deutscher Mädel," 31–2, and Geisler, "Ziel und Wege in der Gesundheitserziehung des Mädels," 200–2.

122 Kuhlo, "Gesundheitsdienst im Bund deutscher Mädel," 194, and Heidepriem-Friedel, "Bericht über die Arbeitstagung der Ober-gauärztinnen des BDM," 198.

123 Koven and Michel, "Womanly Duties," 1079.

124 Burleigh and Wippermann, *The Racial State*, 250.

125 Lower, *Hitler's Furies*, 29–30.

126 Ibid., 61.
127 "Richtlinien des Reichsmütterdienstes im Deutschen Frauenwerk zur Durchführung der Mütterschulung," *Die Ärztin* 10, no. 6 (1934): 106.
128 Erna Röpke, "Die Ärztin im Reichsmütterdienst," *Die Ärztin* 12, no. 2 (1936): 46, and Röpke, "Die Mitarbeit der Ärztin in der deutschen Frauenarbeit, besonders in der Arbeit des Reichsmütterdienstes im Deutschen Frauenwerk," *Die Ärztin* 13, no. 4 (1937): 98–9.
129 Letters from the Deutsches Frauenwerk's Gauabteilungsleiterin für Mütterschulung, Gaustelle Thürigen to Dr Marie-Elise Kayser, June 1937, in StadtA-E 1-2/526-29, S. 32-40.
130 " Richtlinien des Reichsmütterdienstes," 107–8.
131 Burleigh and Wippermann, *The Racial State*, 250.
132 Röpke, "Die Ärztin im Reichsmütterdienst," 43–4, and "Die Mitarbeit der Ärztin in der deutschen Frauenarbeit," 100. By 1937, Röpke stated that there were 1,000 full-time teachers and 2,000 part-time teachers employed in the RMD.
133 Geisler, "Ziel und Wege in der Gesundheitserziehung des Mädels," 201.
134 Röpke, "Die Ärztin im Reichsmütterdienst," 41–2.
135 Ibid., 42.
136 Koonz, *Mothers in the Fatherland*.
137 Kiara Lönnies, "Reichsmütterhilfsamt – Reichsmütterdienst," *Die Ärztin* 10, no. 2 (1934): 35–6.
138 Ibid.
139 Röpke, "Die Ärztin im Reichsmütterdienst," 44.
140 Ibid.
141 Ibid.
142 Röpke, "Die Mitarbeit der Ärztin in der deutschen Frauenarbeit," 97–8.
143 Bluhm, "Aerztin und Rassenhygiene," 209.
144 Thimm, "Agnes Bluhm," 137.
145 Schleiermacher, "Rassenhygienische Mission," 101–2.
146 Peters, *Der Geist von Alt-Rehse*, 30.
147 Ibid., 28–31.
148 Ibid., 34.
149 Ibid., 35.
150 "Alt-Rehse," *Die Ärztin* 12, no. 10 (1936): 187.
151 Ibid.
152 Ibid.
153 "Teilnehmerinnen am 1. Ärztinnenlehrgang Alt-Rehse, herhören!," *Die Ärztin* 12, no. 11 (1936): 218.

154 Dr L. Heidepriem, "Der erste Ärztinnenlehrgang in Alt-Rehse," *Deutsches Ärzteblatt* 66, no. 43 (1936): 1056.
155 "Teilnehmerinnen!," 218.
156 Dr Gertrud Bambach, "Wie wir Alt-Rehse erlebten," *Die Ärztin* 13, no. 11 (1937): 334.
157 Heidepriem, "Der erste Ärztinnenlehrgang in Alt-Rehse," 1056.
158 Bambach, "Wie wir Alt-Rehse erlebten," 335.
159 Hau, *The Cult of Health and Beauty*, 114–24, and Williams, *Turning to Nature in Germany*, 23.
160 "Teilnehmerinnen!" 218.
161 Ibid.
162 Bambach, "Wie wir Alt-Rehse erlebten," 335.
163 Heidepriem, "Der erste Ärztinnenlehrgang in Alt-Rehse," 1056.
164 "Teilnehmerinnen!," 218.
165 Ibid.
166 Kühne, *Belonging and Genocide*, 144.
167 Heidepriem, "Der erste Ärztinnenlehrgang in Alt-Rehse," 1057.
168 Bambach, "Wie wir Alt-Rehse erlebten," 337.
169 Heidepriem also thought the high point of her experience at Alt-Rehse was the farewell party, which she described as "the highest happiness and perfection." See "Der erste Ärztinnenlehrgang in Alt-Rehse," 1057.
170 Dr med. Elisabeth Baecker-Vowinkel, "8. Schulungslehrgang für Ärztinnen in Alt-Rehse vom 5.-15. Juli 1939," *Die Ärztin* 15, no. 8 (1939): 262.
171 Peters, *Der Geist von Alt-Rehse*, 40–1.
172 Heidepriem, "Der erste Ärztinnenlehrgang in Alt-Rehse," 1056.
173 Ibid., 1056–7.
174 "Teilnehmerinnen!," 218.
175 "Alt-Rehse," 188.
176 Peters, *Der Geist von Alt-Rehse*, 7–8.
177 Kater, *Doctors under Hitler*, 109–10.
178 Bambach, "Wie wir Alt-Rehse erlebten," 337.
179 Hoffmann, "Die Aufgaben der Aerztin im Bund Deutscher Mädel," 31.
180 Heidepriem, "Der erste Ärztinnenlehrgang in Alt-Rehse," 1057.
181 For more on this and other Nazi family policies, see Mouton, *From Nurturing the Nation*, 18.
182 Anja Peters has made a similar argument in *Der Geist von Alt-Rehse*, 39–40.

183 Dr med. Else Petri, "Rassenhygienische Verantwortung der Frau," *Die Ärztin* 13, no. 12 (1937): 361–2, and Bluhm, "Aerztin und Rassenhygiene," 209.
184 Grossmann, "Berliner Ärztinnen und Volksgesundheit," 214–15.
185 Bock, "Ordinary Women in Nazi Germany," 85–100. See also Schleiermacher, "Rassenhygienische Mission," 99–100.
186 For more on the fate of Jewish women doctors, see Grossmann, "German Women Doctors from Berlin to New York."

5. Advocating Healthy Infant Nutrition Practices

1 Kater, *Doctors under Hitler*, 93.
2 Hester Vaizey, for example, in *Surviving Hitler's War*, examines the impact of war on everyday life by showing how it affected family relationships.
3 Anna Davin has discussed how an ideology of motherhood developed during the period of colonization when Europeans viewed good motherhood as essential to raising healthy future citizens and soldiers. See "Imperialism and Motherhood."
4 Maureen Healy argues that a striking feature of "total war" on the home front during the First World War was the spread of a war mentality to the mundane sites of everyday life. See *Vienna and the Fall of the Habsburg Empire*.
5 Recent work has examined women as agents, actors, or even perpetrators in implementing Nazi wartime ideology. See Harvey, *Women and the Nazi East*; Kramer, *Volksgenossinnen an der Heimatfront*; Lower, *Hitler's Furies*; Steinbacher, *"Volksgenossinnen"*; and von Saldern, "Innovative Trends in Women's and Gender Studies."
6 von Saldern, "Innovative Trends in Women's and Gender Studies," 104.
7 Kramer, *Volksgenossinnen an der Heimatfront*, 12.
8 Lower, *Hitler's Furies*, 74.
9 Dr Ulla Kuhlo, the leader of the Female Physicians Department within the Reichsärztekammer (Reich Physicians' Chamber), noted that the army granted women doctors very few contracts to do service, namely in hospitals. See "Zum Jahre 1944," *Die Ärztin* 20, no. 1/2 (1944): 1–2.
10 Hagemann, "Rationalizing Family Work," 26–7.
11 Dr Marie-Elise Kayser, "Die Frauenmilchsammelstelle eine öffentliche Einrichtung," *Die Ärztin* 18, no. 5 (1942): 145.
12 Eckardt and Feldweg, *Die Frauenmilchsammelstellen*, 13, and Wülfing, "Frau Dr med. M.-E. Kayser und die Frauenmilchsammelstellen," 9.

13 Schmidt, "Die Geschichte und gesellschaftliche Bedeutung der Fraeunmilch-Sammelstellen," 20.

14 Wülfing, "Frau Dr med. M.-E. Kayser und die Frauenmilch-sammelstellen," 8.

15 Dr Graevinghoff, "Frauenmilchsammelstelle," Ärztliche Nachrichten für die Provinz Sachsen und das Land Anhalt, 1921–2, in StadtA-E 1-2/526-4, S. 20-21.

16 Kayser, "Frauenmilchsammelstellen!," 23.

17 Daniel, *The War from Within*, 160.

18 Kayser, "Frauenmilchsammelstellen!," 23.

19 Ibid.

20 Eckardt and Feldweg, *Die Frauenmilchsammelstellen*, 13–14. The Weckschen method involved boiling jars filled with food and capped with a rubber seal in order to release all the pressure out of the jar to create an airtight seal, which allowed for the longer conservation of food. It was outlined by J. Oeflingen Weck in 1913 in *Koche auf Vorrat!*

21 Dr Marie-Elise Kayser, "Frauenmilchsammelstelle Erfurt," in StadtA-E 1-2/526-6, S. 8.

22 Eckardt and Feldweg, *Die Frauenmilchsammelstellen*, 13–14.

23 "Gründung einer Sammelstelle für Frauenmilch," *Magdeburger Generalanzieger*, 4 June 1919, in StadtA-E 1-2/526-4, S. 5.

24 Statistics in StadtA-E 1-2/526-4, S. 3. See also Dr med. Marie Elise Kayser, "Sammelstelle für Frauenmilch," *Münchener Medizinische Wochenschrift* 66, no. 46 (1919): 1323.

25 Eckardt, "Zum Gedenken an Frau Dr med. Marie-Elise Kayser," 1619. See also: Buchin, "Dokumentation: Ärztinnen aus dem Kaisserreich." Kayser responded to early opposition to breast milk collection facilities in "Sprechsaal," *Magdeburger Generalanzieger*, 15 June 1919, in StadtA-E 1-2/526-4, S. 6.

26 Letter from Marezkaja to Kayser, 2 September 1930, in StadtA-E 1-2/526-34, S. 3.

27 See her numerous lectures, in StadtA-E 1-2/526-26 and 1-2/526-27.

28 Kayser, *Frauenmilchsammelstellen*.

29 Wülfing, "Frau Dr med. M.-E. Kayser und die Frauenmilchsammelstellen," 9.

30 Eckardt and Feldweg, *Die Frauenmilchsammelstellen*, 14. See extensive correspondence between Kayser and Feldweg, in StadtA-E 1-2/526-37 and between Kayser and Eckardt in 1-2/527-39.

31 Letter from Stadtsgesundheitsamt Obermedizinalrat, Dr Ruckert, to Kayser, 8 January 1942, in StadtA-E 1-2/526-30, S. 22.

32 Eckardt and Feldweg, *Die Frauenmilchsammelstellen*, 14.

33 Kara Swanson discusses the medical monitoring of US milk banks in *Banking on the Body*, especially chapter 5, and "Human Milk as Technology and Technologies of Human Milk."

34 Kayser, *Frauenmilchsammelstellen*, 12–13.

35 Ibid.

36 Ibid., 15–16.

37 Ibid.

38 Letter from Lufthansa to the FMS Erfurt, 15 March 1935, and Bericht an die Ständige Tarifkommision über den Antrag Nr 1165 betreffend ermäßigter Expreßguttarif für Frauenmilch, 14 September 1935, in StadtA-E 1-2/526-22, S. 21 and 71a.

39 Letter from Kraftverkehr-Gesellschaft Sachsen to Eckardt, 7 February 1939, in StadtA-E 1-2/526-39, S. 32.

40 Kayser, *Frauenmilchsammelstellen*, 17–18.

41 Eckardt and Feldweg, *Die Frauenmilchsammelstellen*, 24–5.

42 Ibid., 18, 24.

43 Mazower, *Dark Continent*, 77.

44 Whitaker, *Measuring Mama's Milk*, 167. As Tricia Starks demonstrates, the private sphere also disappeared in socialist states like Soviet Russia, where authorities emphasized new ways of mothering at home while women were also "being told to abandon their four walls to mother all of society." See *The Body Soviet*, 160.

45 Goebbels, "Nun, Volk steh auf, und Sturm brich los!"

46 Letters between Marg. Book-Vollrath and Kayser, June 1937, in StadtA-E 1-2/ 526-29, S. 32-40.

47 Kayser, *Frauenmilchsammelstellen*, 23.

48 See correspondence between Kayser and individuals and organizations using the film in StadtA-E 1-2/526-29.

49 Eckardt and Feldweg, *Die Frauenmilchsammelstellen*, 22; Kayser, *Frauenmilchsammelstellen*, 24.

50 Eckardt and Feldweg, *Die Frauenmilchsammelstellen*, 18.

51 Kayser, *Frauenmilchsammelstellen*, 25.

52 Eckardt and Feldweg, *Die Frauenmilchsammelstellen*, 22.

53 Kayser, *Frauenmilchsammelstellen*, 29.

54 Ibid., 28.

55 Ibid., 29.

56 Eckardt and Feldweg, *Die Frauenmilchsammelstellen*, 19.

57 The Erfurt record books for collected milk and delivered milk can be found in StadtA-E 1-2/526-23 and 1-2/526-25.

58   Kayser, *Frauenmilchsammelstellen*, 31.
59   See StadtA-E 1-2/526-23475 for examples of these cards.
60   Kayser, *Frauenmilchsammelstellen*, 33–49; Eckardt and Feldweg, *Die Frauenmilchsammelstellen*, 25–6.
61   Eckardt and Feldweg, *Die Frauenmilchsammelstellen*, 27.
62   Kayser, *Frauenmilchsammelstellen*, 55.
63   Eckardt and Feldweg, *Die Frauenmilchsammelstellen*, 27.
64   "Überblick über 6 Jahre Frauenmilchsammelstelle Erfurt," in StadtA-E 1-2/526-6, S. 18.
65   Eckardt and Feldweg, *Die Frauenmilchsammelstellen*, 28.
66   Letter from Tiedemann to FMS Erfurt, 21 March 1936, in StadtA-E 1-2/526-3, S. 21.
67   Kayser, *Frauenmilchsammelstellen*, 56–7.
68   Eckardt and Feldweg, *Die Frauenmilchsammelstellen*, 25.
69   Dr Marie-Elise Kayser, "Mother's Milk," *Hospital Social Service* 24 (1931): 382–3, in StadtA-E 1-2/526-51.
70   Eckardt and Feldweg, *Die Frauenmilchsammelstellen*, 23–4; Kayser, *Frauenmilchsammelstellen*, 58–9.
71   Dr Emmi Justi, "Entwicklung der Pforzheimer Frauenmilchsammelstelle seit 1935," *Die Ärztin* 20, no. 5/6 (1944): 66.
72   Dr Marie-Elise Kayser, "Ueberblick über die letzten sechs Jahre Frauenmilchsammelstelle Erfurt," *Münchener Medizinische Wochenschrift* 80, no. 48 (1933): 1894.
73   Dr med. Edith von Lölhöffel, "Über die Einrichtung von Frauenmilch-sammelstellen nach Erfurter Muster (Dr Marie-Elise Kayser) und ihre Bedeutung für die Kinderheilkunde," *Die Ärztin* 13, no. 4 (1937): 104.
74   Although Germany did not have a long tradition of wet nursing, in other Western countries wet nursing was an occupation for lower-class women and often became associated with women who gave birth out of wedlock. On the class background of wet nurses in the US and Europe, see: Fuchs, *Poor and Pregnant in Paris*; Golden, *A Social History of Wet Nursing in America*; Miller, *Abandoned*; Sussman, *Selling Mothers' Milk*.
75   Correspondence between Kayser and Astel, December 1935–October 1936, in StadtA-E 1-2/526-30, S. 2-13.
76   Letter from Regierungspräsident to Reichsausschuß für Volks-gesundheitsdienst Haupteilung II: Gesundheitsführung, Reichs-arbeitsgemeinschaft Mutter und Kind, 8 May 1937, in StadtA-E 1-2/526-6, S. 66.

77 Correspondence between Kayser and Wagner via the Hauptamt für Volksgesundheit, September-October 1937, in StadtA-E 1-2/526-6, S. 69-74.

78 Kayser, Art der Sterilisation und Dauer der Aufbewahrung, in StadtA-E 1-2/526-6, S. 89-92.

79 Letters between Kayser and Tießler, January 1936, in StadtA-E 1-2/526-2, S. 4-7.

80 Dr med. Kurt Fenner, deputy dierector of the Reichsarbeitsgemeinschaft für Mutter und Kind, to Tießler, 30 October 1936, in StadtA-E 1-2/526-2, S. 8-9.

81 Letter from A. Schöbel to Kayser, 29 November 1937, in StadtA-E 1-2/526-30, S. 19.

82 See correspondence between Kayser and Reichsgemeinschaft für Mutter und Kind in StadtA-E 1-2/526-2.

83 The guidelines can be found in StadtA-E 1-2/526-2, S. 61.

84 Letter from Dr Ilse Szagunn, editor of *Die Ärztin*, to Kayser, 11 February 1942, in StadtA-E 1-2/526-27, S. 138.

85 See StadtA-E 1-2/526-34, 1-2/526-35, and 1-2/526-41 for correspondence between Kayser and doctors in other countries. See also Eckardt and Feldweg, *Die Frauenmilchsammelstellen*, 28–9.

86 Letters from Feldweg to Kayser, July-November 1935, in StadtA-E 1-2/526-37, S. 2-15.

87 Letter from Eckardt to Kayser, 4 July 1938, in StadtA-E 1-2/526-39, S. 1.

88 Letter from Eckardt to Reichsarbeitsgemeinschaft für Mutter und Kind, 27 November 1938, in StadtA-E 1-2/526-39, S. 18.

89 Letter from Eckardt to Kayser, 19 September 1939, in StadtA-E 1-2/526-39, S. 63.

90 Letter from the Head of the Foreign Department of the Reich Health Leader to Erfurt FMS, 7 November 1944, in StadtA-E 1-2/526-30, S. 31.

91 See correspondence on additional rationing for donors in: StadtA-E 1-2/526-18; BArch, DC 15/981; BArch, DQ 1/956; and BArch, DQ 2/388.

92 Letter from Eckardt to Conti, 20 November 1942, in StadtA-E 1-2/526-18, S. 27-29. Eckardt estimated one litre of milk was equivalent to 700 calories and many women donated 10–12 calories a month.

93 Kayser, *Frauenmilchsammelstellen*, 58–9.

94 Here, she is referring to *Der Stürmer*, Julius Streicher's anti-Semitic weekly tabloid newspaper, published from 1923 until the end of the Second World War.

95 Letter from Feldweg to Kayser, 7 May 1937, in StadtA-E 1-2/526-37, S. 78-79.
96 For example, Rachel Boaz argues that the Nazis sometimes accepted non-Aryan blood, especially during wartime. See *In Search of "Aryan Blood."*
97 Letter from Kayser to Feldweg, 9 May 1937, in StadtA-E 1-2/526-37, S. 80.
98 Volhynia was a region that straddled Poland and the Soviet Union. When the Nazis invaded and subsequently divided Poland with the Soviet Union in September 1939, the latter occupied Volhynia. In the course of Nazi–Soviet population transfers that followed, the Nazis resettled most of the ethnic Germans in Volhynia in resettlement camps in Polish areas annexed by Nazi Germany or they ended up in far eastern regions of Germany, like Plauen.
99 Letter from Eckardt to Kayser, 3 February 1940, in StadtA-E 1-2/526-39, S. 68.
100 See examples in Herf, *The Jewish Enemy.*
101 Whitaker, *Measuring Mama's Milk,* 66.
102 Boak, *Women in the Weimar Republic,* 227–8; Frohman, "Prevention, Welfare, and Citizenship," 438–9, 454; Hagemann, "Rationalizing Family Work," 25–6; Stöckel, "Infant Mortality and Concepts of Hygiene," 611; Stokes, "Contested Conceptions," 154–63. On the effect of the National Youth Welfare Law on the reduction of infant mortality rates for illegitimate children, see Mouton, *From Nurturing the Nation,* 202.
103 In 1905, infant mortality was 20.5 per 100 live births, but then decreased to 16.4 in 1914, 13.1 in 1920, 10.5 in 1925, and 8.5 in 1930. See *Statistsches Jahrbuch* (1934): 46; Stokes, "Pathology, Danger, and Power," 360–1.
104 Crew, *Germans on Welfare,* 119–21.
105 Whitaker, *Measuring Mama's Milk,* 170.
106 For examples from Italy see: de Grazia, *How Fascism Ruled Women*; for France: Offen, "Depopulation, Nationalism, and Feminism"; and for the Soviet Union: Starks, *The Body Soviet.*
107 Stokes, "Contested Conceptions," 156–7.
108 Frohman, "Prevention, Welfare, and Citizenship," 449–66. In Italy, the Fascist regime established a national agency for maternity and infancy (OMNI), which taught courses about the relationship between a mother's ignorance and infant mortality, as infant mortality rates were much higher for infants who received artificial feeding. See Whitaker, *Measuring Mama's Milk,* especially 1–2, 63, 68, 133, 170.
109 Weindling, *Health, Race and German Politics,* 580.
110 Kayser's speech can be found in StadtA-E 1-2/526-26, S. 126.
111 Eckardt and Feldweg, *Die Frauenmilchsammelstellen,* 9–10.

112 The Gesundheitspflege, Sozialfürsorge und Leibesübungen (Gesolei) exhibit that appeared in Düsseldorf in 1927 also highlighted the fact that mother's milk was irreplaceable. See ibid.

113 Ibid., 9.

114 Peukert, "The Genesis of the 'Final Solution' from the Spirit of Science," 236.

115 Kayser, *Frauenmilchsammelstellen*, 64.

116 Feldweg, "Frauenmilchsammelstelle und Säuglingssterblichkeit," 317.

117 "Verlängerung der Stilldauer. Die Erziehungsaufgabe des Hilfswerks 'Mutter und Kind,'" *NS-Volksdienst*, no. 8 (1937), in BArch, NS 5/ VI/4738.

118 "Rückgang der Säuglingssterblichkeit. Vorbildliche Arbeit des Hilfswerks 'Mutter und Kind,'" *Völkisher Beobachter*, 14 February 1937, in BArch, NS 5/VI/4738.

119 "Säuglichssterblichkeit geht zurück. Jahrestagung des Hilfswerks, 'Mutter und Kind,'" *Mitteldeutsche Nationalzeitung*, 22 April 1937, in BArch, NS 5/VI/4738.

120 Kayser to RAfMuK, 21 March 1938, in StadtA-E 1-2/526-37, S. 114-115.

121 Dr Friedrich Eckardt, "25 Jahre Frauenmilchsammelstellen in Deutschland," *Deutsches Ärzteblatt* 74, no. 9 (1944), in StadtA-E 1-2/526-5, S. 178.

122 Eckardt and Feldweg, *Die Frauenmilchsammelstellen*, 34–5. Kayser made this statement in "Sammelstelle für Frauenmilch."

123 Ibid., 16–17.

124 Goebbels, "Nun, Volk steh auf, und Sturm brich los!"

125 Cole, "Feeding the Volk," 11, 14. On the history of food in Nazi Germany, see Gerhard, *Nazi Hunger Politics*. Their work, my own, and others inspired a seminar at the 2016 German Studies Association: "Nourishing the Volk: Food and Foodways in Central Europe."

126 "Die Gesundheitsfürsorge im Kriege," *Die Ärzin* 16, no. 1 (1940): 20.

127 Dr med. Edith von Lölhöffel, "Die Ärztin in der Front der Heimat," *Die Ärztin* 15, no. 9 (1939): 267.

128 Dr Ilse Szagunn, "Wie sollen Schwerkranke ernährt werden," *Die Ärztin* 19, no. 2 (1943): 48–53.

129 Cole, "Feeding the Volk," 238.

130 Stephenson argues that female employment did not increase tremendously during wartime – from about 14 million workers in 1939 to 14.9 million by 1944 – partially because of the importation of several million foreign workers. See Stephenson, *Women in Nazi Germany*, 55. See also Stibbe, *Women in the Third Reich*, especially 36–40 and 84–96 on the

number of women working and the various welfare measures the Nazi regime put in place to try to attract women to work.

131 Cole, "Feeding the Volk," 188–9.

132 Ibid.

133 Boak, *Women in the Weimar Republic*, 17–18, 32, 228; Daniel, *The War from Within*, 158–60; Hagemann, "Rationalizing Family Work," 29; Stöckel, "Infant Mortality and Concepts of Hygeiene," 606; Stokes, "Contested Conceptions," 164–81; Whitaker, *Measuring Mama's Milk*, 82–4. For more on Lüders, see *Das unbekannte Heer*.

134 Whitaker, *Measuring Mama's Milk*, 82–4, 183.

135 Downs, *Manufacturing Inequality*, 169–73.

136 Boak, *Women in the Weimar Republic*, 148, 226.

137 Alice Rilke, "Die Frauenberufs- und Erwerbstätigkeit in der Betrachtung des medizinish-bevölkerungspolitischen Schrifttums," *Die Ärztin* 15, no. 1 (1939): 7.

138 Dr Magda Menzerath, "Zum erweiterten Arbeitseinsatz der Frauen – Aufgaben der Ärztin," *Die Ärztin* 20, no. 9/10 (1944): 125–7.

139 Dr med. Ilse Szagunn, "Stillmöglichkeiten für erwerbstätige Mütter," *Die Ärztin* 17, no. 9 (1941): 392–3.

140 While Timothy Mason includes a discussion of childcare for working-class mothers in his book on workers in the Third Reich, he lacks any discussion of how these mothers would breastfeed after going back to work. See *Nazism, Fascism, and the Working Class*, 189–90.

141 Szagunn, "Stillmöglichkeiten," 393.

142 Dr Margot Noack, "Die erzieherischen Aufgaben der Ärztin beim Stillvorgang," *Die Ärztin* 19, no. 4–6 (1943): 105–6.

143 Szagunn, "Stillmöglichkeiten," 393.

144 Dr med. Cläre Hellpap, "Aus der Arbeit der NSV.-Fraeunmilchsammelstelle Kassel," *Die Ärztin* 17, no. 2 (1941): 49.

145 Ibid., 49–50.

146 Ibid., 47.

147 Kayser responded to Eckardt by hand on 6 February 1940. See StadtA-E 1-2/526-39, S. 68.

148 Foreign troops occupied the Saar from 1920 until 1935, in accordance with the Treaty of Versailles.

149 See, for example, letters between Feldweg and Kayser, April 1936, in StadtA-E 1-2/526-37, S. 34-36.

150 Letters between Bauer and Kayser, January 1944, in StadtA-E 1-2/526-20, S. 50-51.

151 Letter from FMS Magdeburg to Kayser, 30 March 1945, in StadtA-E 1-2/526-4, S. 34.

152 Letters from Urschlitz to Kayser, October 1944, in StadtA-E 1-2/526-33, S. 21-22.

153 Letter from Urschlitz to Kayser, 26 November 1947, in StadtA-E 1-2/526-33, S. 25.

154 Dr Marie-Elise Kayser, Nachrichten aus den Sammelstellen der Ostzone, January 1946, in StadtA-E 1-2/526-5, S. 189. See also letters from Eckardt to Kayser, 1945–6, in StadtA-E 1-2/526-39.

155 Kayser, Nachrichten aus den Sammelstellen der Ostzone, 13 March 1946, in StadtA-E 1-2/526-5, S. 189.

156 Dr med. Kläre Hellpap, "Die Frauenmilch-Spende im Kriege," *Die Ärztin* 15, no. 12 (1939): 337.

157 Dr von Lölhöffel, "Unsere Aufgaben," 3.

158 Noack, "Die erzieherischen Aufgaben," 104–6.

159 Dr med. Cläre Sieberg, "Stillwerbung und Frauenmilchspende," *Die Ärztin* 20, no. 5/6 (1944): 63.

160 Ibid., 64.

161 Ibid., 64–5.

162 Dr Marie Elise-Kayser, "Die Ärztin und die Fraeunmilchsammelstelle," *Die Ärztin* 16, no. 5 (1940): 122.

163 Ibid.

164 Ibid., 123.

165 von Lölhöffel, "Über die Einrichtung von Frauenmilchsammelstellen, " 105–6.

166 Ibid., 106

167 Sieberg, "Stillwerbung und Frauenmilchspende," 65.

168 See table of donors with one child, with two children, and with more than two children in ibid., 64.

169 Dr Friedrich Eckardt, "Über Altergliederung, soziale Schichtung, und Leistungen der Spenderinnen von Muttermilch," *Die Ärztin* 20, no. 5/6 (1944): 72.

170 Justi, "Entwicklung," 66.

171 Eckardt, "Über Altergliederung," 73.

172 Noack, "Die erzieherischen Aufgaben," 104–6.

173 Eckardt, "Über Altergliederung," 73.

174 Sieberg, "Stillwerbung und Frauenmilchspende," 65.

175 Ibid.; Hellpap, "Aus der Arbeit der NSV.-Fraeunmilchsammelstelle Kassel," 50.

176 Feldweg, "Frauenmilchsammelstelle und Säuglingssterblichkeit," 317.

177 See photos in StadtA-E 60/7B1a6.

178 Letter from Dr Ackermann to Kayser, 24 February 1941, in StadtA-E 1-2/526-20, S. 9. See more examples of these letters to Kayser in the same collection.

179 See, for example, letters from the customers of the Magdeburg facility between 1935 and 1936, in StadtA-E 1-2/526-4, S. 9-10.

180 Kayser, *Frauenmilchsammelstellen*, 58–9.

181 Eckardt, "25 Jahre Frauenmilchsammelstelle in Deutschland," 178.

182 Ibid.

6. Conclusion

1 See Mazón's *Gender and the Modern Research University* for a longer discussion of these arguments.

2 See Pauwels, *Women, Nazis, and Universities*, 24.

3 The inclusiveness/exclusiveness of *Volksgemeinschaft*, the Nazis' central social concept, has been recently debated among historians. See: Kühne, *Belonging and Genocide*; Pine, *Hitler's "National Community"*; Steber and Gotto, *Visions of Community in Nazi Germany*; Wildt, *Hitler's Volksgemeinschaft and the Dynamics of Racial Exclusion*; Wildt, *Volksgemeinschaft als Selbstermächtigung*.

4 Steber and Gotto, *Visions of Community in Nazi Germany*, 6–7, 15, 20.

5 Ibid., 7.

6 Schoenbaum, *Hitler's Social Revolution*.

7 For discussions of class in the BDM, see Maschmann, *Account Rendered*, and Mouton, "Sports, Song, and Socialization."

8 Swanson, *Banking on the Body*, 4.

9 Kayser, *Frauenmilchsammelstellen*, 55; Hellpap, "Aus der Arbeit der NSV.-Fraeunmilchsammelstelle Kassel," 49–50; Eckardt, "Über Altergliederung," 70–2.

10 Childers and Caplan highlight the historiography of class perspectives of National Socialism in the introduction to *Reevaluating the Third Reich*, 3. For a recent discussion of the historiographical trend of class and class analysis in German history, see an article in *German History* from 2012: "Forum: Class in German History." For a discussion of gender and class as important, relational analytical categories of Germany in the 1920s, see Ziemann, "Weimar Was Weimar," and for a practical application of this type of analysis, see Harris, *Selling Sex in the Reich*.

11 Swanson, *Banking on the Body*, 13.

12 Letters between Bauer and Kayser, January 1944, in StadtA-E 1-2/526-20, S. 50-51.

13 See examples of these letters to Kayser, in StadtA-E 1-2/526-20.

14 Rieger, "'Fast Couples,'" 366.

15 Herf, *Reactionary Modernism*.

16 Brüggemeier, Cioc, and Zeller, *How Green Were the Nazis?*; Lekan and Zeller, *Germany's Nature*; Proctor, *The Nazi War on Cancer*.

17 Eckardt, "25 Jahre Frauenmilchsammelstelle in Deutschland," 178.

18 Usborne, *The Politics of the Body*, 123. Kristine von Soden talks about the atmosphere of clinics in *Sexualberatungsstellen der Weimarer Republik*, especially 125–44. Michelle Mouton argues that it was precisely *because* of this female solidarity in clinic waiting rooms that the Nazis found Weimar marriage and sex counselling centres reprehensible and lashed out against them. See *From Nurturing the Nation*, 49.

Bibliography

Archival Sources

Berlin

ARCHIV FÜR DIAKONIE UND ENTWICKLUNG (ADE)
Central-Ausschuß für die Innere Mission der deutschen evangelischen Kirche,
   Referat Gesundheitsfürsorge (CA/G)
Central-Ausschuß für die Innere Mission der deutschen evangelischen Kirche,
   Referat Gefährdetenfürsorge und Straffälligenhilfe (CA/GfSt)

BUNDESARCHIV (BARCH)
Deutsche Arbeitsfront-Zentralbüro, Arbeitswissenschaftliches Institut
   (NS 5 VI)
Deutsche Wirtschaftskommission (DC 15)
Hauptamt für Volkswohlfahrt der NSDAP (NS 37)
Hauptarchiv der NSDAP (NS 26)
Ministerium für Arbeit und Berufsausbildung (der DDR) (DQ 2)
Ministerium für Gesundheitswesen (der DDR) (DQ 1)
Reichsgesundheitsamt (R 86)
Reichsministerium des Innern (R 1501)
Reichsministerium für Wissenschaft, Erziehung und Volksbildung (R 4901)
Reichsstelle für Speisefette (R 8840)

LANDESARCHIV (LARCH-BERLIN)
Bund Deutscher Frauenvereine, Helene-Lange Archiv (B Rep.235-01)
Deutscher Akademikerinnenbund, Helene-Lange Archiv (B Rep.235-05)
Deutscher Ärztinnenbund, Helene-Lange Archiv (B Rep.235-08)

Nachlass Anna Pappritz (B Rep.235-13)
Nachlass Helene Lange (B Rep.235-11)
Nachlass Hermine Heusler-Edenhuizen (E Rep.300-52)
Zeitungsausschnitssammlung, Helene-Lange Archiv (B Rep.235-20)

Dresden

DEUTSCHES HYGIENE MUSEUM

Erfurt

STADTARCHIV ERFURT (STADTA-E)

Journals

Die Ärztin
Monatsschrift deutscher Ärztinnen
Reichsmedizinalkalendar für Deutschland
Statistik des Deutschen Reichs
Vierteljahrsschrift deutscher Ärztinnen

Books, Articles, Dissertations (Primary)

Adams-Lehmann, Hope Bridges. *Das Frauenbuch. Ein ärztlicher Ratgeber für die Frau in der Familie und bei Frauenkrankheiten.* Stuttgart: Süddeutsches Verlags-Institut, 1897.
Adelsberger, Lucie. "Die Frau als Ärztin." In *Die Kultur der Frau. Eine Lebenssymphonie der Frau des XX. Jahrhunderts,* edited by Ada Schmidt-Beil, 198–205. Berlin: Verlag für Kultur und Wissenschaft GmbH, 1931.
"Aus der Kriegsarbeit der Ärztinnen." *Deutsches Ärzteblatt* 70, no. 18 (1940): 213.
Bäumer, Gertrud. *Krisis des Frauenstudiums.* Leipzig: Voigtlanders, 1932.
Benz, Wolfgang, ed. *Das Tagebuch der Hertha Nathorff. Berlin-New York Augzeichnungen 1933 bis 1945.* Frankfurt am Main: Fischer Taschenbuch, 1988.
Bischoff, Theodore. *Das Studium und die Ausübung der Medizin durch Frauen.* Munich: Literarisch-artistische Anstalt, 1872.
Bluhm, Agnes. "Sind Alkoholschäden vererbbar?" *Internationale Zeitschrift gegen den Alkohlismus* 38, no. 6 (1930), 297–308.
– *Die rassenhygienischen Aufgaben des weiblichen Arztes.* Berlin: Alfred Metzner, 1936.

– "Wie behüten wir die Familie vor dem Einfluß des Alkoholismus?" *Das Kommende Geschlecht* 2, no. 2 (1922): 94–109.

– *Zum Problem "Alkohol und Nachkommenschaft." Eine experimentelle Studie.* Munich: Lehmann, 1930.

Broecker, Anne. "Gesundheitsfürsorge." In *Die Kultur der Frau. Eine Lebenssymphonie der Frau des XX. Jahrhunderts*, edited by Ada Schmidt-Beil, 333–9. Berlin: Verlag für Kultur und Wissenschaft GmbH, 1931.

Busse-Wilson, Elisabeth. "Das moralische Dilemma in der modernen Mädchenerziehung." In *Die Kultur der Frau. Eine Lebenssymphonie der Frau des XX. Jahrhunderts*, edited by Ada Schmidt-Beil, 589–96. Berlin: Verlag für Kultur und Wissenschaft GmbH, 1931.

Darwin, Charles. *On the Origin of Species by Means of Natural Selection, or the Preservation of Favoured Races in the Struggle for Life.* London: John Murray, 1859.

Dreuw, Wilhelm Heinrich. "Gesetzliche Bekämpfung der Geschlechtskrankheiten." *Zeitschrift für Medizinalbeamte* 35, no. 10 (1922): 249–56.

Durand-Wever, Anne-Marie. "Die ärztliche Erfahrungen über medizinisch indizierte Konzeptionsverhütung." *Die Medizinische Welt* 5, no. 21 (1931): 759–60.

– "Die ärztliche Erfahrungen über medizinisch indizierte Konzeptionsverhütung." *Die Medizinische Welt* 5, no. 23 (1931): 826–7.

– "Die ärztliche Erfahrungen über medizinisch indizierte Konzeptionsverhütung." *Die Medizinische Welt* 5, no. 26 (1931): 936–7.

– "Ehe und Erziehungsberatung." In *Die Kultur der Frau. Eine Lebenssymphonie der Frau des XX. Jahrhunderts*, edited by Ada Schmidt-Beil, 573–80. Berlin: Verlag für Kultur und Wissenschaft GmbH, 1931.

– *Der Frauenkörper in gesunden und kranken Tagen.* Berlin: Asklepios, 1930.

– "Für und wider den § 218." *Die Medizinische Welt* 4, no. 31 (1930): 1121.

– "Der Kampf um den § 218 auf der Bühne." *Die Medizinische Welt* 4, no. 22 (1930): 785–6.

– "Umfang und Ursache der Geburtenbeschränkung." *Die Medizinische Welt* 7, no. 7 (1931): 243–5.

– "Umfang und Ursache der Geburtenbeschränkung." *Die Medizinische Welt* 7, no. 9 (1931): 315–17.

Eckardt, Dr Friedrich. "Zum Gedenken an Frau Dr med. Marie-Elise Kayser, die Gründerin der 1. Frauenmilchsammelstelle." *Das Deutsche Gesundheitswesen* 5 (1950): 1619–21.

Eckardt, Dr Friedrich, and Dr Irma Feldweg. *Die Frauenmilchsammelstellen. Bedeutung und Entwicklung der Fraeunmilchsammelstellen.* Köln: Deutsches Gesundheits-Museum, 1954.

Feldweg, Irma, "Frauenmilchsammelstelle und Säuglingssterblichkeit," *Medizinische Klinik* 40, no. 21/22 (1944): 316-18.

Fischer, Max. "Ärzteschaft und organisierte Arbeit gegen den Alkoholismus," *Deutsches Ärzteblatt* 60, no. 12 (1931): 157–8.

Fischer-Dückelmann, Anna. *Die Frau als Hausärztin.* Stüttgart: Süddeutsches Verlags-Institut, 1905.

Fraenkel, Marta. "Die Frauengruppe auf der Internationalen Hygiene-Ausstellung." *Mutter und Kind* 8, no. 7 (1930): 97–8.

– "Hygiene-Ausstellung, eine Hochschule für jedermann!" In *Das Deutsche Hygiene-Museum: Festschrift zur Eröffnung des Museums und der Internationale Hygiene-Ausstellung Dresden 1930,* edited by Heinrich Zerkaulen, 15–23. Dresden: Wolfgang Jess, 1930.

– "Das Kind auf der Internat. Hygiene-Ausstellung." *Kleine Kinder* 3, no. 9 (1930): 161–5.

– "Eine 'Kinderwoche' in der Hygiene-Ausstellung." *Kleine Kinder* 4, no. 10 (1931): 182–3.

– "Ziel und Wesen einer Hygiene-Ausstellung." *Hygiene-Sonderheft der Zeitschrift für Desinfektions- und Gesundheitswesen* 22, no. 5 (1930): 259–64.

– "Zur Kinderwoche!" *Internationale Hygiene-Ausstellung. Offizielle Ausstellungzeitung,* 15 June 1931.

Frankenthal, Käte. "Ärzteschaft und Faschismus." *Der sozialistische Arzt* 8, no. 6 (1932): 101–7.

– *Der dreifache Fluch: Jüdin, Intellektuelle, Sozialistin. Lebenserinnerungen einer Ärztin in Deutschland und Exil.* Edited by Kathleen M. Pearle und Stephan Leibfried. New York: Basic Books, 1981.

– "Zur Frage der Geburtenregelung." *Die Genossin* 6, no. 9 (1929): 388–92.

Gläsmer, Erna. *Eheberatungsstellen und Geburtenverhütung.* Stuttgart: Ferdinand Enke, 1932.

Goebbels, Joseph. "Nun, Volk steh auf, und Sturm brich los! Rede im Berliner Sportpalast." *Der steile Aufstieg.* Munich: Zentralverlag der NSDAP, 1944.

Grotjahn, Alfred. "Soziale Hygiene (Definition)." In *Handwörterbuch der Sozialen Hygiene,* edited by A. Grotjahn and J. Kaup, 410–12. Leipzig: F.C.W. Vogel, 1912.

Heidepriem, L. "Der erste Ärztinnenlehrgang in Alt-Rehse." *Deutsches Ärzteblatt* 66, no. 43 (1936): 1056–7.

Heusler, Otto. "Der Beruf der Ärztin im Lichte 'nationaler, sozialer und ethischer Erkenntnis. Eine Erwiderung.'" *Deutsches Ärzteblatt* 61, no. 20 (1932): 271–2.

– "Der Beruf der Ärztin im Lichte 'nationaler, sozialer und ethischer Erkenntnis. Eine Erwiderung.'" *Deutsches Ärzteblatt* 61, no. 21 (1932): 285–6.

Heusler-Edenhuizen, Hermine. "Der Bund Deutscher Aerztinnen." *Die Studentin* 4, no. 7 (1928): 106–8.

– "Eheberatungsstellen," *Soziale Praxis* 37, no. 8 (1928): 187.

– "§ 218 vom Standpunkt der Frau," *Deutsches Ärzteblatt* 60, no. 13 (1931): 173–5.

– "Die sexuelle Not unserer Jugend," *Die Frau* 35, no. 10 (1928): 605–11.

Hirsch, Max. "Das Chaos der Eheberatung." *Deutsche Medizinische Wochenschrift* 18, no. 57 (1931): 764–7.

Höber, Josephine. "Zweck, Erfahrungen und Ziele der Eheberatung." *Die Frau* 36, no. 3 (1928): 142–8.

Kaufmann-Wolf, Marie. "Die Reglementierung der Prostitution." In *Einführung in das Studium der Prostitutionfrage*, edited by Anna Papritz, 99–106. Leipzig: Johann Ambrosius Barth, 1919.

– "Zur Bekämpfung der Geschlechtskrankheiten." *Die Frau* 27, no. 8 (1920): 233–5.

Kayser, Dr Marie-Elise. *Frauenmilchsammelstellen: Ein Leitfaden für deren Einrichtung und Betrieb*. Jena: Gustav Fischer, 1940.

Kelchner, Mathilde. *Die Frau und der weibliche Arzt: Eine psychologische Untersuchung auf Grund einer Umfrage*. Leipzig: Adolph Klein, 1934.

Kienle, Elsa. *Frauen. Aus dem Tagebuch einer Ärztin*. Berlin: Schmetterling Verlag, 1932.

Laroe, Else K. *Mit Skalpell und Nadel. Das abenteuerliche Leben eine Chirurgin*. Rüschilkon-Zürich: Albert Müller Verlag, 1968.

Lüders, Marie Elisabeth. *Das unbekannte Heer*. Berlin: Mittler, 1937.

Mayer, Anna. "Jugendamt und Jugendwohlfahrt." In *Die Kultur der Frau. Eine Lebenssymphonie der Frau des XX. Jahrhunderts*, edited by Ada Schmidt-Beil, 339–45. Berlin: Verlag für Kultur und Wissenschaft GmbH, 1931.

Mitscherlich, Alexander, and Fred Mielke. *The Death Doctors*. Translated by James Cleugh. London: Elek Books, 1962.

– "Epilogue: Seven Were Hanged." In *The Nazi Doctors and the Nuremberg Code: Human Rights in Human Experimentation*, edited by George J. Annas and Michael A. Grodin, 105–8. New York: Oxford University Press, 1992.

Müller, P. *Ueber die Zulassung der Frauen zum Studium der Medizin*. Hamburg: A.G., 1894.

Nathorff, Hertha. "Zum Problem der Geburtenregelung." *Die Medizinische Welt* 4, no. 24 (1930): 862–3.

Neisser-Schroeter, Lotte. *Enquete über die Ehe- und Sexualberatungsstellen in Deutschland mit Berücksichtigung der Geburtenregelung.* Berlin: Verlag der neuen Generation, 1928.

Niedermeyer, Albert Dr. "Die Aufgaben des Frauenarztes bei der Eheberatung." In *Veröffentlichungen aus dem Gebiete der Medizinalverwaltung,* edited by Otto Lenz, 258–88. Berlin: Richard Schoetz, 1929.

Prinz, Elizabeth. "Ehe- und Sexualreform. Zur Frage der Ethik und Diätetik des Sexuallebens." *Die Neue Generation* 27, no. 7/8/9 (1931): 159–62.

Profé, Alice. "Frauensport aus Ärztliche Sicht [1928]." In *Frau und Sport,* edited by Gertrud Pfister, 113–15. Frankfurt am Main: Fischer Taschenbuch, 1980.

– "Die körperliche Erziehung unsere Mädchen." *Körper und Geist* 14 (1905/1906): 135–9.

– "Mädchen – Kinder Zweiter Klasse? [1912]" In *Frau und Sport,* edited by Gertrud Pfister, 105–9. Frankfurt am Main: Fischer Taschenbuch, 1980.

– "Soll auch die Frau Leistungssport treiben? [1928]" In *Frau und Sport,* edited by Gertrud Pfister, 124–5. Frankfurt am Main: Fischer Taschenbuch, 1980.

– "Unser Mädchenturnen." *Körper und Geist* 14 (1905/1906): 404–9.

– "Unsinn in Mädchenturnen [1908]." In *Frau und Sport,* edited by Gertrud Pfister, 84–7. Frankfurt am Main: Fischer Taschenbuch, 1980.

– "Zur Hygiene der Frauen- und Mädchenkleidung." *Medizinische Klinik* 10, no. 22 (1914): 1–4.

Riderer-Kleemann, Margarete. "Die gesundheitlicher Erziehung in der Mädchenschule." *Gesundheit und Erziehung* 47, no. 2 (1934): 59–65.

Riegger, Luise. "Die Frau in der Jugendbewegung." In *Die Kultur der Frau. Eine Lebenssymphonie der Frau des XX. Jahrhunderts,* edited by Ada Schmidt-Beil, 237–45. Berlin: Verlag für Kultur und Wissenschaft GmbH, 1931.

Riese, Hertha. "Erfahrungen der Sexualberatungsstelle Frankfurt A.M. nebst Grundsätzlichen Bemerkungen über Geburtensregelungspolitik." *Die Neue Generation* 21, no. 10 (1925): 250–5.

– *Die sexuelle Not unserer Zeit.* Leipzig: Hesse & Becker, 1927.

– "Soll der Staat Heiratsvermittler werden? Ueber die Notwendigkeit der Einrichtung staatlicher Ehevermittlungsstellen." *Berliner Tageblatt,* 8 January 1928.

Sachs, Bertha. "Neuartige Körperpflege." In *Die Kultur der Frau. Eine Lebenssymphonie der Frau des XX. Jahrhunderts,* edited by Ada Schmidt-Beil, 427–33. Berlin: Verlag für Kultur und Wissenschaft GmbH, 1931.

Scheffin-Döring, "Die Mutterschaftsaufgabe der Frau." In *Die Kultur der Frau. Eine Lebenssymphonie der Frau des XX. Jahrhunderts*, edited by Ada Schmidt-Beil, 557–63. Berlin: Verlag für Kultur und Wissenschaft GmbH, 1931.

Schlossmann, Arthur. "Zur Eröffnung der Kinderwoche der Internationalen Hygiene- Ausstellung in Dresden." *Kleine Kinder* 4, no. 10 (1931): 181.

Schwerin, Ludwig. *Die Zulassung der Frauen zur Ausübung des ärztlichen Berufes*. Berlin: Carl Habel, 1880.

Staunder. "Die Standespolitik der deutschen Ärzte im Dienst der Volksgemeinschaft." *Deutsches Ärzteblatt* 61, no. 3 (1932): 41–2.

Stelzner, Helenefriederike. "Die Ärztin." In *Das Frauenbuch: eine allgemeinverständliche Einführung in alle Gebiete des Frauenlebens in der Gegenwart*, edited by Eugenie von Soden, 82–7. Stuttgart: Franckh'sch Verlagshandlung, 1913.

– "Die Hygiene in der Entwicklungsjahre." *Die Welt der Frau* 38 (1908): 593–5.

– "Soziale Medizin und Hygiene. Ein Beitrag zur Materie von der Verhütung unwerten Lebens." *Münchener Medizinische Wochenschrift* 72, no. 28 (1925): 1165–8.

– *Weibliche Fürsorgezöglinge: ihre psychologische und psychopathologische Wertung*. Berlin: Karger, 1929.

– "Zur Hygiene der weiblichen Seele." *Die Welt der Frau* 34 (1906): 529–31.

Szagunn, Ilse. "Der Arbeitsdienst für die weibliche Jugend. Aus der Arbeit einer Lagerärztin." *Gesundheit und Erziehung* 47, no. 7 (1934): 262–6.

– "Die Aufgaben der Mutter als Hüterin der Gesundheit." *Gesundheit und Eziehung* 47, no. 2 (1934): 49–58.

– "Gesundheitsfürsorge für die schulentlassene Jugend." *Hamburger Correspondent*, 18 April 1926.

– "Die Kommunal- und Fürsorgeärztin." *Die Studentin* 4, no. 7 (1928): 104–6.

– "Schulärztliche Untersuchungen an Lyzeen und Studienanstalten." *Zeitschrift für Schulgesundeitspflege* 39 (1926): 459–60.

– "Über die schulärztliche Tätigkeit an Fortbildungscchulen." *Zeitschrift für Schulgesundheitspflege* 34 (1921): 84–9.

– "Vita von Ise Szagunn. Ein Lebensbild in der Zeit." *Berliner Medizin* 12, no. 11 (1961): 261–6.

– "Warum Ärztinnenbund?" *Berliner Ärzteblatt* 64, no. 2 (1951): 27.

Többen, Dr. "Gefährdung, Verwahrlosung und Kriminalität der Jugend in ihren Beziehungen zum Alkoholismus." In *Alkoholfreies Jugendleben: Wege der Pädagogik und Selbsterziehung*, edited by Heinrich Czeloth and Erich Reisch. Berlin: Hoheneck-Verlag, 1930.

Turnau, Laura. *Die Ärztin. (Merkblätter für Berufsberatung der Deutschen Zentralstelle für Berufsberatung der Akademiker)*. Berlin: Trowitzsch, 1928.

- "Der Beruf der Aerztin." *Die Studentin* 4, no. 7 (1928): 97–9.
- "Meine Autobiographie." *Mitteilungsblatt des Deutschen Ärztinnenbundes* 18, no. 2 (1971): 8–13.
- "Meine Autobiographie." *Mitteilungsblatt des Deutschen Ärztinnenbundes* 18, no. 4 (1971): 2–4.
van Kann, Edmund. "Die Zahl der Ärzte 1942 und ein Rückblick bis 1937." *Deutsches Ärzteblatt* 72, no. 26/27 (1942): 300–3.
- "Zahl und Gliedergung der Fachärzte Deutschlands im Jahre 1940." *Deutsches Ärzteblatt* 70, no. 26 (1940): 283–6.
von Lölhoffel, Edith. "Die Frau im Sport." In *Die Kultur der Frau. Eine Lebenssymphonie der Frau des XX. Jahrhunderts*, edited by Ada Schmidt-Beil, 449–53. Berlin: Verlag für Kultur und Wissenschaft GmbH, 1931.
von Renthe-Fink, Barbara. *So alt wie das Jahrhundert. Lebensbericht einer Berliner Ärztin*. Frankfurt: R.G. Fischer, 1982.
Weber, Mathilde. *Ärztinnen für Frauenkrankheiten: eine ethische und sanitäre Notwendigkeit*. Tübingen: Franz Fues Verlag, 1888.
Weck, J. Oeflingen. *Koche auf Vorrat! Handbuch fuer die Frischhaltung aller Nahrungsmittel mit den "Weckschen Einrichtungen."* Baden: J. Weck GmbH., Öflingen, 1913.
Wolff, Charlotte. *Augenblicke verändern uns mehr als die Zeit. Eine Autobiographie*. Translated by Michaela Huber. Frankfurt am Main: Fischer Taschenbuch, 1990.
- *Hindsight. An Autobiography*. London: Quartet Books, 1980.

Books, Articles, Dissertations (Secondary)

Abrams, Lynn. "Prostitutes in Imperial Germany, 1870-1918: Working Girls or Social Outcasts?" In *The German Underworld: Deviants and Outcasts in German History*, edited by Richard Evans, 189–209. New York: Routledge, 1988.
Adams, Julia, and Tasleem Padamsee. "Signs and Regimes: Rereading Feminist Work on Welfare States." *Social Politics* 9, no. 2 (2002): 187–202.
Albisetti, James. "The Fight for Female Physicians in Imperial Germany." *Central European History* 15, no. 2 (1982): 99–123.
Allen, Ann Taylor. "Feminism and Eugenics in Germany and Britain, 1900–1940: A Comparative Perspective." *German Studies Review* 23, no. 3 (2000): 477–506.
- *Feminism and Motherhood in Germany, 1800–1914*. New Brunswick, NJ: Rutgers University Press, 1991.
- "Feminism, Venereal Diseases, and the State in Germany, 1890–1918." *Journal of the History of Sexuality* 4, no. 1 (1993): 27–50.

- "German Radical Feminism and Eugenics, 1900-1908." *German Studies Review* 11, no. 1 (1988): 31–56.

Aly, Götz. *Hitler's Beneficiaries: Plunder, Racial War, and the Nazi Welfare State*. Translated by Jefferson Chase. New York: Metropolitan Books, 2007.

Andréolle, Donna Spalding, and Véronique Molinari, eds. *Women and Science, 17th Century to Present: Pioneers, Activists and Protagonists*. Newcastle upon Tyne: Cambridge Scholars, 2011.

Annas, George J., and Michael A. Grodin, eds. *The Nazi Doctors and the Nuremberg Code: Human Rights in Human Experimentation*. New York: Oxford University Press, 1992.

Aschenbrenner, Susanne. "Marta Fraenkel (1896–1976). Ärztin, Museumspädagogin und Public Health Officer." Med. diss., Rheinisch-Westfälischen Technischen Hochschule, 2000.

Baranowski, Shelly. *Strength through Joy: Consumerism and Mass Tourism in the Third Reich*. New York: Cambridge University Press, 2004.

Barinaga, Marcia. "Is There a Female Style of Doing Science?" *Science* 260, no. 5106 (1993): 384–91.

Berger, Uta, ed. *Ärztin in Vergangenheit-Gegenwart-Zukunft, 1924–1999. Festschrift des Deutschen Ärztinnebundes e.V.* Greven: WWF Verl.-Ges., 1999.

Berning, Cornelia. "Die Einbindung der Ärztinnen in das frauenpolitische Konzept des Nationalsozialismus unter besonderer Berücksichtigung ihrer Studien- und Berufsituation." Med. diss., Westfälische Wilhelms-Universität Münster, 1994.

Bessel, Richard. *Germany after the First World War*. New York: Oxford University Press, 1993.

Blackbourn, David. "Germans Abroad and Auslandsdeutsche: Places, Networks, and Experiences from the Sixteenth Century to the Twentieth Century." *Geschichte und Gesellschaft* 41, no. 2 (2015): 321–46.

Blackbourn, David, and James Retallack, eds. *Localism, Landscape, and Ambiguities of Place: German-Speaking Central Europe, 1860–1930*. Toronto: University of Toronto Press, 2007.

Bleker, Johanna. "Agnes Bluhm, die Wissenschaftlerin unter den Rassenhygienikerin, und die Frauenbewegung." *Acta Historica Leopoldina* 48 (2007): 89–111.

- "Anerkennung durch Unterordnung? Ärztinnen und Nationalsozialismus." In *Weibliche Ärzte: Die Durchsetzung des Berufsbildes in Deutschland*, edited by Eva Brinkschulte, 126–39. Berlin: Edition Hentrich, 1993.

- "Die Frau als Weib: Sex und Gender in der Medizingeschichte." In *Geschlechterverhältnisse in Medizin, Naturwissenschaft und Technik*, edited by Christoph Meinel and Monika Renneberg, 15–29. Bassum: Verlag für Geschichte der Naturwissenschaften und der Technik, 1996.

Bleker, Johanna, and Christine Eckelmann. "'Der Erfolg der Gleichschaltungsaktion kann als durchschlagend bezeichnet werden' – 'Der Bund Deutscher Ärztinnen' 1933 bis 1936." In *Medizin im "Dritten Reich,"* edited by Johanna Bleker and Norbert Jachertz, 87–96. Köln: Deutscher Ärzte-Verlag, 1993.

Bleker, Johanna, and Sabine Schleiermacher. *Ärztinnen aus dem Kaiserreich: Lebensläufe einer Generation.* Weinheim: Deutscher Studien Verlag, 2000.

Bleker, Johanna, and Svenja Ludwig. *Emanzipation und Eugenik: die Briefe der Frauenrechtlerin, Rassenhygienikerin und Genetikerin Agnes Bluhm an den Studienfreund Alfred Ploetz aus den Jahren 1901–1938.* Husum: Matthiesen, 2007.

Boak, Helen. *Women in the Weimar Republic.* Manchester: Manchester University Press, 2013.

Boaz, Rachel. *In Search of "Aryan Blood": Serology in Interwar and National Socialist Germany.* Budapest: Central European University Press, 2014.

Bock, Gisela. "Antinatalism, Maternity and Paternity in National Socialist Racism." In *Nazism and German Society, 1933–1945,* edited by David Crew, 110-40. New York: Routledge, 1994.

– "Ganz normale Frauen. Täter, Opfer, Mitläufer, und Zuschauer im Nationalsozialismus." In *Zwischen Karriere und Verfolgung: Handlungsräume von Frauen im nationalsozialistischen Deutschland,* edited by Kirsten Heinsohn, Barbara Vogel, and Ulrike Weckel, 245–77. Frankfurt am Main: Campus, 1997.

– "Ordinary Women in Nazi Germany: Perpetrators, Victims, Followers, and Bystanders." In *Women in the Holocaust,* edited by Dalia Ofer and Lenore J. Weitzman, 85–100. New Haven, CT: Yale University Press, 1998.

– "Racism and Sexism in Nazi Germany: Motherhood, Compulsory Sterilization, and the State." In *Different Voices: Women and the Holocaust,* edited by Carol Rittner and John K. Roth, 161–86. New York: Paragon House, 1993.

– *Zwangssterilisation im Nationalsozialismus: Studien zur Rassenpolitik und Frauenpolitik.* Opladen: Westdeutscher Verlag, 1986.

Bridenthal, Renate. "Beyond Kinder, Küche, Kirche: Weimar Women at Work." *Central European History* 6, no. 2 (1973): 148–66.

Bridenthal, Renate, Atina Grossmann, and Marion Kaplan, eds. *When Biology Became Destiny: Women in Weimar and Nazi Germany.* New York: Monthly Review Press, 1984.

Bridenthal, Renate, and Claudia Koonz. "Beyond Kinder, Küche, Kirche: Weimar Women in Politics and Work." In *When Biology Became Destiny:*

Women in Weimar and Nazi Germany, edited by Renate Bridenthal, Atina Grossmann, and Marion Kaplan, 33–65. New York: Monthly Review Press, 1984.

Briggs, Laura. "Discourses of 'Forced Sterilization' in Puerto Rico: The Problem with the Speaking Subaltern." *Differences* 10, no. 2 (1998): 30–67.

– *Reproducing Empire: Race, Sex, Science, and U.S. Imperialism in Puerto Rico*. Berkeley: University of California Press, 2002.

Brinkschulte, Eva, ed. *Weibliche Ärzte: Die Durchsetzung des Berufsbildes in Deutschland*. Berlin: Edition Hentrich, 1993.

Brüggemeier, Franz-Josef, Mark Cioc, and Thomas Zeller, eds. *How Green Were the Nazis? Nature, Environment, and Nation in the Third Reich*. Athens: Ohio University Press, 2005.

Buchin, Jutta. "Dokumentation: Ärztinnen aus dem Kaiserreich." Berlin: Institute für Geschichte der Medizin, 2003. https://geschichte.charite.de/aeik/.

Burleigh, Michael, and Wolfgang Wippermann. *The Racial State: Germany, 1933–1945*. New York: Cambridge University Press, 1991.

Cahn, Susan K. *Coming on Strong: Gender and Sexuality in Twentieth-Century Women's Sport*. New York: Free Press, 1994.

Campbell, Annily. *Childfree and Sterilized: Women's Decisions and Medical Responses*. New York: Cassell, 1999.

Childers, Thomas, ed. *The Formation of the Nazi Constituency, 1919–1933*. London: Croom Helm, 1986.

– *The Nazi Voter: The Social Foundations of Fascism in Germany, 1919–1933*. Chapel Hill: University of North Carolina Press, 1983.

Childers, Thomas, and Jane Caplan, eds. *Reevaluating the Third Reich*. New York: Holmes and Meier, 1993.

Cocks, Geoffrey. "The Old as New: The Nuremberg Doctors' Trial and Medicine in Modern Germany." In *Medicine and Modernity: Public Health and Medical Care in Nineteenth-and Twentieth-Century Germany*, edited by Manfred Berg and Geoffrey Cocks, 173–92. Washington, DC: German Historical Institute, 1997.

Cocks, Geoffrey, and Konrad H. Jarausch, eds. *German Professions, 1800–1950*. New York: Oxford University Press, 1990.

Cole, Mark B. "Feeding the Volk: Food, Culture, and the Politics of Nazi Consumption, 1933–1945." PhD diss., University of Florida, 2011.

Collins, Patricia Hill. "Defining Black Feminist Thought." In *Feminist Theory Reader: Local and Global Perspectives*, edited by Carole R. McCann and Seung-Kyung Kim, 379–94. New York: Routledge, 2013.

Connelly, Matthew. *Fatal Misconception: The Struggle to Control World Populations*. Cambridge, MA: Belknap Press of Harvard University Press, 2008.

Corbin, Alain. *Women for Hire: Prostitution and Sexuality in France after 1850*. Translated by Alan Sheridan. Cambridge, MA: Harvard University Press, 1990.

Cowan, Ruth Schwartz. *More Work for Mother: The Ironies of Household Technology from the Open Hearth to the Microwave*. New York: Basic Books, 1983.

Crew, David. *Germans on Welfare: From Weimar to Hitler*. New York: Oxford University Press, 1998.

Daniel, Ute. *The War from Within: German Working-Class Women in the First World War*. Translated by Margaret Ries. New York: Berg, 1997.

Davin, Anna. "Imperialism and Motherhood." *History Workshop Journal* 5, no. 1 (1978): 9–65.

de Grazia, Victoria. *How Fascism Ruled Women: Italy, 1922–1945*. Berkeley: University of California Press, 1992.

Dickinson, Edward Ross. "Biopolitics, Fascism, Democracy." *Central European History* 37, no. 1 (2004): 1–48.

– *The Politics of German Child Welfare from the Empire to the Federal Republic*. Cambridge, MA: Harvard University Press, 1996.

Doerry, Martin. *Mein verwundetes Herz. Das Leben der Lilli Jahn 1900–1944*. Munich: Deutscher Taschenbuch Verlag, 2002.

Donson, Andrew. *Youth in the Fatherless Land: War Pedagogy, Nationalism, and Authority in Germany, 1914–1918*. Cambridge, MA: Harvard University Press, 2010.

Downs, Laura Lee. *Manufacturing Inequality: Gender Division in the French and British Metalworking Industries, 1914–1939*. Ithaca, NY: Cornell University Press, 1995.

Eckelmann, Christine. *Ärztinnen in der Weimarer Zeit und im Nationalsozialismus: eine Untersuchung über den Bund Deutscher Ärztinnen*. Wermelskirchen: Verlag für Wissenschaft, Forschung und Technik, 1992.

Eifert, Christiane. "Coming to Terms with the State: Maternalist Politics and the Development of the Welfare State in Weimar Germany." *Central European History* 30, no. 1 (1997): 25–47.

Erben, Ulrike. "'Die Ärztin gehört mit an die vorderste Front.' Das Berufsbild der deutschen Ärztin im Nationalsozialismus im Spiegel der Zeitschrfit *Die Ärztin*." In *"Im Dienste der Volksgesundheit": Frauen, Gesundheitswesen, Nationalsozialismus*, edited by Ingrid Arias, 3–15. Vienna: Verlagshaus der Ärzte, 2006.

Evans, Richard J. *The Feminist Movement in Germany, 1894–1933*. London: Sage, 1976.

– "Prostitution, State and Society in Imperial Germany." *Past & Present* 70, no. 1 (1976): 106–29.

Evans, Sara M. *Born for Liberty: A History of Women in America.* New York: Simon & Schuster, 1997.

Fallwell, Lynne Anne. "Nazism Delivered: The Ethos and Legacy of Midwifery in 20th Century Germany." PhD diss., Pennsylvania State University, 2003.

"Forum: Class in German History." *German History* 30, no. 3 (2012): 429–51.

Foucault, Michel. *The Archaeology of Knowledge: And the Discourse on Language.* Translated by Alan Sheridan. New York: Pantheon Books, 1972.

– *The Birth of Biopolitics: Lectures at the Collège de France, 1978–79.* Edited by Michel Senellart. Translated by Graham Burchell. New York: Palgrave Macmillan, 2008.

– *The History of Sexuality,* vol. 1: *An Introduction.* New York: Vintage, 1990.

Freund-Widder, Michaela. *Frauen unter Kontrolle: Prostitution und ihre Staatliche Bekämpfung in Hamburg vom Ende des Kaiserreichs bis zu den Anfängen der Bundesrepublik.* Münster: LIT, 2003.

Frevert, Ute. *Women in German History: From Bourgeois Emancipation to Sexual Liberation.* Oxford: Berg, 1989.

Frohman, Larry. "Prevention, Welfare, and Citizenship: The War on Tuberculosis and Infant Mortality in Germany, 1900–1930." *Central European History* 39, no. 3 (2006): 431–81.

Fuchs, Rachel. *Poor and Pregnant in Paris: Strategies for Survival in the Nineteenth Century.* New Brunswick, NJ: Rutgers University Press, 1992.

Fuchs-Heinritz, Werner, Martin Kohli, and Fritz Schütze, eds. *Wiebke Lohfeld Im Dazwischen. Porträt der jüdischen und deutschen Ärztin Paula Tobias (1886–1970).* Opladen: Leske + Budrich, 2003.

Gallin, Alice. *Midwives to Nazism: University Professors in Weimar Germany, 1925–1933.* Macon, GA: Mercer University Press, 1986.

Gamper, Martina. "'Du hast die Pflicht gesund zu sein.' BDM-Ärztinnen in Wien." In *Im Dienste der Volksgesundheit: Frauen, Gesundheitswesen, Nationalsozialismus,* edited by Ingrid Arias, 15–30. Vienna: Verlagshaus der Ärzte, 2006.

Gerhard, Gesine. *Nazi Hunger Politics: A History of Food in the Third Reich.* Lanham: Rowman & Littlefield, 2015.

Gibson, Mary. *Prostitution and the State in Italy, 1860–1915.* New Brunswick, NJ: Rutgers University Press, 1986.

Glaser, Edith. *Hindernisse, Umwege, Sackgassen. Die Anfänge des Frauenstudiums in Tübingen (1904–1934).* Weinheim: Deutscher Studien Verlag, 1992.

Golden, Janet Lynne. *A Social History of Wet Nursing in America: From Breast to Bottle*. New York: Cambridge University Press, 1996.

Goltermann, Svenja. *Körper der Nation: Habitusformierung und die Politik des Turnens: 1860–1890*. Göttingen: Vandenhoeck & Ruprecht, 1998.

Gordon, Linda. *Woman's Body, Woman's Right: A Social History of Birth Control in America*. New York: Grossman, 1976.

Grant, Susan. *Physical Culture and Sport in Soviet Society: Propaganda, Acculturation, and Transformation in the 1920s and 1930s*. New York: Routledge, 2013.

Gregor, Neil, Nils Roemer, and Mark Roseman, eds. *German History from the Margins*. Bloomington: Indiana University Press, 2006.

Grossmann, Atina. "Abortion and Economic Crisis: The 1931 Campaign against Paragraph 218." In *When Biology Became Destiny: Women in Weimar and Nazi Germany*, edited by Renate Bridenthal, Atina Grossmann, and Marion Kaplan, 66-86. New York: Monthly Review Press, 1984.

– "Berliner Ärztinnen und Volksgesundheit in der Weimarer Republik: Zwischen Sexualreform und Eugenik." In *Unter allen Umständen: Frauengeschichte(n) in Berlin*, edited by Christiane Eifert and Susanne Rouette, 183–217. Berlin: Rotation, 1986.

– "Feminist Debates about Women and National Socialism." *Gender and History* 3, no. 3 (1991): 350–8.

– "Gender and Rationalization: Questions about the German/American Comparison." *Social Politics* 4, no. 1 (1997): 6–18.

– "German Women Doctors from Berlin to New York: Maternity and Modernity in Weimar and in Exile." *Feminist Studies* 19, no. 1 (1993): 65–88.

– "*Girlkultur* or Thoroughly Rationalized Female: A New Woman in Weimar Germany?" *Women in Culture and Politics: A Century of Change*, edited by Judith Friedlander et al., 62–80. Bloomington: Indiana University Press, 1986.

– "The New Woman and the Rationalization of Sexuality in Weimar Germany." In *Powers of Desire: The Politics of Sexuality*, edited by Ann Snitow, Christine Stansell, and Sharon Thompson, 153–71. New York: Monthly Review Press, 1983.

– *Reforming Sex: The German Movement for Birth Control and Abortion Reform, 1920–1950*. New York: Oxford University Press, 1995.

Hackett, Amy. "Helene Stöcker: Left-Wing Intellectual and Sex Reformer." *When Biology Became Destiny: Women in Weimar and Nazi Germany*, edited by Renate Bridenthal, Atina Grossmann, and Marion Kaplan, 109–30. New York: Monthly Review Press, 1984.

Hagemann, Karen. *Frauenalltag und Männerpolitik: Alltagsleben und gesellschaftliches Handeln von Arbeiterfrauen in der Weimarer Republik.* Bonn: J.H.W. Dietz, 1990.

– "Rationalizing Family Work: Municipal Family Welfare and Urban Working-Class Mothers in Germany." *Social Politics* 4, no. 1 (1997): 19–48.

Hamilton, Richard F. *Who Voted for Hitler?* Princeton, NJ: Princeton University Press, 1982.

Harris, Victoria. *Selling Sex in the Reich: Prostitutes in German Society, 1914–1945.* New York: Oxford University Press, 2010.

Hartsock, Nancy C.M. "The Feminist Standpoint: Toward a Specifically Feminist Historical Materialism." In *Feminist Theory Reader: Local and Global Perspectives*, edited by Carole R. McCann and Seung-Kyung Kim, 354–69. New York: Routledge, 2013.

Harvey, Elizabeth. *Women and the Nazi East: Agents and Witnesses of Germanization.* New Haven, CT: Yale University Press, 2003.

– *Youth and the Welfare State in Weimar Germany.* Oxford: Clarendon Press, 1993.

Hau, Michael. *The Cult of Health and Beauty: A Social History, 1890–1930.* Chicago: University of Chicago Press, 2003.

Healy, Maureen. *Vienna and the Fall of the Habsburg Empire: Total War and Everyday Life in World War I.* New York: Cambridge University Press, 2004.

Herf, Jeffrey. *The Jewish Enemy: Nazi Propaganda during World War II and the Holocaust.* Cambridge, MA: Harvard University Press, 2008.

– *Reactionary Modernism: Technology, Culture, and Politics in Weimar and the Third Reich.* New York: Cambridge University Press, 1984.

Hering, Sabine, and Kurt Schilde. *Das BDM-Werk "Glaube und Schönheit." Die Organisation junger Frauen im Nationalsozialismus.* Berlin: Metropol, 2000.

Hoesch, Kristin. *Ärztinnen für Frauen. Kliniken in Berlin, 1877–1914.* Stuttgart: Metzler, 1995.

Hoffmann, David, and Annette Timm. "Utopian Biopolitics: Reproductive Policies, Gender Roles, and Sexuality in Nazi Germany and the Soviet Union." In *Beyond Totalitarianism: Stalinism and Nazism Compared*, edited by Michael Geyer and Sheila Fitzpatrick, 87–129. New York: Cambridge University Press, 2008.

Hong, Young-Sun. "Gender, Citizenship, and the Welfare State: Social Work and the Politics of Femininity in the Weimar Republic." *Central European History* 30, no. 1 (1997): 1–24.

– *Welfare, Modernity, and the Weimar State, 1919–1933.* Princeton, NJ: Princeton University Press, 1998.

Huerkamp, Claudia. "Frauen, Universitäten, und Bildungsbürgertum: Zur Lage studierender Frauen." In *Bürgerliche Berufe: Zur Sozialgeschichte der freien und akademischen Berufe im internationalen Vergleich*, edited by Hannes Siegrist, 200–22. Göttingen: Vandenhoek & Ruprecht, 1988.

- "The Making of the Modern Medical Profession, 1800–1914: Prussian Doctors in the Nineteenth Century." In *German Professions, 1800–1950*, edited by Geoffrey Cocks and Konrad H. Jarausch, 66–84. New York: Oxford University Press, 1990.

Jacob, Wilson Chacko. "Working Out Egypt: Masculinity and Subject Formation between Colonial Modernity and Nationalism, 1870–1940." PhD diss., New York University, 2005.

Jarausch, Konrad H. "The Crisis of German Professions, 1918–1933." *Journal of Contemporary History* 20, no. 3 (1985): 379–98.

- "The German Professions in History and Theory." In *German Professions, 1800–1950*, edited by Geoffrey Cocks and Konrad H. Jarausch, 9–24. New York: Oxford University Press, 1990.

- *The Transformation of Higher Learning: Expansion, Diversification, Social Opening, and Professionalization in England, Germany, Russia, and the United States*. Chicago: University of Chicago Press, 1983.

- *The Unfree Professions: German Lawyers, Teachers, and Engineers, 1900–1950*. New York: Oxford University Press, 1990.

Jenders, Andrea, and Andreas Müller. *"Nur die Dummen sind eingeschrieben": Dortmunder Dirnen und Sittengeschichte zwischen 1870 und 1927*. Dortmund: Geschichtswerkstatt Dortmund, 1993.

Jensen, Erik N. *Body by Weimar: Athletes, Gender, and German Modernity*. New York: Oxford University Press, 2010.

Jürgens, Birgit. *Zur Geschichte des BDM (Bund Deutscher Mädel) von 1923 bis 1939*. Frankfurt am Main: P. Lang, 1994.

Kaplan, Marion. *Between Dignity and Despair: Jewish Life in Nazi Germany*. New York: Oxford University Press, 1998.

- *The Making of the Jewish Middle Class: Women, Family, and Identity in Imperial Germany*. New York: Oxford University Press, 1991.

Kater, Michael H. "Ärzte und Politik in Deutschland, 1848–1945." *Jahrbuch des Instituts für Geschichte der Medizin der Robert Bosch Stiftung* 5 (1987): 34–48.

- "The Burden of the Past: Problems of a Modern Historiography of Physicians and Medicine in Nazi Germany." *German Studies Review* 10, no. 1 (1987): 31–56.

- *Doctors under Hitler*. Chapel Hill: University of North Carolina Press, 1989.

- "Hitler's Early Doctors: Nazi Physicians in Predepression Germany." *Journal of Modern History* 59, no. 1 (1972): 207–55.

- "Krisis des Frauenstudiums in der Weimarer Republik." *Vierteljahrsschrift für Sozial-und Wirtschaftsgeschichte* 59, no. 2 (1972): 207–55.
- "Medizin und Mediziner im Dritten Reich. Eine Bestandsaufnahme" *Historische Zeitschrift* 244, no. 2 (1987): 299–352.
- *The Nazi Party: A Social Profile of Members and Leaders, 1919–1945.* Cambridge, MA: Harvard University Press, 1983.
- "The Nazi Physicians' League of 1929: Causes and Consequences." In *The Formation of the Nazi Constituency, 1919–1933,* edited by Thomas Childers, 147–81. London: Croom Helm, 1986.
- "Physicians in Crisis at the End of the Weimar Republic." In *Unemployment and the Great Depression in Weimar Germany,* edited by Peter D. Stachura, 49–77. Basingstoke: Palgrave Macmillan, 1986.
- "Professionalization and Socialization of Physicians in Wilhelmine and Weimar Germany." *Journal of Contemporary History* 20, no. 4 (1985): 677–701.
Kaufmann, Doris. *Geschichte der Kaiser-Wilhelm-Gesellschaft im Nationalsozialismus.* Göttingen: Wallstein, 2000.
Kavčič, Silvija. "Dr. Herta Oberheuser-Karriere einer Ärztin." In *Frauen als Täterinnen und Mittäterinnen im Nationalsozialismus. Gestaltungsspielräume und Handlungsmöglichkeiten: Beiträge zum 5. Tag der Frauen- und Geschlechterforschung an der Martin-Luther-Universität Halle-Wittenberg,* edited by Viola Schubert-Lehnhardt and Sylvia Korch, 99–113. Halle: Martin-Luther-Universität, 2006.
Keller, Evelyn Fox. "The Anomaly of a Woman in Physics." In *Women, Science and Technology: A Reader in Feminist Science Studies,* edited by Mary Wyer, 23–30. New York: Routledge, 2001.
- *A Feeling for the Organism: The Life and Work of Barbara McClintock.* New York: W.H. Freeman and Company, 1983.
Kevles, Daniel. "Eugenics Then and Genetics Now – Avoiding the Pitfalls of the Past." In *The Implications of Genetics for Health Professional Education: Proceedings of a Conference,* edited by Mary Hager, 187–204. New York: Macy Foundation, 1999.
- *In the Name of Eugenics: Genetics and the Uses of Human Heredity.* Cambridge, MA: Harvard University Press, 1995.
Kinz, Gabriele. *Der Bund Deutscher Mädel. Ein Beitrag zur außerschulischen Mädchenerziehung im Nationalsozialismus.* Frankfurt am Main: P. Lang, 1990.
Klaus, Martin. *Mädchen im Dritten Reich. Der Bund Deutscher Mädel (BDM).* Cologne: Pahl- Rugenstein, 1983.
- *Mädchen in der Hitlerjugend: Die Erziehung zur "deutschen Frau."* Cologne: Pahl-Rugenstein, 1980.

Knodel, John. *The Decline of Fertility in Germany, 1871–1939*. Princeton, NJ: Princeton University Press, 1974.

Koblitz, Ann Hibner. "Science, Women, and the Russian Intelligentsia: The Generation of the 1860s." In *History of Women in the Sciences: Readings from Isis*, edited by Sally Gregory Kohlstedt, 208–26. Chicago: University of Chicago Press, 1999.

Kohlstedt, Sally Gregory. "Nature, Not Books: Scientists and the Origins of the Nature-Study Movement in the 1890s." *Isis* 96, no. 3 (2005): 324–52.

– "Parlors, Primers, and Public Schooling: Education for Science in Nineteenth-Century America." *Isis* 81, no. 3 (1990): 424–45.

Koonz, Claudia. "Eugenics, Gender, and Ethics in Nazi Germany: The Debate about Involuntary Sterilization, 1933–1936." In *Reevaluating the Third Reich*, edited by Thomas Childers and Jane Caplan, 66–85. New York: Holmes and Meier, 1993.

– "Mothers in the Fatherland: Women in Nazi Germany." In *Becoming Visible: Women in European History*, edited by Renate Bridenthal and Claudia Koonz, 445–73. Boston: Houghton Mifflin, 1977.

– *Mothers in the Fatherland: Women, The Family, and Nazi Politics*. New York: St Martin's Press, 1987.

Koven, Seth, and Sonya Michel, eds. *Mothers of a New World: Maternalist Politics and the Origins of Welfare States*. New York: Routledge, 1993.

– "Womanly Duties: Maternalist Politics and the Origins of Welfare States in France, Germany, Great Britain, and the United States, 1880–1920." *American Historical Review* 95, no. 4 (1990): 1076–108.

Kramer, Nicole. *Volksgenossinnen an der Heimatfront: Mobilisierung, Verhalten, Erinnerung*. Göttingen: Vandenhoeck & Ruprecht, 2011.

Krauss, Martina. *Die Frau der Zukunft. Dr. Hope Bridges Adams Lehmann, 1855–1916: Ärztin und Reformerin*. Munich: Buchendorfer, 2002.

Kravetz, Melissa. "Finding a Space in Schools: Female Doctors and the Reform of Girls' Physical Education in Weimar Germany." *Journal of Women's History* 29, no. 1 (Spring 2017): 38–62.

– "Promoting Eugenics and Maternalism: Women Doctors and Marriage Counselling in Weimar Germany." In *Women and Science, 17th Century to Present: Pioneers, Activists and Protagonists*, edited by Donna Spalding Andréolle and Véronique Molinari, 69–86. Newcastle upon Tyne: Cambridge Scholars, 2011.

Kühl, Stefan. *The Nazi Connection: Eugenics, American Racism, and German National Socialism*. New York: Oxford University Press, 1994.

Kühne, Thomas. *Belonging and Genocide: Hitler's Community, 1918–1945*. New Haven, CT: Yale University Press, 2010.

– *Kameradschaft: Die Soldaten des nationalsozialistischen Krieges und das 20. Jahrhundert.* Göttingen: Vandenhoeck & Ruprecht, 2006.

Kurlander, Eric. *Living with Hitler: Liberal Democrats in the Third Reich.* New Haven, CT: Yale University Press, 2009.

Lamberti, Marjorie. *The Politics of Education: Teachers and School Reform in Weimar Germany.* New York: Berghahn Books, 2002.

– *State, Society, and the Elementary School in Imperial Germany.* New York: Oxford University Press, 1989.

Lansing, Charles B. *From Nazism to Communism: German Schoolteachers under Two Dictatorships.* Cambridge, MA: Harvard University Press, 2010.

Laquer, Walter Z. *Young Germany: A History of the German Youth Movement.* New York: Basic Books, 1962.

Lekan, Thomas, and Thomas Zeller, eds. *Germany's Nature: Cultural Landscapes and Environmental History.* New Brunswick, NJ: Rutgers University Press, 2005.

Lifton, Robert Jay. *The Nazi Doctors: Medical Killing and the Psychology of Genocide.* New York: Basic Books, 1986.

Lower, Wendy. *Hitler's Furies: The Uncovered Story of German Women in the Nazi Killing Fields.* Boston: Houghton Mifflin Harcourt, 2013.

Ludwig, Karl-Heinz. *Technik, Ingenieure und Gesellschaft: Geschichte des Vereins Deutscher Ingenieure, 1856–1981.* Düsseldorf: VDI-Verlag, 1981.

Mahlendorf, Ursula. *The Shame of Survival: Working through a Nazi Childhood.* University Park, PA: Pennsylvania State University, 2009.

Mahler, Stefanie. "Die eugenische Argumentation der Ärzte und Ärztinnen in der Bewegung gegen den §218 in der Weimarer Republik." MA thesis, Freie Universität, 1996.

Mangan, J.A., and Roberta J. Park. *From "Fair Sex" to Feminism: Sport and the Socialization of Women in the Industrial and Post-Industrial Eras.* London: Frank Cass, 1987.

Manthorpe, Catherine. "Science or Domestic Science? The Struggle to Define an Appropriate Science Education for Girls in Early Twentieth-Century England." *History of Education* 15, no. 3 (1986): 195–213.

Marhoefer, Laurie. *Sex and the Weimar Republic: German Homosexual Emancipation and the Rise of the Nazis.* Toronto: University of Toronto Press, 2015.

Maschmann, Melita. *Account Rendered: A Dossier on My Former Self.* Translated by Geoffrey Strachan. London: Abelard-Schuman, 1964.

Mason, Timothy. *Nazism, Fascism, and the Working Class.* New York: Cambridge University Press, 1995.

Mazón, Patricia M. *Gender and the Modern Research University: The Admission of Women to German Higher Education, 1865–1914.* Stanford, CA: Stanford University Press, 2003.

Mazower, Mark. *Dark Continent: Europe's Twentieth Century*. New York: Alfred A. Knopf, 1999.

McClive, Cathy. *Menstruation and Procreation in Early Modern France*. New York: Routledge, 2015.

McFarland-Icke, Bronwyn Rebekah. *Nurses in Nazi Germany: Moral Choice in History*. Princeton, NJ: Princeton University Press, 1999.

McIntosh, Peter C. *Physical Education in England since 1800*. London: G. Bell & Sons, 1968.

Meinander, Heinrik. *Towards a Bourgeois Manhood: Boys' Physical Education in Nordic Secondary Schools, 1880–1940*. Helsinki: Finnish Society of Sciences and Letters, 1994.

Merton, Robert K. "The Matthew Effect in Science." *Science* 159, no. 3810 (1968): 56–63.

Michalczyk, John J., ed. *Medicine, Ethics, and the Third Reich: Historical and Contemporary Issues*. Kansas City, MO: Sheed and Ward, 1994.

Michel, Sonya. "Maternalism and Beyond." In *Maternalism Reconsidered: Motherhood, Welfare and Social Policy in the Twentieth Century*, edited by Marian van der Klein, Rebecca Jo Plant, Nichole Sanders, and Lori R. Weintrob, 22–37. New York: Berghahn Books, 2012.

Miller, Julie. *Abandoned: Foundlings in Nineteenth-Century New York City*. New York: New York University Press, 2008.

Miller-Kipp, Gisela, ed. *"Auch du gehörst dem Führer": Die Geschichte des Bundes Deutscher Mädel (BDM) in Quellen und Dokumenten*. Weinheim: Juventa, 2001.

Mitterauer, Michael. *A History of Youth*. Translated by Graeme Dunphy. Cambridge, MA: Blackwell, 1992.

Morantz-Sanchez, Regina. *Sympathy and Science: Women Physicians in American Medicine*. New York: Oxford University Press, 1985.

Mouton, Michelle. *From Nurturing the Nation to Purifying the Volk: Weimar and Nazi Family Policy, 1918–1945*. New York: Cambridge University Press, 2007.

– "Sports, Song, and Socialization: Women's Memories of Youthful Activity and Political Indoctrination in the BDM." *Journal of Women's History* 17, no. 2 (2005): 62–86.

Müller, Manfried. "Mörder von zwölf Millionen. Die Ärzteschule in Alt-Rehse am Tollensesee." *Freie Erde* 217 (1982): 4.

Müller-Hill, Benno. "Eugenics: The Science and Religion of the Nazis." In *When Medicine Went Mad: Bioethics and the Holocaust*, edited by Arthur L. Caplan, 43–52. Totowa, NJ: Humana Press, 1992.

Nelson, Jennifer A. "'Abortions under Community Control': Feminism, Nationalism, and the Politics of Reproduction among New York City's Young Lords." *Journal of Women's History* 13, no. 1 (2001): 157–80.

Noakes, Jeremy. "Nazism and Eugenics: The Background to the Nazi Sterilization Law of 14 July 1933." In *Ideas into Politics: Aspects of European History, 1880–1950*, edited by R.J. Bullen, H. Pogge von Strandmann, and A.B. Polonsky, 75–94. London: Croom Helm, 1984.

O'Donnell, Krista, Renate Bridenthal, and Nancy Reagin. *Heimat Abroad: The Boundaries of Germanness*. Ann Arbor: University of Michigan Press, 2005.

Offen, Karen. "Defining Feminism: A Comparative Historical Approach." *Signs* 14, no. 1 (1998): 119–57.

– "Depopulation, Nationalism, and Feminism in Fin-de-siècle France." *American Historical Review* 89, no. 3 (1984): 648–76.

– "Liberty, Equality, and Justice for Women: The Theory and Practice of Feminism in Nineteenth-Century Europe." In *Becoming Visible: Women in European History*, 2nd ed., edited by Renate Bridenthal, Claudia Koonz, and Susan Stuard, 335–73. Boston: Houghton Mifflin, 1987.

Oldenziel, Ruth. "Man the Maker, Woman the Consumer: The Consumption Junction Revisited." In *Feminism in Twentieth Century Science, Technology and Medicine*, edited by Angela N.H. Creager, Elizabeth Lunbeck, and Londa Schiebinger, 128–48. Chicago: University of Chicago Press, 2001.

Oreskes, Naomi. "Objectivity or Heroism? On the Invisibility of Women in Science." *Osiris* 11 (1996): 87–113.

Pauwels, Jacques R. *Women, Nazis, and Universities: Female University Students in the Third Reich, 1933–1945*. Westport, CT: Greenwood Press, 1984.

Penny, H. Glenn. "Historiographies in Dialogue: Beyond Categories of Germans and Brazilians." *German History* 33, no. 3 (2015): 347–66.

– "Respatializing Historical Narrative." *Geschichte und Gesellschaft* 41, no. 2 (2015): 173–196.

Petchesky, Rosalind Pollack. *Global Prescriptions: Gendering Health and Human Rights*. London: Zed Books, 2003.

Peters, Anja. *Der Geist von Alt-Rehse. Die Hebammenkurse an der Reichsärzteschule, 1935–1941*. Frankfurt am Main: Mabuse-Verlag, 2005.

Peukert, Detlev J.K. "The Genesis of the 'Final Solution' from the Spirit of Science." In *Reevaluating the Third Reich*, edited by Thomas Childers and Jane Caplan, 234–52. New York: Holmes and Meier, 1993.

– *The Weimar Republic: The Crisis of Classical Modernity*. Translated by Richard Deveson. New York: Hill and Wang, 1987.

Pine, Lisa. "Creating Conformity: The Training of Girls in the Bund Deutscher Mädel." *European History Quarterly* 33, no. 3 (2003): 367–85.

– *Hitler's "National Community": Society and Culture in Nazi Germany*. London: Hodder Arnold, 2007.

Plant, Rebecca Jo, and Marian van der Klein, "Introduction: A New Generation of Scholars on Maternalism." In *Maternalism Reconsidered: Motherhood, Welfare and Social Policy in the Twentieth Century*, edited by Marian van der Klein, Rebecca Jo Plant, Nichole Sanders, and Lori R. Weintrob, 1–21. New York: Berghahn Books, 2012.

Plotkin, Diane M. "Medicine in the Shadow of Nuremberg." In *Problems Unique to the Holocaust*, edited by Harry James Cargas, 83–97. Lexington: University Press of Kentucky, 1999.

Prahm, Heyo. *Hermine Heusler-Edenhuizen. Die erste deutsche Frauenärztin: Lebenserinnerungen im Kampf um den ärztlichen Beruf der Frau*. Opladen: Verlag Barbara Budrich, 2006.

Proctor, Robert. *The Nazi War on Cancer*. Princeton, NJ: Princeton University Press, 1999.

– "The Nazi War on Tobacco: Ideology, Evidence, and Public Health Consequences." *Bulletin of the History of Medicine* 71, no. 3 (1997): 435–88.

– *Racial Hygiene: Medicine under the Nazis*. Cambridge, MA: Harvard University Press, 1988.

Pross, Christian. "Nazi Doctors, German Medicine, and Historical Truth." In *The Nazi Doctors and the Nuremberg Code: Human Rights in Human Experimentation*, edited by George J. Annas and Michael A. Grodin, 32–52. New York: Oxford University Press, 1992.

Pycior, Helena M. "Marie Curie's 'Anti-Natural Path': Time Only for Science and Family." In *Uneasy Careers and Intimate Lives: Women in Science, 1789–1979*, edited by Pnina G. Abir-Am and Dorinda Outram, 190–215. New Brunswick, NJ: Rutgers University Press, 1987.

Rabinow, Paul, ed. *The Foucault Reader*. New York: Pantheon, 1984.

Rabkin, Yakob M., and Elena Z. Mirskaya. "Science and Totalitarianism: Lessons for the Twenty-First Century." In *Science and Ideology: A Comparative History*, edited by Mark Walker, 17–34. New York: Routledge, 2003.

Ras, Marion E.P. *Body, Femininity, and Nationalism: Girls in the German Youth Movement. 1900–1934*. New York: Routledge, 2008.

Read, Sara. *Menstruation and the Female Body in Early-Modern England*. Hampshire: Palgrave Macmillan, 2013.

Reese, Dagmar. "Bund Deutscher Mädel – Zur Geschichte der weiblichen deutschen Jugend im Dritten Reich." In *Mutterkreuz und Arbeitsbuch: Zur Geschichte der Frauen in der Weimarer Republik und im Nationalsozialismus*, edited by Frauengruppe Faschismusforschung, 163–87. Frankfurt am Main: Fischer, 1981.

– *Growing Up Female in Nazi Germany*. Translated by William Templer. Ann Arbor: University of Michigan Press, 2006.

– *'Straff, aber nicht stramm – herb, aber nicht derb'. Zur Vergesellschaftung der Mädchen durch den Bund Deutscher Mädel im sozialkulturellen Vergleich zweier Milieus*. Weinheim: Beltz, 1989.

Reinert, Kirsten. *Frauen und Sexualreform: 1897–1933*. Herbolzheim: Centaurus, 2000.

Remy, Steven P. *The Heidelberg Myth: The Nazification and Denazification of a German University*. Cambridge, MA: Harvard University Press, 2002.

Renneberg, Monika, and Mark Walker, eds. *Science, Technology, and National Socialism*. New York: Cambridge University Press, 1994.

Richards, Eveleen. "Huxley and Woman's Place in Science: The 'Woman Question' and the Control of Victorian Anthropology." In *History, Humanity, and Evolution: Essays for John C. Greene*, edited by James Moore, 253–84. New York: Cambridge University Press, 1989.

Rieger, Bernhard. "'Fast Couples': Technology, Gender and Modernity in Britain and Germany during the Nineteen-Thirties." *Historical Research* 76, no. 193 (2003): 364–88.

Roberts, Mary Louise. *Civilization without Sexes: Reconstructing Gender in Postwar France, 1917–1927*. Chicago: University of Chicago Press, 1994.

Roos, Julia. "Backlash against Prostitutes' Rights: Origins and Dynamics of Nazi Prostitution Policies." *Journal of the History of Sexuality* 11, no. 1/2 (2002): 67–94.

– *Weimar through the Lens of Gender: Prostitution Reform, Woman's Emancipation, and German Democracy, 1919–1933*. Ann Arbor: University of Michigan Press, 2010.

– "Weimar's Crisis through the Lens of Gender: The Case of Prostitution." PhD diss., Carnegie Mellon University, 2001.

Rosser, Sue V. *Female-Friendly Science: Applying Women's Studies Methods and Theories to Attract Students*. New York: Pergamon Press, 1990.

Rossiter, Margaret W. "The Matthew Matilda Effect in Science." *Social Studies of Science* 23, no. 2 (1993): 325–41.

– "Which Women? Which Science?" *Osiris* 12 (1997): 169–85.

Sach, Louisa. "Gedenke, daß du eine deutsche Frau bist! Die Ärztin und Bevölkerungspolitikerin Ilse Szagunn (1887–1971) in der Weimarer Republik und im Nationalsozialismus." Med. diss., Freie Universität, 2006.

Sauerteig, Lutz. "'The Fatherland Is in Danger, Save the Fatherland!' Venereal Disease, Sexuality and Gender in Imperial and Weimar Germany." In *Sex,*

Sin and Suffering: Venereal Disease and European Society since 1870, edited by Richard Davidson and Lesley Hall, 76–92. London: Routledge, 2001.

– "Sex Education in Germany from the Eighteenth to the Twentieth Century." In *Sexual Cultures in Europe: Themes in Sexuality*, edited by Franz X. Eder, Lesley A. Hall, and Gert Hekma, 9–33. New York: Manchester University Press, 1999.

Sauerteig, Lutz, and Roger Davidson, eds. *Shaping Sexual Knowledge: A Cultural History of Sex Education in Twentieth Century Europe.* New York: Routledge, 2009.

Schiebinger, Londa. *Has Feminism Changed Science?* Cambridge, MA: Harvard University Press, 1999.

– "Maria Winkelmann at the Berlin Academy: A Turning Point for Women in Science." *Isis* 78, no. 2 (1987): 174–200.

Schleiermacher, Sabine. "Ärztinnen zwischen Sozialhygiene und Eugenik in der Weimarer Republik." In *Medizin und Gewissen. 50 Jahre Medizin nach dem Nürnberger Ärzteprozeß*, edited by Stephan Kolb and Horst Seithe. CD-ROM. Berlin, 1998.

– "Die Frau als Hausärztin und Mutter: Das Frauenbild in der Gesundheitsaufklärung." In *Hauptsache gesund! Gesundheitsaufklärung zwischen Disziplinierung und Emanzipation*, edited by Susanne Roessiger and Heidrun Merk, 48–58. Marburg: Jonas Verlag, 1998.

– "Gesundheitsfürsorge und Gesundheitswissenschaft. Der Aufbau weiblicher Kompetenz außerhalb der traditionellen scientific community." In *Der Eintritt der Frauen in die Gelehrtenrepublik: Zur Geschlechterfrage im akademischen Selbstverständnis und in der wissenschaftlichen Praxis am Anfang des 20. Jahrhunderts*, edited by Johanna Bleker, 101–15. Husum: Matthiesen, 1998.

– "Racial Hygiene and Deliberate Parenthood: Two Sides of Demographer Hans Harmsen's Population Policy." *Issues in Reproductive and Genetic Engineering* 3, no. 3 (1990): 201–10.

– "Rassenhygienische Mission und berufliche Diskriminierung: Übereinstimmung zwischen Ärztinnen und Nationalsozialismus." In *Ärztinnen – Patientinnen: Frauen im deutschen und britischen Gesundheitswesen des 20. Jahrhunderts*, edited by Ulrike Lindner and Merith Niehuss, 95–109. Köln: Böhlau Verlag, 2002.

– *Sozialethik im Spannungsfeld von Sozial- und Rassenhygiene. Der Mediziner Hans Harmsen im Centralausschuß für die Innere Mission.* Husum: Matthiesen, 1998.

Schmidt, Dr phil. Helmut. "Die Geschichte und gesellschaftliche Bedeutung der Frauenmilch Sammelstellen in Deutschland sowie ihres Erfurter Zentrums in den Jahren 1926 bis 1950." PhD diss., Leipzig, 1983.

Schoen, Johanna. "Between Choice and Coercion: Women and the Politics of Sterilization in North Carolina, 1929–1975." *Journal of Women's History* 13, no. 1 (2001): 132–56.

Schoenbaum, David. *Hitler's Social Revolution: Class and Status in Nazi Germany, 1933–1939.* Garden City, NY: Doubleday, 1966.

Schwoch, Rebecca. *Ärztliche Standespolitik im Nationalsozialismus: Julius Hadrich und Karl Haedenkamp als Beispiele.* Husum: Mattiesen, 2001.

– "'Ich glaube, damals immer eine einwandfreie Haltung gehabt zu haben.' Die Kinderärztin und Neurologin Gertrud Soeken und der Nationalsozialismus." *Medizin Historisches Journal* 41, no. 3/4 (2006): 315–53.

Scott, Joan Wallach. "Deconstructing Equality-versus-Difference: Or, The Uses of Poststructuralist Theory for Feminism." *Feminist Studies* 14, no. 1 (1988): 32–50.

– *Gender and the Politics of History*, rev. ed. New York: Columbia University Press, 1999.

– *Only Paradoxes to Offer: French Feminists and the Rights of Man.* Cambridge, MA: Harvard University Press, 1996.

Shteir, Ann B. "Botany in the Breakfast Room: Women and Early Nineteenth-Century British Plant Study." In *Uneasy Careers and Intimate Lives: Women in Science, 1789–1979*, edited by Pnina G. Abir-Am and Dorinda Outram, 31–44. New Brunswick, NJ: Rutgers, 1987.

Skocpol, Theda. *Protecting Mothers and Soldiers: The Political Origins of Social Policy in the United States.* Cambridge, MA: Harvard University Press, 1992.

Smith, Helmut Walser. *The Continuities of German History: Nation, Religion, and Race Across the Long Nineteenth Century.* New York: Cambridge University Press, 2008.

Smith, Jill Suzanne. *Berlin Coquette: Prostitution and the New German Woman, 1890–1933.* Ithaca, NY: Cornell University Press, 2013.

Solomon, Susan Gross. "The Demographic Argument in Soviet Debates over the Legalization of Abortion in the 1920s." In *Doctors, Politics, and Society: Historical Essays*, edited by Dorothy Porter and Ray Porter, 140–73. Atlanta, GA: Rodopi, 1993.

– "The Expert and the State in Russian Public Health: Continuities and Changes Across the Revolutionary Divide." In *The History of Public Health and the Modern State*, edited by Dorothy Porter, 183–223. Atlanta, GA: Rodopi, 1994.

– "The Limits of Government Patronage of Sciences: Social Hygiene and the Soviet State, 1920–1930." *Social History of Medicine* 3, no. 3 (1990): 405–35.

Starks, Tricia. *The Body Soviet: Propaganda, Hygiene, and the Revolutionary State.* Madison: University of Wisconsin Press, 2008.

Steber, Martina, and Bernhard Gotto, eds. *Visions of Community in Nazi Germany: Social Engineering and Private Lives*. Oxford: Oxford University Press, 2014.

Steinbacher, Sybille. *"Volksgenossinnen": Frauen in der NS-Volksgemeinschaft*. Göttingen: Wallstein, 2007.

Steinecke, Verena. *Ich musste zuerst Rebellin werden. Trotz Bedrohung und Gefahr – das gute und wunderbare Leben der Ärztin Else Kienle*. Stuttgart: Schmetterling Verlag, 1992.

Stepan, Nancy Leys. *"The Hour of Eugenics": Race, Gender, and Nation in Latin America*. Ithaca, NY: Cornell University Press, 1991.

Stephenson, Jill. "Girls' Higher Education in Germany in the 1930s." *Journal of Contemporary History* 10, no. 1 (1975): 41–69.

– *The Nazi Organization of Women*. London: Croom Helm, 1980.

– "Women and the Professions in Germany, 1900–1945." In *German Professions, 1800–1950*, edited by Geoffrey Cocks and Konrad H. Jarausch, 270–88. New York: Oxford University Press, 1990.

– *Women in Nazi Germany*. London: Pearson, 2001.

– *Women in Nazi Society*. New York: Harper & Row, 1975.

Stibbe, Matthew. *Women in the Third Reich*. New York: Oxford University Press, 2003.

Stöckel, Sigrid. "Infant Mortality and Concepts of Hygiene. Strategies and Consequences in the Kaiserreich and the Weimar Republic: The Example of Berlin." *History of the Family* 7, no. 4 (2002): 601–16.

– *Säuglingsfürsorge zwischen sozialer Hygiene und Eugenik: Das Beispiel Berlins im Kaiserreich und in der Weimarer Republik*. Berlin: Walter de Gruyter, 1996.

Stokes, Patricia. "Contested Conceptions: Experiences and Discourses of Pregnancy and Childbirth in Germany, 1914–1933." PhD diss., Cornell University, 2003.

– "Pathology, Danger, and Power: Women's and Physicians' Views of Pregnancy and Childbirth in Weimar Germany." *Social History of Medicine* 13, no. 3 (2000): 359–80.

Stommer, Rainer, ed. *Medizin im Dienste der Rassenideologie: die "Führerschule der Deutschen Ärzteschaft" in Alt Rehse*. Berlin: Links, 2008.

Sussman, George D. *Selling Mothers' Milk: The Wet-Nursing Business in France, 1715–1914*. Urbana: University of Illinois Press, 1982.

Svenja, Ludwig. "Agnes Bluhm (1862–1943). Briefe an Alfred Ploetz (1860–1940) aus den Jahren 1901–1938." Med. diss., Freie Universität, 1998.

Swanson, Kara W. *Banking on the Body: The Market in Blood, Milk, and Sperm in Modern America*. Cambridge, MA: Harvard University Press, 2014.

– "Human Milk as Technology and Technologies of Human Milk: Medical Imaginings in the Early 20th Century United States." *Women's Studies Quarterly* 37, no. 1/2 (2009): 20–37.

Terrall, Mary. "Salon, Academy and Boudoir: Generation and Desire in Maupertuis's Science of Life." *Isis* 87, no. 2 (1996): 217–29.

Timm, Annette. *The Politics of Fertility in Twentieth-Century Berlin*. New York: Cambridge University Press, 2010.

– "The Politics of Fertility: Population Politics and Health Care in Berlin, 1919–1972." PhD diss., University of Chicago, 1999.

– "Sex with a Purpose: Prostitution, Venereal Disease and Militarized Masculinity in the Third Reich." *Journal of the History of Sexuality* 11, no. 1/2 (2002): 223–55.

Trischler, Helmuth. "Self-Mobilization or Resistance? Aeronautical Research and National Socialism." In *Science, Technology, and National Socialism*, edited by Monika Renneberg and Mark Walker, 72–87. New York: Cambridge University Press, 1994.

Tyrrell, Ian. *Woman's World/Woman's Empire: The Woman's Christian Temperance Union in International Perspective, 1880–1930*. Chapel Hill: University of North Carolina Press, 1991.

Usborne, Cornelie. "Abortion in Weimar Germany – The Debate amongst the Medical Profession." *Continuity and Change* 5, no. 2 (1990): 199–224.

– "Body Biological to Body Politic: Women's Demands for Reproductive Self-Determination in World War I and Early Weimar Germany." In *Citizenship and National Identity in Twentieth-Century Germany*, edited by Geoff Eley and Jan Palmowski, 129–45. Stanford, CA: Stanford University Press, 2008.

– *Cultures of Abortion in Weimar Germany*. New York: Berghahn, 2007.

– "The New Woman and Generational Conflicts: Perceptions of Young Women's Sexual Mores in the Weimar Republic." In *Generations in Conflict: Youth Revolt and Generation Formation in Gemrany, 1770–1968*, edited by Mark Roseman, 137–63. New York: Cambridge University Press, 1995.

– *The Politics of the Body in Weimar Germany: Women's Reproductive Rights and Duties*. London: Macmillan Press, 1992.

– "Women Doctors and Gender Identity in Weimar Germany (1918–1933)." In *Women and Modern Medicine*, edited by Lawrence Conrad and Anne Hardy, 109–26. New York: Editions Rodopi, 2001.

Vaizey, Hester. *Surviving Hitler's War: Family Life in Germany, 1939–1948*. New York: Palgrave Macmillan, 2010.

Verbrugge, Martha H. *Active Bodies: A History of Women's Physical Education in Twentieth-Century America*. New York: Oxford University Press, 2012.

von Oertzen, Monika. "'Nicht nur fort sollst du dich pflanzen, sondern hinauf.' Die Ärztin und Sexualreformerin Anne-Marie Durand-Wever (1889–1970)." In *Weibliche Ärzte: Die Durchsetzung des Berufsbildes in Deutschland*, edited by Eva Brinkschulte, 140–55. Berlin: Edition Hentrich, 1993.

von Saldern, Adelheid. "Innovative Trends in Women's and Gender Studies of the National Socialist Era." *German History* 27, no. 1 (2009): 84–112.

– "Victims or Perpetrators? Controversies about the Role of Women in the Nazi State." In *Nazism and German Society, 1933–1945*, edited by David Crew, 141–65. New York: Routledge, 1994.

von Soden, Kristine. *Die Sexualberatungsstellen der Weimarer Republik, 1919–1933*. Berlin: Edition Hentrich, 1988.

Walker, Mark. *Nazi Science: Myth, Truth, and the German Atomic Bomb*. New York: Plenum Press, 1995.

Walkowitz, Judith. *Prostitution and Victorian Society: Women, Class and the State*. New York: Cambridge University Press, 1980.

Walther, Daniel J. *Sex and Control: Venereal Disease, Colonial Physicians, and Indigenous Agency in German Colonialism, 1884–1914*. New York: Berghahn Books, 2015.

Weinbaum, Alys Eve, Lynn M. Thomas, Priti Ramamurthy, Uta G. Poiger, Madeleine Yue Dong, and Tani E. Barlow, eds. *The Modern Girl around the World: Consumption, Modernity, and Globalization*. Durham, NC: Duke University Press, 2008.

Weindling, Paul. "Bourgeois Values, Doctors and the State: The Professionalization of Medicine in Germany, 1848–1933." In *The German Bourgeoisie: Essays on the Social History of the German Middle Class from the Late Eighteenth to the Early Twentieth Century*, edited by David Blackbourn and Richard J. Evans, 198–223. New York: Routledge, 1991.

– "Eugenics and the Welfare State During the Weimar Republic." In *The State and Social Change in Germany, 1880–1980*, edited by W.R. Lee and Eve Rosenhaft, 131–60. New York: Berg, 1990.

– *Health, Race and German Politics between National Unification and Nazism, 1870–1945*. New York: Cambridge University Press, 1989.

– "The Medical Profession, Social Hygiene and the Birth Rate in Germany, 1914-18." In *The Upheaval of War: Family, Work and Welfare in Europe, 1914–1918*, edited by Richard Wall and Jay Winter, 417–38. New York: Cambridge University Press, 1988.

– *Nazi Medicine and the Nuremberg Trials: From Medical War Crimes to Informed Consent*. New York: Palgrave Macmillan, 2004.

Weiss, Sheila Faith. "German Eugenics, 1890–1933." In *Deadly Medicine: Creating the Master Race*, edited by Susan Bachrach and Dieter Kuntz, 15–39. Chapel Hill: University of North Carolina Press, 2004.

– *Race Hygiene and National Efficiency: The Eugenics of Wilhem Schallmayer*. Berkeley: University of California Press, 1987.

– "The Race Hygiene Movement in Germany, 1904–1945." In *The Wellborn Science: Eugenics in Germany, France, Brazil, and Russia*, edited by Mark B. Adams, 8–68. New York: Oxford University Press, 1990.

– "Die Rassenhygienische Bewegung in Deutschland, 1904–1933." In *Der Wert des Menschen. Medizin in Deutschland, 1918–1945*, edited by Christian Pross und Götz Aly, 153–73. Berlin: Edition Hentrich, 1989.

Weingart, Peter, Jürgen Kroll, and Kurt Bayertz. *Rasse, Blut und Gene: Geschichte der Eugenik und Rassenhygiene in Deutschland*. Frankfurt: Suhrkamp, 1992.

Weitz, Eric D. *Weimar Germany: Promise and Tragedy*. Princeton, NJ: Princeton University Press, 2007.

Whitaker, Elizabeth Dixon. *Measuring Mama's Milk: Fascism and the Medicalization of Maternity in Italy*. Ann Arbor: University of Michigan Press, 2000.

Widdig, Bernd. *Culture and Inflation in Weimar Germany*. Berkeley: University of California Press, 2001.

Wildt, Michael. *Hitler's Volksgemeinschaft and the Dynamics of Racial Exclusion: Violence against Jews in Provincial Germany, 1919–1939*. New York: Berghahn Books, 2012.

– *Volksgemeinschaft als Selbstermächtigung. Gewalt gegen Juden in der deutschen Provinz 1919 bis 1939*. Hamburg: Hamburger Edition, 2007.

Williams, John Alexander. *Turning to Nature in Germany: Hiking, Nudism, and Conservation, 1900–1940*. Stanford, CA: Stanford University Press, 2007.

Wülfing, Karin. "Frau Dr med. M.-E. Kayser und die Frauenmilchsammelstellen in Deutschland." Med. diss., Universität Düsseldorf, 1989.

Zegenhagen, Evelyn. "'The Holy Desire to Serve the Poor and Tortured Fatherland': German Women Motor Pilots of the Inter-War Era and Their Political Mission." *German Studies Review* 30, no. 3 (2007): 579–610.

Ziemann, Benjamin. "Weimar Was Weimar: Politics, Culture, and the Emplotment of the German Republic." *German History* 28, no. 4 (2010): 542–71.

Zweiniger-Bargielowska, Ina. *Managing the Body: Beauty, Health, and Fitness in Britain, 1880–1939*. New York: Oxford University Press, 2010.

Index

GERMAN AND EUROPEAN STUDIES

General Editor: Jennifer J. Jenkins

Printed and bound by CPI Group (UK) Ltd, Croydon, CR0 4YY

27/10/2024

14580702-0004